# Stress Management

## *Developing Resilience in an Evolving World*

# Stress Management

## *Developing Resilience in an Evolving World*


**Pardess Mitchell, EdD, MCHES**

Professor

Harper College

Palatine, Illinois



HUMAN KINETICS

**Library of Congress Cataloging-in-Publication Data**

Names: Mitchell, Pardess, author.
Title: Stress management : developing resilience in an evolving world / Pardess Mitchell, EdD, MCHES, Professor, Harper College, Palatine, Illinois.
Description: Champaign, IL : Human Kinetics, [2025] | Includes bibliographical references and index.
Identifiers: LCCN 2023020320 (print) | LCCN 2023020321 (ebook) | ISBN 9781718213180 (paperback) | ISBN 9781718213197 (epub) | ISBN 9781718213203 (pdf)
Subjects: LCSH: Stress management. | Stress (Psychology)
Classification: LCC RA785 .M58 2025 (print) | LCC RA785 (ebook) | DDC 155.9/042--dc23/eng/20230828
LC record available at https://lccn.loc.gov/2023020320
LC ebook record available at https://lccn.loc.gov/2023020321

ISBN: 978-1-7182-1318-0 (paperback)
ISBN: 978-1-7182-1423-1 (loose-leaf)



**Acquisitions Editor:** Bethany J. Bentley; **Developmental Editor:** Judy Park; **Managing Editor:** Anna Lan Seaman; **Copyeditor:** Heather Gauen Hutches; **Proofreader:** Karin Kipp; **Indexer:** Nancy Ball; **Permissions Manager:** Laurel Mitchell; **Graphic Designers:** Sean Roosevelt and Julie L. Denzer; **Cover Designer:** Keri Evans; **Cover Design Specialist:** Susan Rothermel Allen; **Photograph (cover):** SDI Productions/E+/Getty Images; **Photo Asset Manager:** Laura Fitch; **Photo Production Manager:** Jason Allen; **Senior Art Manager:** Kelly Hendren; **Illustrations:** © Human Kinetics, unless otherwise noted; **Printer:** Walsworth

Printed in the United States of America 10 9 8 7 6 5 4 3 2 1

The paper in this book was manufactured using responsible forestry methods.

**Human Kinetics**
1607 N. Market Street
Champaign, IL 61820
USA

*United States and International*
Website: **US.HumanKinetics.com**
Email: info@hkusa.com
Phone: 1-800-747-4457

*Canada*
Website: **Canada.HumanKinetics.com**
Email: info@hkcanada.com

E8618 (paperback) / E8695 (loose-leaf)

I dedicate this textbook to my abba, אבא, Yehuda Kahnovitch—
a courageous, funny, great dad, who left us way too early.
You are loved and missed dearly.

# CONTENTS

# PART II Managing Stress Using Dimensions of Wellness

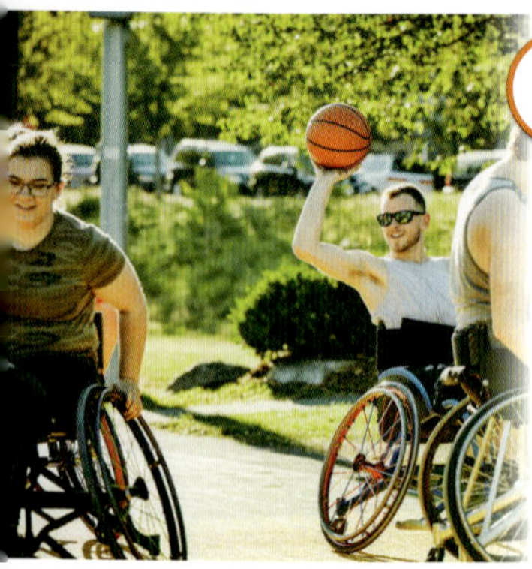



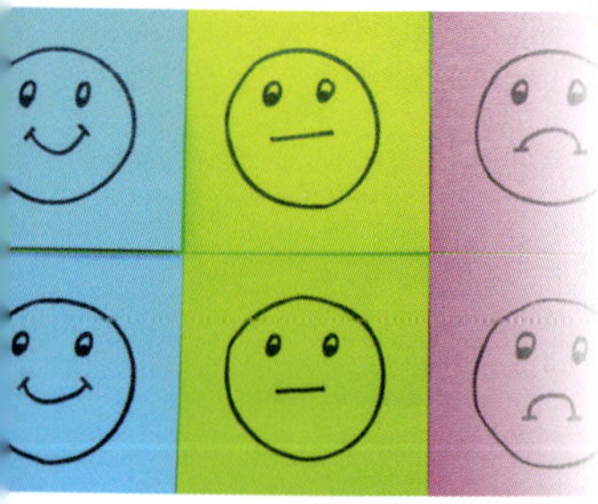



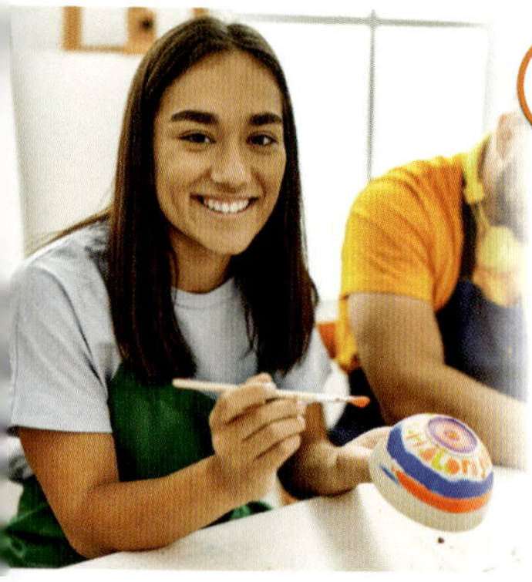

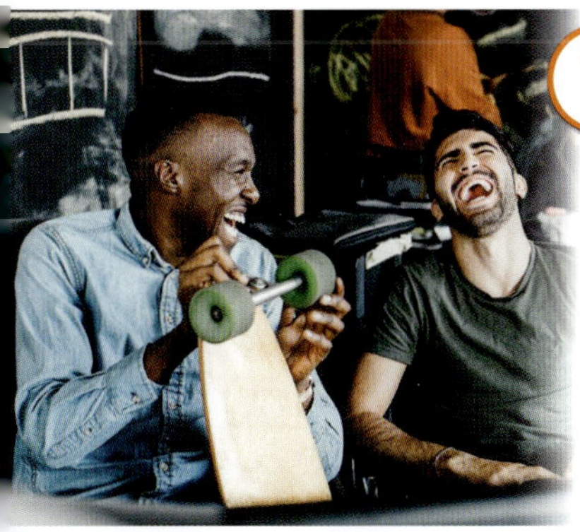



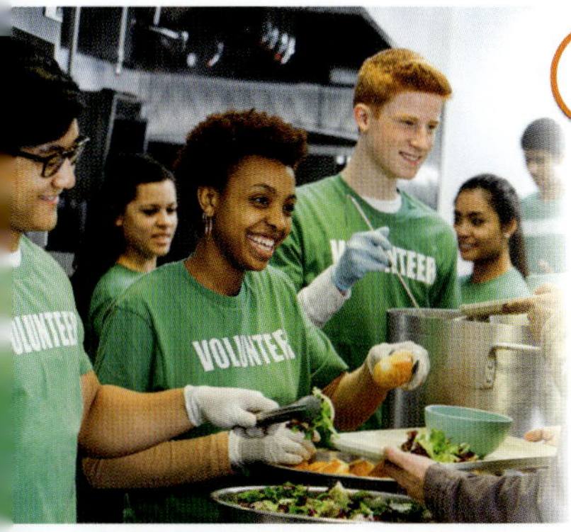



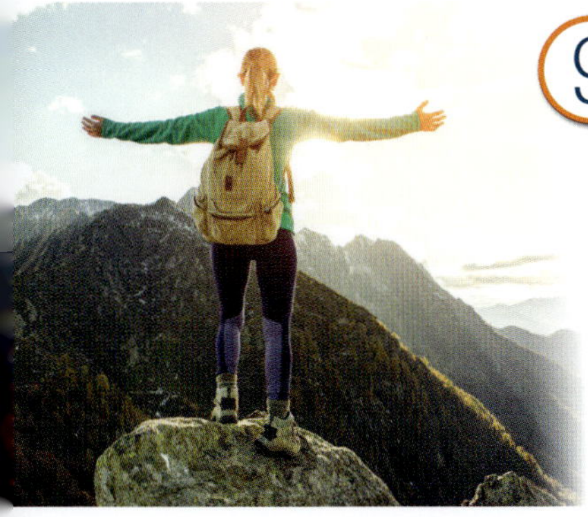

# PART III Practical Strategies for Managing Stress

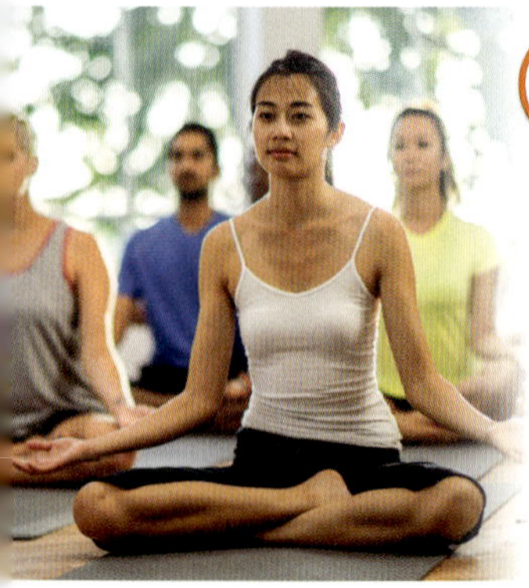



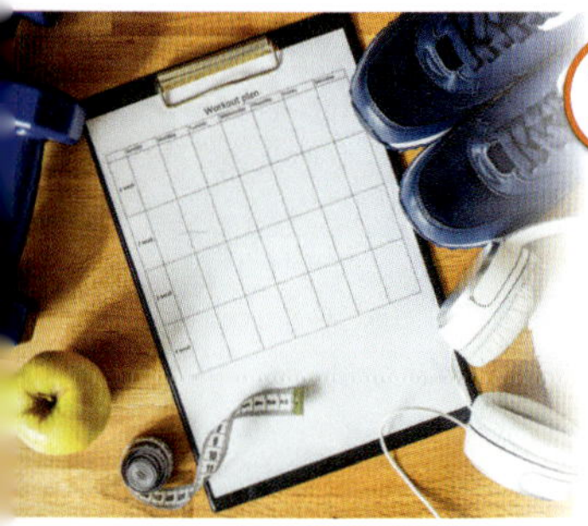

# PREFACE

Over the past 25 years of teaching, I have noticed an exponential increase in the stress my students experience. For the past few years, I have heard many stories about the impact stress has had on their academic careers and personal lives. This planted the seed in me to write a book about stress management for college students. I hope to help them gain the skills to manage their stress and lead healthier lives.

As stress increases at alarming rates, the mental health of our nation is at risk. Stress is related to all areas of wellness—physical, emotional, intellectual, social, spiritual, and environmental.

Part I, Introduction to Stress and Well-Being, provides general information on the dimensions of wellness, the physiological responses to stress, and the impact of stress on the body. Part II, Managing Stress Using Dimensions of Wellness, highlights the different dimensions of wellness and the ways they affect and are affected by stress. Lastly, part III, Practical Strategies for Managing Stress, provides a plethora of strategies to help prevent and manage stress.

Students will find the following features as they navigate the chapters:

- Case Study sidebars in each chapter to help highlight key concepts
- Research Spotlight sidebars in each chapter with up-to-date studies
- Engaging text with real-life examples to help with understanding and retention
- Explanations about the importance of stress management
- A variety of tools and techniques to better manage stress
- Discussion questions to encourage critical thinking at the end of each chapter

Tools for instructors include the following:

- Engaging instructor resources
- Classroom activities
- Teaching tips

The goal of a good stress management plan is to tackle stress from all sides—before it occurs, while it is occurring, and after it occurs. Having a well-rounded plan can help you avoid stress and better cope with stress when it occurs. Robert Epstein (2011) proposes a model to combat stress using multiple approaches:

- *Source management.* This seeks to reduce or eliminate stress at its source. For example, if you are working too many hours to focus on school, source management would mean either reducing your hours at work or reducing your workload at school.
- *Relaxation.* These techniques are intended to focus the mind and relax the body (decrease heart rate, lower heart blood pressure, and reduce muscle tension). They include breathing, meditation, and rest.
- *Thought management.* These techniques have you actively change your thought process to better manage the stressor. For example, if you procrastinate on a big paper, telling yourself you are a bad writer, what do you think will happen? You will probably wait until the last minute and end up turning in a paper that is not your best work. Instead of focusing on you hate writing, focus on a part of the writing process you enjoy. Change your negative thoughts to positive ones.
- *Prevention.* This component refers to avoiding stress when possible. For example, if you experience stress when you go to dance clubs, don't go to dance clubs. If you experience stress when performing onstage, don't audition for a play.

Not all approaches are appropriate for all types of stressors—for example, prevention may not be a viable option if your classes are stressing you out. Although dropping out may reduce your stress in the moment, it would ultimately cause more stress when you are unable to obtain your degree. These approaches can be thought of as different checkpoints in the stress management timeline and can help you before, during, and after stressful events. Examples of these approaches will be discussed throughout this text.

# STUDENT AND INSTRUCTOR RESOURCES

Visit HK*Propel* to access a wealth of study activities and resources.

## Student Resources

Students, visit HK*Propel* for interactive learning activities and materials to aid your learning. You'll find a vocabulary flash card activity and quiz along with an audio mini lecture for each chapter. HK*Propel* is also where you'll find materials assigned by your instructor for this course, such as worksheets and additional quizzes. Student access codes are included with the purchase of a print book or ebook through Human Kinetics. Student access codes are also sold separately on the Human Kinetics website.

Review key terms

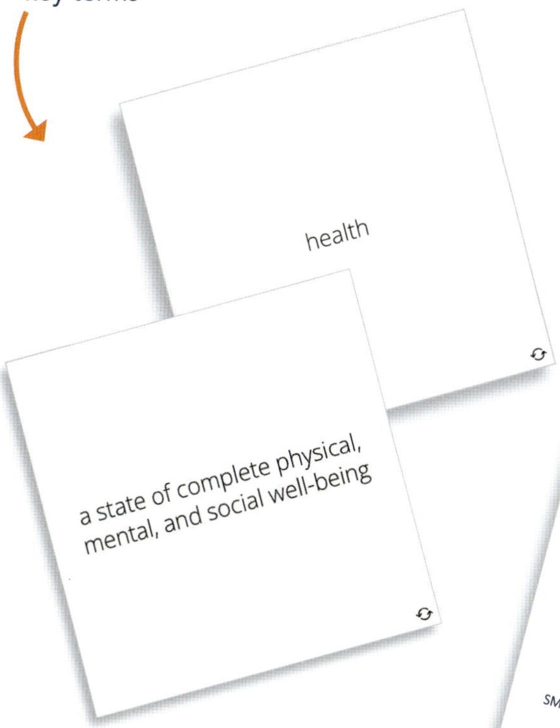
health
a state of complete physical, mental, and social well-being

Complete self-discovery activities

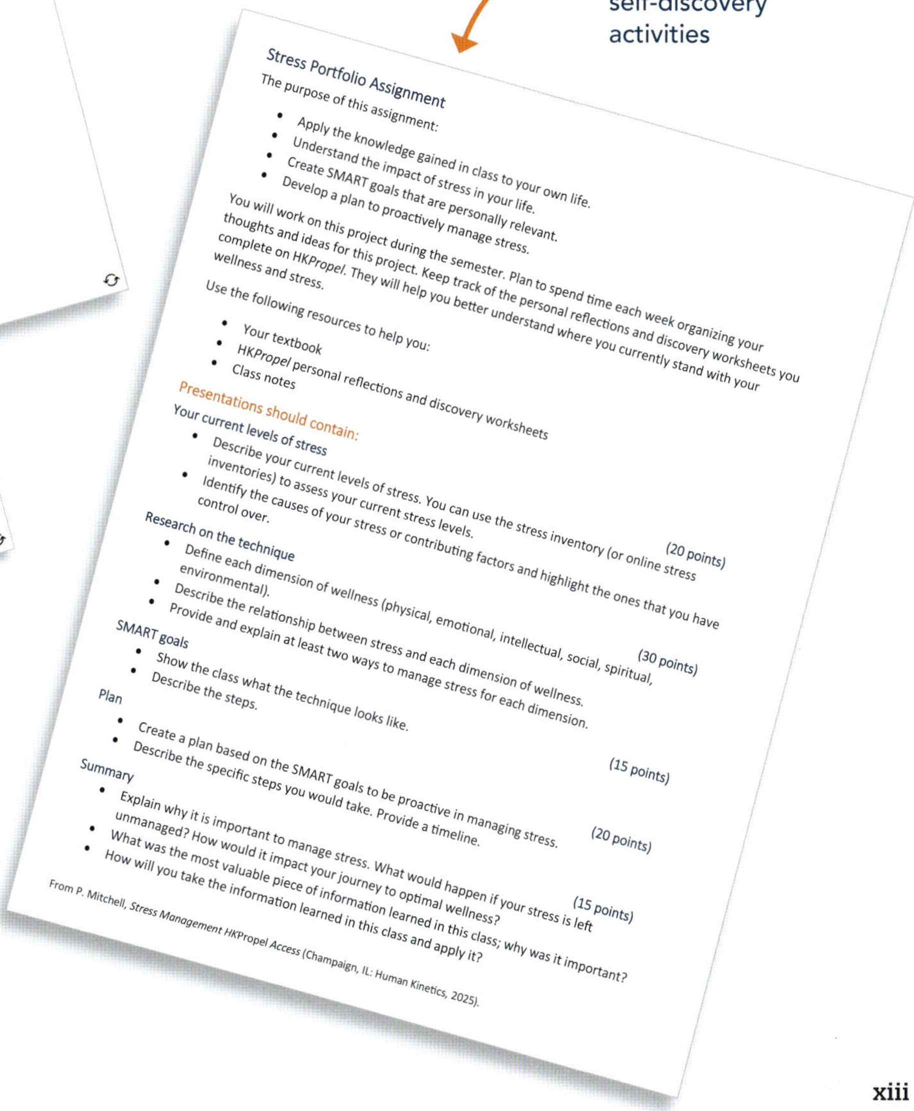

Stress Portfolio Assignment

The purpose of this assignment:

- Apply the knowledge gained in class to your own life.
- Understand the impact of stress in your life.
- Create SMART goals that are personally relevant.
- Develop a plan to proactively manage stress.

You will work on this project during the semester. Plan to spend time each week organizing your thoughts and ideas for this project. Keep track of the personal reflections and discovery worksheets you complete on HKPropel. They will help you better understand where you currently stand with your wellness and stress.

Use the following resources to help you:

- Your textbook
- HKPropel personal reflections and discovery worksheets
- Class notes

Presentations should contain:

Your current levels of stress (20 points)

- Describe your current levels of stress. You can use the stress inventory (or online stress inventories) to assess your current stress levels.
- Identify the causes of your stress or contributing factors and highlight the ones that you have control over.

Research on the technique (30 points)

- Define each dimension of wellness (physical, emotional, intellectual, social, spiritual, environmental).
- Describe the relationship between stress and each dimension of wellness.
- Provide and explain at least two ways to manage stress for each dimension.

SMART goals (15 points)

- Show the class what the technique looks like.
- Describe the steps.

Plan (20 points)

- Create a plan based on the SMART goals to be proactive in managing stress.
- Describe the specific steps you would take. Provide a timeline.

Summary (15 points)

- Explain why it is important to manage stress. What would happen if your stress is left unmanaged? How would it impact your journey to optimal wellness?
- What was the most valuable piece of information learned in this class; why was it important?
- How will you take the information learned in this class and apply it?

From P. Mitchell, *Stress Management HKPropel Access* (Champaign, IL: Human Kinetics, 2025).

# Instructor Resources

Instructors using this text in their courses will find a wealth of updated ancillary materials available in HK*Propel*, including an instructor guide, a presentation package, a test package, chapter quizzes, mini lecture quizzes, and chapter essay questions.

The instructor ancillaries are free to course adopters.

## Instructor Guide

Specifically developed for instructors who have adopted *Stress Management*, the instructor guide includes a sample syllabus, chapter summaries, teaching tips, activities, projects, assignment guides, web links for further exploration, a list of student materials assignable in HK*Propel*, essay questions and answer guides, citations for articles mentioned in the audio mini lectures, and printable classroom materials.

## Test Package

The test package includes more than 330 questions created especially for *Stress Management*. Various question types are included: multiple-choice, multiple-response, true-false, fill-in-the-blank, and matching questions. The files may be downloaded for integration with a learning management system or printed for use as paper-based tests. Instructors may also create their own customized quizzes or tests from the test bank questions to assign to students directly through HK*Propel*. Multiple-choice and true-false questions are automatically graded, and instructors can easily review student scores in the platform.

## Chapter Quizzes

These ready-to-use 10-question quizzes test students' understanding of the most important concepts in each chapter. Each quiz may be downloaded or assigned to students within HK*Propel*. The chapter quizzes are automatically graded, with scores available for review in the platform.

## Presentation Package

The presentation package includes a comprehensive series of more than 245 PowerPoint slides. These can be used directly in PowerPoint or printed to make transparencies or handouts for students. Instructors can easily add to, modify, or rearrange the order of the slides as well as search for slides based on key words. Access the presentation package by visiting HK*Propel*.

# ACKNOWLEDGMENTS

I would like to extend my sincere thanks to the team at Human Kinetics: Bethany Bentley, who provided me with the opportunity to write this textbook; Judy Park, who offered invaluable insights and feedback; and Heather Gauen Hutches, who provided clarity throughout the text.

I am forever grateful to my husband, Jack, who was so supportive in my venture to write a textbook. Thank you for watching the kids, giving me time to write this textbook.

Thank you to my three lovely children, Devin, Jase, and Arieanne, for providing me the motivation to research many different ways to manage stress.

# PHOTO CREDITS

**Table of contents photos in chronological order:** Jacobs Stock Photography Ltd/Digital Vision/Getty Images; skynesher/E+/Getty Images; Jasmin Merdan/Moment RF/Getty Images; Thomas Barwick/Digital Vision/Getty Images; jayk7/Moment RF/Getty Images; AaronAmat/iStockphoto/Getty Images; Maskot/Digital Vision/Getty Images; Ariel Skelley/Getty Images/Getty Images; swissmediavision/E+/Getty Images; FatCamera/E+/Getty Images; sergio_kumer/iStockphoto/Getty Images

**Page xiii:** © Human Kinetics; © Human Kinetics
**Page 3:** Jacobs Stock Photography Ltd/Digital Vision/Getty Images
**Page 5:** Jonathan Knowles/Stone RF/Getty Images
**Page 7:** Peter Cade/Stone RF/Getty Images
**Page 9:** Portra/Digital Vision/Getty Images
**Page 10:** kali9/E+/Getty Images
**Page 12:** Getty Images/iStockphoto/monkeybusinessimage
**Page 15:** BJI / Blue Jean Images/blue jean images RF/Getty Images
**Page 16:** gbh007/iStockphoto/Getty Images
**Page 17:** Henn Photography/Cultura RF/Getty Images
**Page 19:** skynesher/E+/Getty Images
**Page 21:** Ariel Skelley/Digital Vision/Getty Images
**Page 24:** william87/iStockphoto/Getty Images
**Page 27:** Peter Stark/fStop/Getty Images
**Page 30:** uschools/E+/Getty Images
**Page 33:** PeopleImages/iStockphoto/Getty Images
**Page 34:** Newsday LLC/Newsday RM/Getty Images
**Page 35:** Westend61/Westend61/Getty Images
**Page 36:** UpperCut Images/Uppercut RF/Getty Images
**Page 41:** Jasmin Merdan/Moment RF/Getty Imagesv
**Page 45:** FatCamera/Getty Images/iStockphoto
**Page 46:** Universal History Archive/Universal Images Group Editorial/Getty Images
**Page 49:** krisanapong detraphiphat/Moment RF/Getty Images
**Page 50:** Getty Images/Westend61
**Page 51:** martin-dm/E+/Getty Images
**Page 54:** CocoSan/E+/Getty Images
**Page 59:** Thomas Barwick/Digital Vision/Getty Images
**Page 63:** AntonioGuillem/iStockphoto/Getty Images
**Page 64:** Kolostock/Blend Images/Getty Images
**Page 65:** miljko/E+/Getty Images
**Page 67:** Maskot/Getty Images
**Page 70:** Yulia Naumenko/Moment RF/Getty Images
**Page 73:** PeopleImages/Digital Vision/Getty Images
**Page 74:** PhotoDisc
**Page 77:** jayk7/Moment RF/Getty Images
**Page 79:** Elena Zaretskaya/Moment RF/Getty Images
**Page 80:** Wavebreakmedia/iStockphoto/Getty Images
**Page 82:** Image_Source/Getty Images
**Page 85:** iStockphoto/Juan Monino
**Page 87:** Jacob Ammentorp Lund/iStockphoto/Getty Images
**Page 90:** PeopleImages/E+/Getty Images
**Page 94:** skynesher/E+/Getty Images
**Page 96:** kali9/E+/Getty Images
**Page 97:** AaronAmat/iStockphoto/Getty Images
**Page 99:** kali9/E+/Getty Images
**Page 101:** Luis Alvarez/Digital Vision/Getty Images
**Page 103:** Stockbyte
**Page 104:** PeopleImages/iStockphoto/Getty Images
**Page 108:** monkeybusinessimages/iStockphoto/Getty Images
**Page 109:** James Woodson/Photodisc/Getty Images
**Page 112:** Cavan Images/Cavan Images RF/Getty Images
**Page 117:** Maskot/Digital Vision/Getty Images
**Page 119:** Ariel Skelley/Getty Images/Getty Images
**Page 121:** Justin Case/Digital Vision/Getty Images
**Page 123:** skynesher/E+/Getty Images
**Page 124:** Alistair Berg/Digital Vision/Getty Images

**Page 127:** Hero Images/Getty Images/Getty Images
**Page 128:** Maskot/Getty Images
**Page 131:** MediaNews Group/Reading Eagle via Getty Images/MediaNews Group RM/Getty Images
**Page 133 (from left to right):** Pascal Broze/Onoky/Getty Images; © Human Kinetics; Banana Stock; © Human Kinetics; SDI Productions/E+/Getty Images; © Human Kinetics; © Human Kinetics; Luis Alvarez/Digital Vision/Getty Images; Photodisc; skynesher/E+/Getty Images; Weedezign/iStockphoto/Getty Images
**Page 139:** Ariel Skelley/Getty Images/Getty Images
**Page 141:** Gina Sanders - Fotolia
**Page 143 (clockwise from top left):** Alfian Widiantono/Moment RF/Getty Images; Simon Lehmann/Getty Images/Getty Images; ipopba/iStockphoto/Getty Images; FangXiaNuo/E+/Getty Images; Kamonwan Wankaew/iStockphoto/Getty Images
**Page 145:** © Michael Pettigrew - Fotolia.com
**Page 146:** Alex Vasilev - Fotolia
**Page 148:** Brian Weed/fotolia.com
**Page 151:** kali9/E+/Getty Images
**Page 153:** swissmediavision/E+/Getty Images
**Page 155:** Yellow Dog Productions/Photodisc/Getty Images
**Page 157:** Tanya Paton/iStockphoto/Getty Images
**Page 158:** franckreporter/E+/Getty Images
**Page 159:** SDI Productions/E+/Getty Images
**Page 163:** Pete Saloutos/Image Source/Getty Images
**Page 166:** Marcos Homem/iStockphoto/Getty Images
**Page 171:** FatCamera/E+/Getty Images
**Page 172:** fizkes/iStockphoto/Getty Images
**Page 173:** ljubaphoto/E+/Getty Images
**Page 175:** © Human Kinetics
**Page 178:** Layland Masuda/Moment RF/Getty Images
**Page 182:** © Human Kinetics
**Page 185:** Alexandra Ekdahl / EyeEm/EyeEm/Getty Images
**Page 187:** sergio_kumer/iStockphoto/Getty Images
**Page 190:** nito100/iStockphoto/Getty Images
**Page 192:** Ong-ad Nuseewor/iStockphoto/Getty Images
**Page 195:** AlessandroZocc/iStockphoto/Getty Images
**Page 196:** Jacob Ammentorp Lund/iStockphoto/Getty Images
**Page 197:** AsiaVision/E+/Getty Images
**Page 198:** Maskot/Getty Images
**Page 201:** Tom Merton/iStockphoto/Getty Images

PART I

# Introduction to Stress and Well-Being

1

# Understanding Health and Wellness

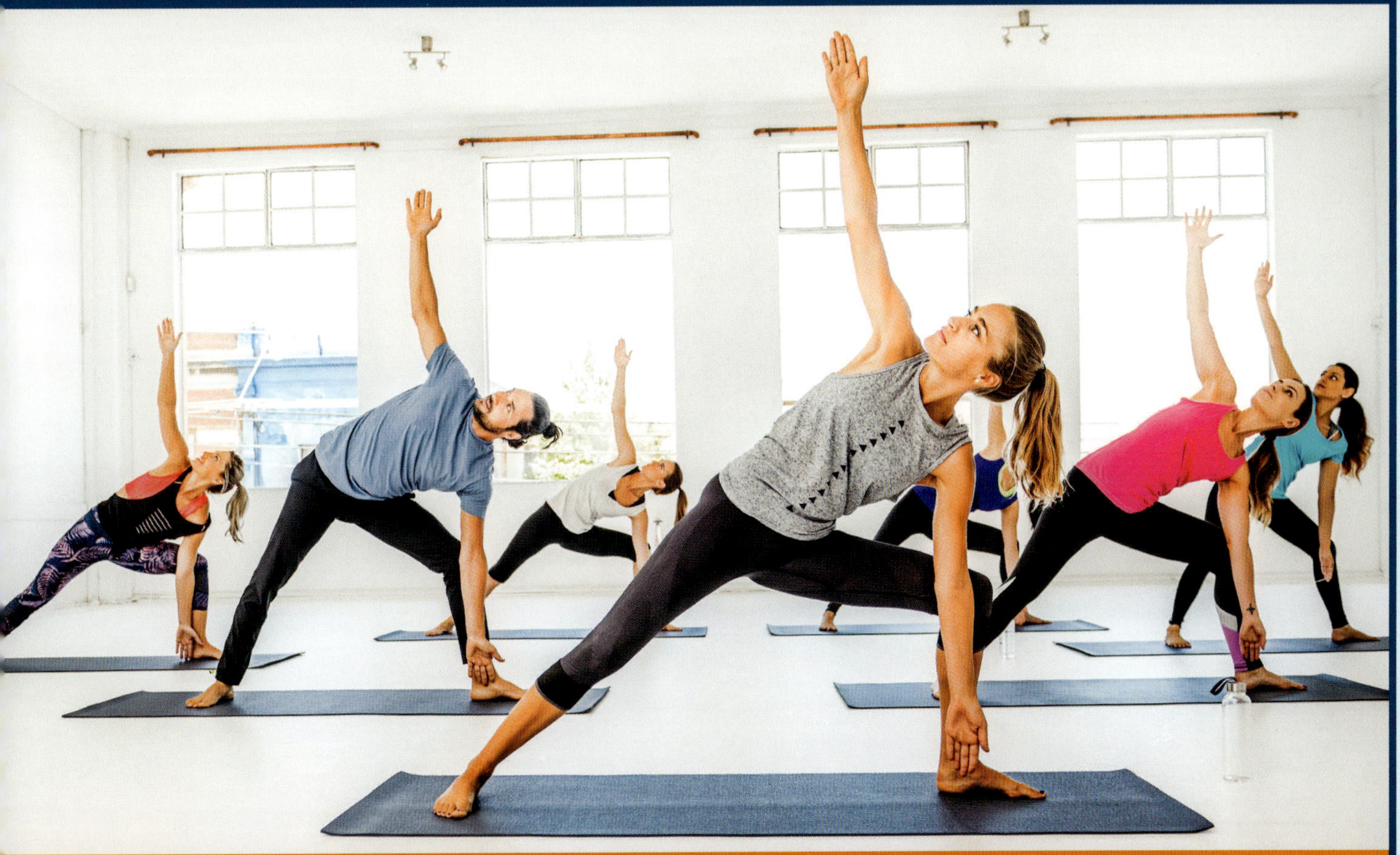

## LEARNING OBJECTIVES

After reading this chapter, you will be able to do the following:

- Define health and wellness
- Identify influences on wellness
- Explain the six dimensions of wellness
- Summarize the mind–body connection
- Examine the strengths-based approach to wellness

# KEY TERMS

emotional wellness
environmental wellness
genetics
health
intellectual wellness
physical wellness
self-care
self-regulation
social wellness
spiritual wellness
wellness

Stress is experienced by all people and closely linked to all areas of health. Stress and wellness are highly interrelated: To effectively manage stress, you need to work toward attaining high levels of wellness, and to maintain high levels of wellness, you must be able to effectively manage stress. Learning to effectively cope with stress will therefore help improve other areas of health. In this chapter, you will learn about health and wellness and the relationship between stress and overall well-being.

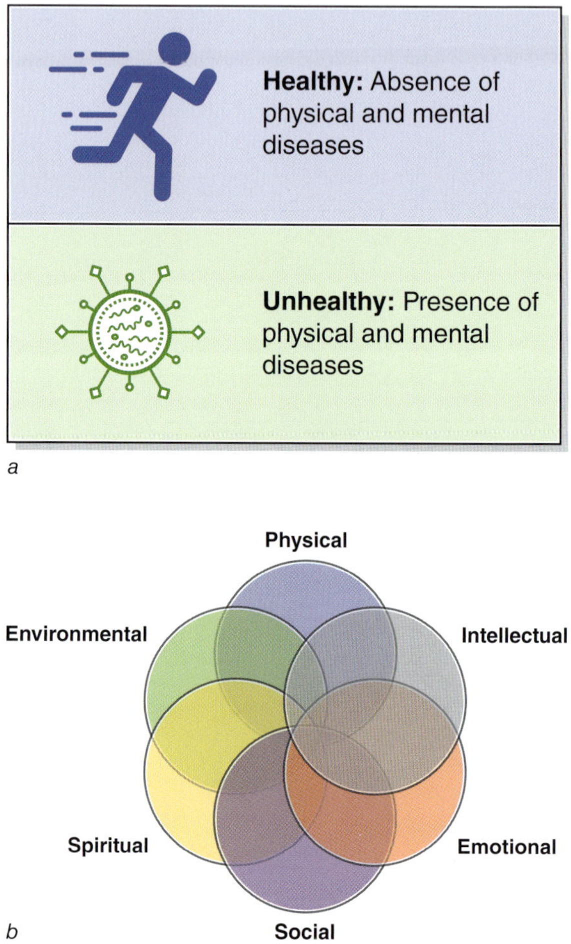


**Figure 1.1** *(a)* The limited view of health is binary and does not consider the full aspects of health. *(b)* The updated view of health is multifaceted and includes multiple dimensions.

## Defining Health and Wellness

**Health** was initially defined as simply as the absence of physical and mental diseases. This definition is limited and tends to view health as a static condition: One either has health or does not. It does not take into account the management of chronic conditions—for example, although a person with diabetes might be able to effectively manage it with relatively few health effects, they would not be considered healthy according to this definition.

To define health from a more comprehensive standpoint, the World Health Organization (WHO) has defined health as "complete physical, mental, and social well-being, not merely as the absence of disease or infirmity" (Grad, 2002). This definition positions health as a condition in the moment or a state of being. Under this definition, a person who is effectively managing a chronic disease can be considered healthy if it is not interfering with their overall well-being. Figure 1.1 displays the differences between the limited and updated definition of health.

**Wellness** expands the previous definition of health to describe the active process an individual goes through to achieve an optimal state of well-being, including their choices and thought processes related to their health. Because most people will, at some point in their lives, become ill, struggle, and have bad days, *wellness* refers to the ability to adapt and make choices to support health throughout a lifetime.

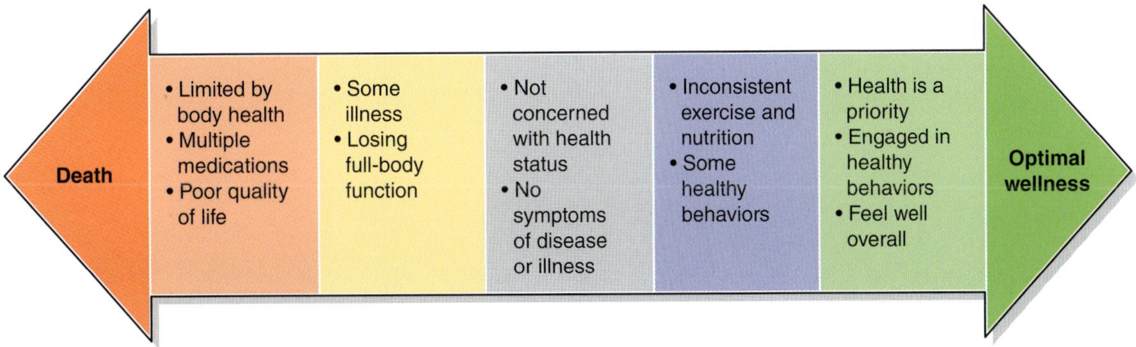


**Figure 1.2** Wellness as a continuum.

We can think of wellness as a continuum with optimal wellness at one end and death at the other (figure 1.2). As such, your position on the continuum changes as you make daily decisions that affect your health. If you feel like your current circumstance isn't supporting your wellness and health, you can change your behavior. As your wellness and health improve, you move closer to optimal wellness on the continuum.

Because your wellness changes over a lifetime, it is important to remember that your decisions today can have a large impact on your life in 5, 10, or even 20 years. Think of health as a savings account. The more you are able to deposit now (in healthy behaviors), the more savings you will have in the future (in health benefits). For instance, although eating a healthy diet right now will help you maintain a healthy weight and feel good, it may be difficult to imagine the long-term reward. However, eating a healthy and balanced diet as a young adult reduces the risk of developing cardiovascular disease and diabetes later in life. Consider depositing healthy habits into your savings account to make a greater impact later in life.

> Wellness is the complete integration of body, mind, and spirit—the realization that everything we do, think, feel, and believe has an effect on our state of well-being.
>
> **Greg Anderson**

Continually working toward wellness helps support efforts in stress management. A person who has poor physical health may find it difficult to focus their energy on stress management techniques.

## Managing Chronic Conditions and Wellness

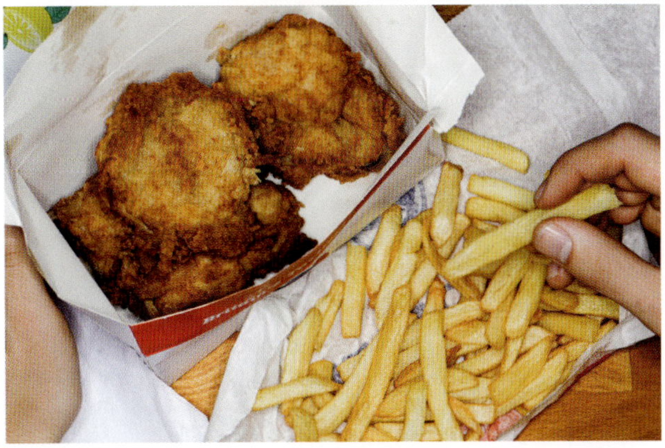

James has type 1 diabetes, a chronic health condition in which the body doesn't make enough insulin to break down the sugar in blood, which can lead to more serious complications (e.g., vision loss and kidney disease). James is taking five college classes and has two term papers due and a midterm exam the same week. The stress has been building up, and James is constantly worrying about his performance in classes. This has made it more difficult for James to find time to manage his other needs (proper diet, regular testing of blood sugar, and getting enough sleep at night). As a result, James' diabetes is not being well managed. This is a classic example of how stress—and the inability to manage it—can take away the focus and energy needed to maintain wellness.

## Influences on Wellness

Optimal wellness is an individual pursuit, but it is influenced by genetics, access to health care, interpersonal relationships, and the surrounding environment. These influences can either make it easier or more difficult to move toward optimal wellness.

### Self-Regulation

If we think of wellness as an ever-changing state of being, it becomes clear that being able to manage our own health and adapt to life circumstances is critical to our wellness (Yu, Tou, & Low, 2022). **Self-regulation**, or the ability to monitor and modify behavior to achieve a goal, is an important task to improve health outcomes. Self-regulation helps you control impulses, manage time and stress, and cope with emotions (Bub, Robinson, Curtis, & Kazak, 2016). For example, when you procrastinate, you are likely to experience more stress as the deadline for the task draws near, which can affect your health. Learning strategies to manage your time, such as starting earlier and planning short-term deadlines to keep you on track, can prevent stress and move you closer to optimal wellness on the continuum. Another example of a self-regulation habit is to always wear a seat belt in the car. Although the act of wearing a seat belt may not be stress relieving, it reduces the likelihood of injury in the event of an accident—an important health outcome.

Self-regulating theory defines the process one goes through to achieve a desired behavior. This process has four components (Baumeister & Vohs, 2007):

1. Standards: A well-defined desired behavior or result
2. Motivation: Motivation to meet the standard
3. Monitoring: Keeping track of the current behavior and situation
4. Willpower: Being able to control one's urges

Because there is a relationship between stress and willpower, these techniques also work for stress reduction. Willpower is a limited resource that can become depleted when under stress (Bernecker & Jon, 2020). Thus, in order to invoke and maintain willpower, you can engage in strategies to minimize stress.

One strategy is through rest: When you feel yourself feeling overwhelmed, take a break. Distracting yourself from something that is draining your willpower can stop it from doing so. This can include taking a walk, removing yourself from the situation, or just performing a separate task. This time away from the task is time that your body uses to restore willpower. Another way to restore willpower is to maintain a positive attitude: Setting out to conduct a stressful task with a positive attitude will make the task less draining.

Planning ahead in order to reduce last-minute decision making can also help maintain willpower. Imagine you need to start studying for an exam. After a long day, it is now 7 p.m., you're hungry

#### Self-Regulation During COVID-19

In 2020, most colleges and universities pivoted to online classes in response to the COVID-19 pandemic, and students who didn't sign up for online classes had to abruptly transition from traditional instruction to virtual instruction. Although many factors influenced academic performance at this time—some students lost their jobs, others were parents whose own children were now learning from home, some had to care for family members who became ill, and some didn't have sufficient technology to keep up with their schoolwork—many students struggled from a lack of self-regulation. For many, the online environment was a new learning arena, and the flexibility proved to be a hindrance rather than a benefit. Many students struggled with the lack of structured class meetings; others had trouble meeting deadlines. Learning to self-regulate behavior is therefore a useful skill, especially for online students. For example, creating a schedule for when to complete readings and assignments and breaking down large projects into smaller tasks will largely diminish stress.

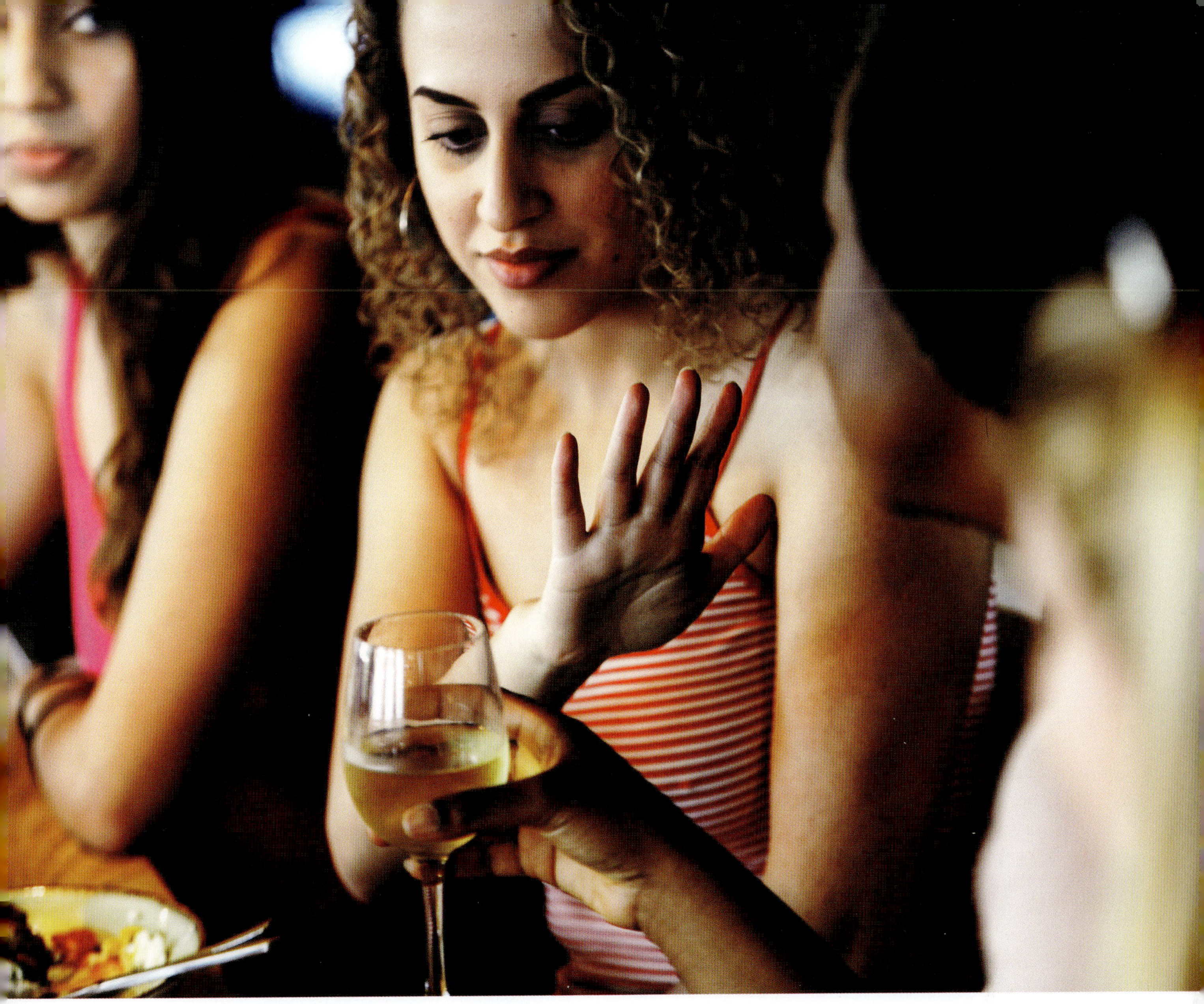

and haven't eaten yet, and you don't even know where your textbook is. It may feel like you have to climb a huge mountain before you can actually start to study. However, if you had set a plan to study at 7 p.m., it would be easier for you to follow through. During the day, you put your textbook on your desk and set aside a snack to eat while studying. Now when you get home from a long day, you are ready to start.

Lastly, having a toolbox of refusal skills allows you to say no without depleting your willpower. When you have a variety of refusal skills that you are comfortable using, it becomes automatic and habitual, which makes it easier to say no—even when you want to say yes. Willpower is like a gas tank. When the tank is getting close to empty, it is important to stop and refill it to allow yourself to go farther.

## Self-Efficacy

When you engage in some type of behavior change to improve wellness, it can be a scary venture. One component that can support your efforts in behavior change is self-efficacy, or a belief in your capability in a particular skill (Bandura, 1995). Self-efficacy is situational—for example, you may have high self-efficacy in one area of your life but not in another. In light of behavior change, self-efficacy is the confidence you have in yourself to change your behavior and continue the changed behavior.

## Transtheoretical Model of Behavior Change

The transtheoretical model (TTM) of behavior change has six stages:

1. *Precontemplation.* You are unaware of the problem or do not see the behavior as problematic.
2. *Contemplation.* You are thinking about their problem behavior with the intention of changing the behavior in the foreseeable future.
3. *Preparation.* You begin to create a plan for behavior change.
4. *Action.* The behavior change takes place; you modify or eliminate the problematic behavior.
5. *Maintenance.* You have made the desired behavior change and are working to prevent relapse.
6. *Termination.* The behavior change is now permanent and not at risk for relapse.

For each stage, different strategies can help you move to the next stage. For example, decisional balance is a strategy most often used in the early stages of TTM (precontemplation or contemplation) that measures the pros and cons of a potential behavior change (Janis & Mann, 1979). For example, if you were considering starting yoga to help manage stress, the cons may include the additional time needed to fit yoga into your schedule, the cost of classes, and your nervousness about learning a new skill. On the other hand, the pros may include reduced stress, increased mental clarity, and increased physical fitness. After weighing both sides, you may decide the pros outweigh the cons and register for yoga classes. Part III of this textbook will introduce other stress management strategies.

Self-efficacy is a skill that you can build. Let's say that after considering the pros and cons of creating a new time management plan for completing your schoolwork, you decide to do it. However, you don't feel confident in your skills to follow through. To improve your chances of success, you can work on building self-efficacy. One way to do so is to model success through small achievements (Bandura, 1997). For example, you create a calendar with all the due dates for this semester's assignments. You begin to feel more competent with everything planned out. As you use the calendar, your self-efficacy builds because you feel more confident managing your time. You begin to expand your use of the calendar to other items, including work schedules, social events, and free time plans. Self-efficacy was built by starting with the small task of creating a calendar for academic success and expanding its use to other areas of your life.

**When you achieve success, it helps you feel capable and can increase your sense of self-efficacy.**

Another way to build self-efficacy is to see people who are similar to yourself succeed in the behavior. When we watch others be successful, we begin to believe that if they can do it, so can we (Bandura, 1995). Having support from others also leads us to believe we can do it—consider how cheering on the other players on your team can help them perform better. Having someone tell us we can succeed makes us feel as though we can.

Lastly, your mood can impact your self-efficacy. Experiencing stress or feeling negative about a behavior can reduce levels of self-efficacy, whereas having a positive attitude about a behavior change can enhance your own level of confidence (Bandura, 1995).

## Genetics

**Genetics** refers to traits that are passed down from a parent to a child. Sometimes these traits can be risk factors that make a person more susceptible to certain diseases and illnesses. For example, your risk of cardiovascular disease increases if you have a parent with cardiovascular disease. Some research suggests that genetic scores may be a better indicator for cardiovascular disease than a risk assessment (Knowles & Ashley, 2018).

Another example of the influence of genetics on health is the increased breast cancer risk for people carrying mutations of the genes BRCA1 and BRCA2, which normally function to repair

Case Study

## Transtheoretical Model of Behavior Change and Willpower

Emily is a full-time college student in her first year. As many students do, Emily is finding college more difficult than high school. Emily was active in high school and finds that she misses working out. As such, she is struggling with finding time to exercise. Emily has exercised a couple of times over the past few months, but it hasn't become part of her routine. Emily is ready to start a program; she just isn't sure how to get started and make it sustainable. She knows she needs to work on willpower but doesn't know how.

### Discussion Questions

1. In which stage of the transtheoretical model of change is Emily? What clues in the passage support your answer?
2. What advice would you give Emily to help her get started on an exercise program?
3. In what ways can Emily prepare and plan for exercise?

damaged cells (particularly in the breast and ovaries). However, BRCA1 and BRCA2 mutations diminish the cells' ability to repair the damage and increase the risk of cancer; it is estimated that these mutations increase the cumulative lifetime risk up to 75 percent for breast cancer and 76 percent for ovarian cancer (Wiggins, Walker, & Pearson, 2020). These BRCA1 and BRCA2 mutations can be passed down from one generation to the next.

## Health Care Access

Access to health care is another important factor in health outcomes. *Access* can mean different things to different people: For some, it may mean the nearest medical clinic is two hours away; for others, it may mean the cost of medical care is prohibitive. Regardless of the barrier, many people simply do not have access to quality medical care and thus have poorer health outcomes. For

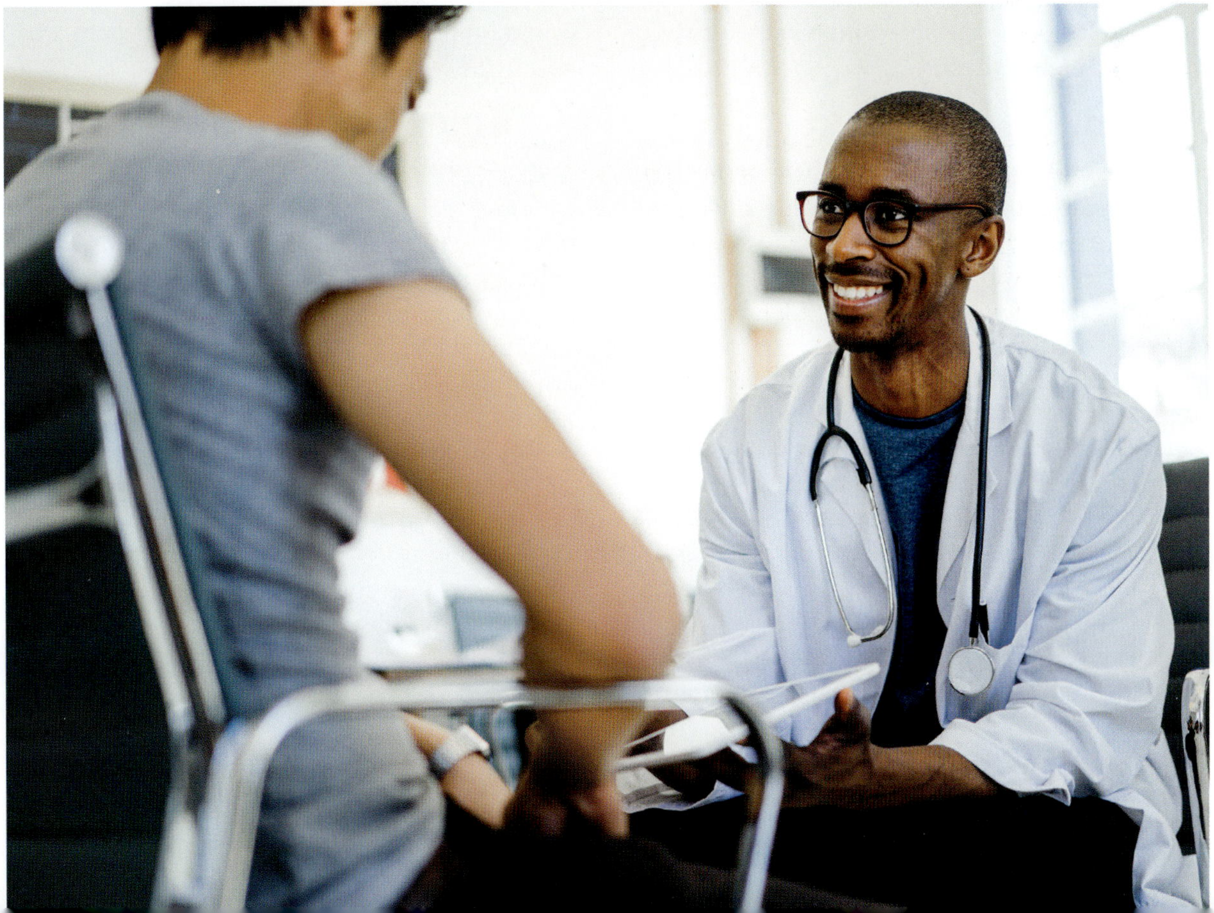

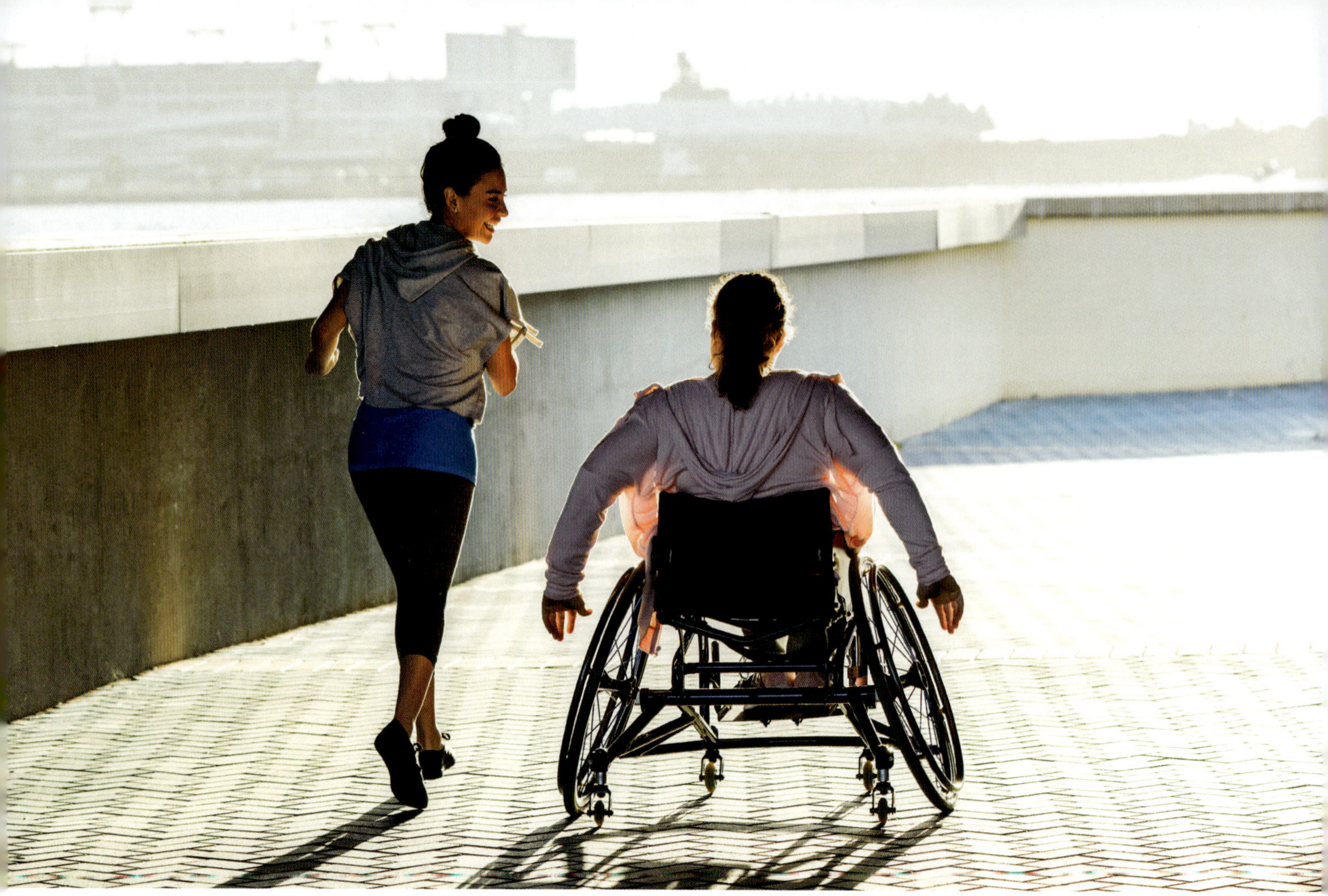

someone with a sick child and no car, for example, it could be very difficult to navigate the public transportation system just to seek help. Barriers to health care not only impact physical health but create additional stress.

### Physical Environment

The places we live and work also have an impact on our health and wellness (Centers for Disease Control, 2011). Positive influences in the built environment may include access to parks, hospitals, and green spaces as well as a general sense of safety. It can include good schools, libraries, and high employment rates. A positive environment has access to fresh fruits and vegetables and a variety of community resources that bring people together. Negative community influences may include few or no grocery stores, high levels of unemployment, and no community resources. It can also mean living in areas with a high crime rate and no or limited access to libraries.

How much control we have over where we live can depend on certain factors, such as employment, income, housing, and family. For example, if you do not have access to reliable transportation, you may need to live close to work, even if you would not prefer to live in this area.

## Dimensions of Wellness

As discussed earlier, wellness is the active process an individual goes through to obtain an optimal state of well-being. There are six dimensions of wellness: physical, emotional, intellectual, social, spiritual, and environmental. These dimensions are interrelated, as shown in figure 1.3. For example, if you love to exercise a few times a week, it will improve your physical health. However, there is also an association between physical activity and improved mental health. Additionally, those who engage in physical activity have stronger social connections with friends and family and feel less isolated compared to people who live a sedentary lifestyle, improving social wellness as well (Iannotti et al., 2009).

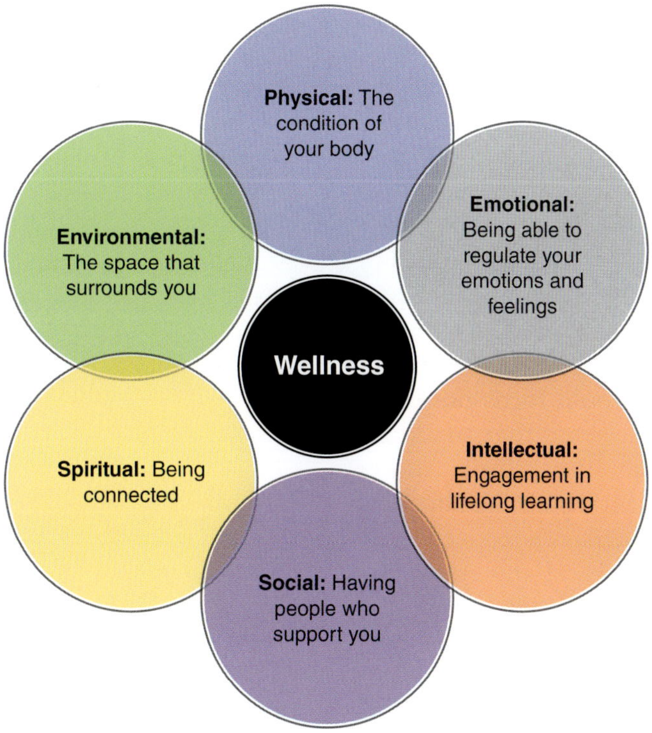
Physical: The condition of your body
Emotional: Being able to regulate your emotions and feelings
Intellectual: Engagement in lifelong learning
Social: Having people who support you
Spiritual: Being connected
Environmental: The space that surrounds you
Wellness

**Figure 1.3** The dimensions of wellness are connected and interrelated. They are often presented as overlapping parts of a circle to represent that there is no beginning and no end to wellness; it is an ongoing journey.

Working toward wellness in each dimension is how you can strive to achieve optimal wellness. Stress can take the focus away from wellness by placing us in a state of duress that makes it very difficult to focus on improving other areas of our lives. On the other hand, when you can achieve balance in the dimensions of wellness, you reduce stress by placing yourself in the best possible position to take care of your health. The goal is not to balance an equal amount of wellness in each dimension but rather a mix of each that works well for you. Ignoring one part of wellness can lead to an imbalance that affects the other parts. It is important to be able to reflect on your own wellness to consider which areas to work on improving.

Creating a balance among these dimensions of wellness is an important task (Substance Abuse and Mental Health Services Administration, 2016). Each person has different needs, traits, and preferences, and each person's balance will look different. In the following section, you will be introduced to the different components of wellness. Part II of this textbook will explore each of these dimensions in greater depth.

## Physical Wellness

**Physical wellness** includes caring for your body. Optimal levels of physical wellness are achieved through nutrition, exercise, following safety protocols, and getting enough sleep. Maintaining optimal levels of physical wellness can help you better manage your stress. When you are healthy, your body and mind are strong and ready to deal with anything.

**Self-care** is the first defense against stress. Taking time out of the day to focus on yourself and ensure your own health status can not only make you a better and more productive person but also help you achieve your health goals while increasing your happiness. When we are under stress, our physical health tends to be placed on the back burner. This can further increase stress and strain our physical well-being. Caring for your physical health should be a priority each day. Self-care will be further discussed in chapter 11.

**The components of physical wellness include fitness, healthy eating, sleep, and rest.**

Fitness and exercise have tremendous health benefits at any age. Regular exercise can improve your cognition and memory while reducing your risk of chronic illness. Currently, only half of adults get the physical activity needed to reduce chronic diseases (Centers for Disease Control, 2020). A balanced diet is an important component of physical health. You should focus on eating a variety of foods and beverages that support a healthy weight and prevent disease (United States Dietary Association, 2019). Obtaining adequate sleep each night is associated with reduced levels of stress and improved physical and emotional wellness (Taylor et al., 2017). In addition to sleep, periods of rest are equally important to help improve physical and overall wellness.

Stress can affect your physical health by placing an increased demand on the energy and resources the body uses to fight disease. For this reason, high levels of stress can increase the risk of illness (Slavich & Auerbach, 2018). Being able to effectively manage your stress can improve your physical health by improving your immune system functioning.

Stress can manifest itself in the body in many ways. For example, it is not uncommon to engage in tensing movements when under stress: Have you ever been stressed and found yourself clenching your jaw? Having a better understanding of your physical health and how to recognize symptoms of stress can help you manage it before it becomes a bigger problem. Some examples of physical symptoms of stress include the following:

- Frequent headaches (Anyeyer, Leach, Klose, Dobos, & Cramer, 2019)
- Jaw grinding (Vlagutu et al., 2022)
- Neck pain (Jahre, Grotle, Smedbraten, Dunn, & Oiestad, 2020) and backache (Ben-Ami, 2020)
- Frequent blushing and sweating (Welnitzova, 2021)
- Dry mouth (Redondo-Florez, Tornero-Aguilera, Ramos-Campo, & Clemente-Suarez, 2020)
- Diminished sexual desire (Tavares, Schlagintweit, Nobre, & Rosen, 2019)
- Chest pain, palpitations, or rapid pulse (Bae et al., 2019)

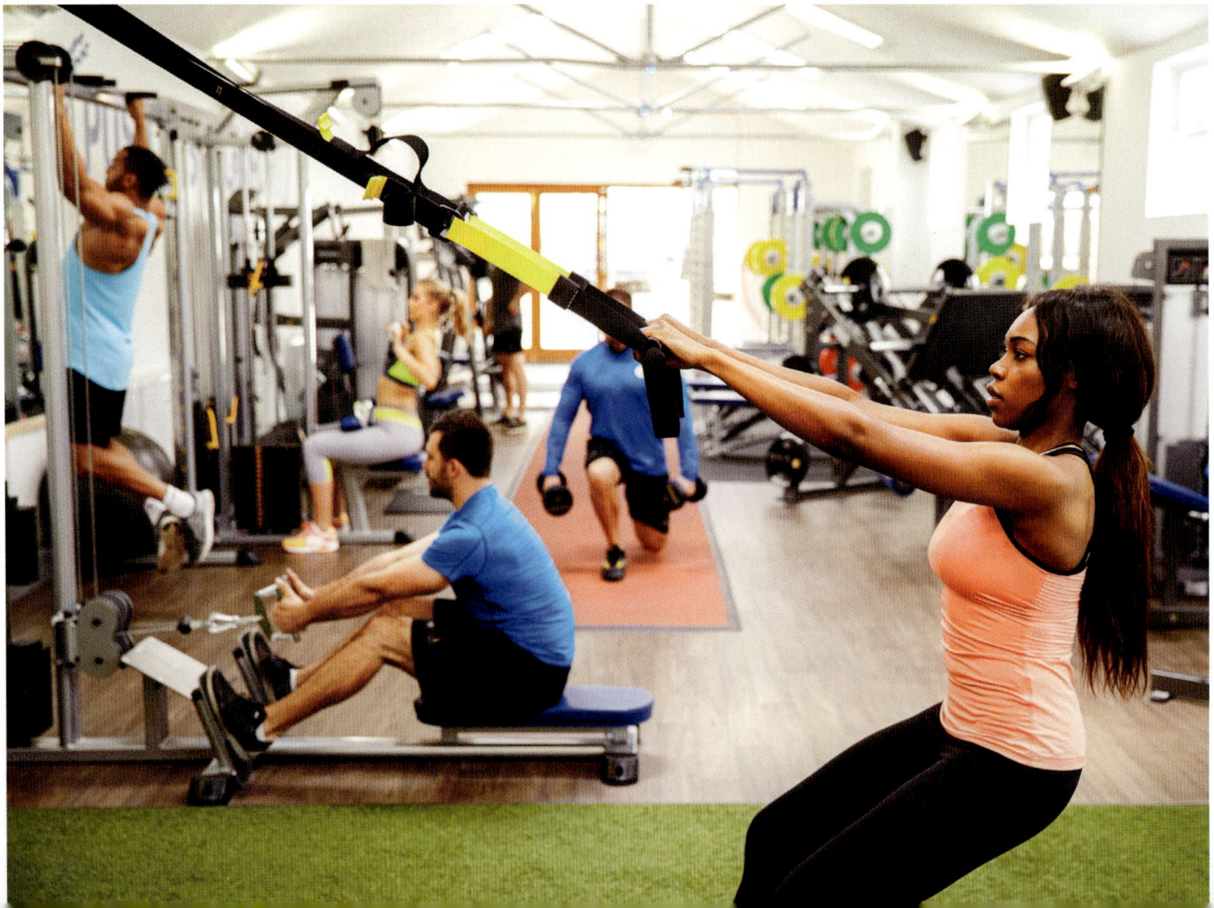

## Stress-Prone and Stress-Resistant Personality Traits

One element that determines how a person manages stress is personality, or individual differences in thinking, feeling, and behaving (Cervone & Pervin, 2018).

- *Thinking* refers to the way a person thinks about life. Is the person optimistic? Pessimistic? Future oriented? Traditional?
- *Feeling* refers to how a person feels emotions. Does the person tend to be happy or sad most of the time? Does the person have extreme emotions or are they more mellow?
- *Behaving* refers to behaviors and actions. Is the person outgoing or shy? Does the person tend to be more comfortable alone or with people? Is the person neat or messy?

Personality tends to be stable over a lifetime (Specht, Egloff, & Schmukle, 2011). Many different theories pertain to personality; however, one common theory pertains to personality types A and B.

People with a type A personality generally tend to be very driven, self-critical, and easily excited (Ilyas, Naseem, & Bibi, 2019). They can be workaholics and like to keep busy, scheduling many tasks throughout the day and working hard to accomplish them all. They are also impatient and competitive and don't feel rewarded when they accomplish tasks and projects. As a result, people with these personality traits have a harder time managing stress and tend to ignore or delay self-care. Additionally, type A personalities tend to be easily angered, which can lead to hostility. These factors contribute to higher risks of heart disease, hypertension, job stress, and social isolation (Ilyas, Naseem, & Bibi, 2019).

On the other hand, people with type B personalities tend to be more relaxed, noncompetitive, and carefree (Uzum, Ozdemir, Kose, Ozkan, & Seneldir, 2022). They adapt better to change and have a tendency to be more flexible. As a result, they may also have better stress management skills compared to those with type A personalities (Shaygannejad, Dahnavi, & Ashtari, 2013).

Regardless of your personality type, it is important to remember that everyone has control over how they manage their stress levels. Although your personality traits may contribute to stress, there are techniques you can use to help manage stress and ultimately lead to better health outcomes.

## Emotional Wellness

**Emotional wellness** refers to the awareness and understanding of one's emotions and the ability to effectively manage those emotions. Negative attitudes and emotions can contribute to and make it difficult to effectively cope with stress, leading to poorer health outcomes and decreased healthy functioning. Learning to focus on positive emotions can help you become more resilient when you encounter a stressful event.

Many assume that having high levels of emotional wellness translates to being happy all the time. This is not the case. Having high levels of emotional wellness means one is attuned to their emotions and can cope with life's challenges (Papanagnou et al., 2017). Think about the last time you were disappointed in something. How did you handle your feelings? Did you dwell on it and allow it to bring you down? Or did you come up with a plan to overcome your disappointment? The initial emotional response is the same, but what is important is how you handle the emotion and plan for the future.

People who have high levels of emotional wellness have the following characteristics:

- Regard for self and others
- Contentment with who they are
- Open-mindedness and flexibility
- Ability to talk about emotions
- Ability to relax
- A purpose in life

Research Spotlight

## Mental Health Disparities

Approximately 21 percent of U.S. adults—or one in five—have a mental illness (Substance Abuse and Mental Health Services Administration, 2021). Among those, less than half utilize any type of mental health service (Substance Abuse and Mental Health Services Administration, 2021). Although mental health services are becoming more widespread, these services remain underused, particularly among people of color.

*Mental health disparities* refer to the differences in mental health outcomes between different groups of people based on factors such as age, sex, gender, race, ethnicity, and geography (Substance Abuse and Mental Health Services Administration, 2021). For example, those who identify as part of a sexual minority group experience higher rates of depression (Marshal et al., 2011), with gay males experiencing depression at rates three times higher than the general adult population (Lee, Oliffe, & Kelly, 2017). Hispanic American females also experience some of the highest depression rates in the United States at almost 40 percent (De Oliveira, Cianelli, Gattamorta, Kowalski, & Peragallo, 2016). Latino youth also have higher rates of depression compared to other ethnic groups, with first-generation youth and those who are undocumented having the highest rates of depression among Latinos/as (Cobb, Xie, Meca, & Schwartz, 2017; Potochnick & Perreira, 2010). Black Americans experience lower rates of depression compared to white Americans, but when depression does occur, it is more likely to be severe and persistent (Budhwani, Hearld, & Chavez-Yenter, 2015).

One of the theories used to explain these disparities is the impact of social stress, which refers to one's relationship with others and their social environment. Because social systems in the United States are based on Eurocentric views of the world that may not include all cultures or groups of people, those identifying with groups outside this social mainstream feel additional strain or stress (Safran et al., 2009). Although these groups hold different ideas, beliefs, and cultures, they share a common history of oppression (Safran et al., 2009).

Another theory that has been used to explain mental health disparities is the impact of racial discrimination. This refers to the systems in place that devalue certain racial groups and provide different societal opportunities and resources based on racial group identity (Williams, 2018). Those affected experience this discrimination as a chronic stressor, which can lead to negative changes in mental and physical health (Williams, 2018).

Mental health disparities may also be attributed to a lack of treatment options and increased barriers to obtaining treatment. In a recent study, almost 25 percent of adults with a mental illness were not able to receive treatment (Substance Abuse and Mental Health Services Administration, 2021). The most common reported barriers to receiving care include lack of insurance, lack of available treatment, undersized mental health workforce, and inability to afford health care (Reinert, Fritze, & Nguyen, 2021). There is also a stigma associated with depression and mental illness. In one study, when asked about perceptions of mental illness, Black Americans were more likely to perceive individuals with a mental illness as dangerous (Abdullah, Brown, & Corrigan, 2020). A stigma associated with a condition acts as a barrier to receiving treatment by discouraging a person from seeking help (Clement et al., 2014).

Income may also play a role in mental health disparities. Treatment for mental health issues can be costly. Those from lower-income households are less likely to know where to go for mental health treatment (Planey, Smith, Moore, & Walker, 2019), and youth from low-income households are more likely to only use services that are available in the educational system (Ali et al., 2019).

Lack of access to quality treatment may contribute to more negative outcomes from a mental illness. For example, Black youth have the lowest utilization rate of mental health services, but the highest attempted suicide rate compared to white and Hispanic students (Ivey-Stephenson et al., 2020). Binge drinking, illicit drug use, and tobacco use are also more frequent among youth with mental illnesses (Substance Abuse and Mental Health Services Administration, 2021). In general, quality of life is decreased when mental illness is left untreated.

In conclusion, mental health disparities tend to derive from barriers to accessing mental health treatment, whether material (not having a treatment center in the area), financial (not having the money to pay for treatment), or informational (not knowing where and how to find help). One mechanism to reduce mental health disparities may be to increase mental health treatment options across the United States. It is safe to assume improved access to mental health treatment will improve mental health for all.

## Intellectual Wellness

**Intellectual wellness** is the ability and desire to continue learning throughout a lifetime. It includes creative and cognitive development. A person who is intellectually well is constantly challenging themselves to experience new things, learn new ideas, and engage in activities that promote thinking and foster growth.

You can practice behaviors to enhance your own levels of intellectual wellness. These include taking in other people's perspectives, learning new hobbies, experiencing other cultures, and being aware of current events. Focusing on improving intellectual health can provide benefits later in life. For example, older people who participate in brain-building activities such as reading, crossword puzzles, or sudoku reduce a variety of short-term and long-term (i.e., Alzheimer's) memory problems" (Kitko, 2001).

Intellectual symptoms of stress include the following:

- Worrying thoughts and increased anxiety (Garfin, Poulin, Blum, & Silver, 2018)
- Pessimistic outlook (Arsian, Yildirim, Tanhan, Bulus, & Allen, 2022)
- Inability to focus and memory problems (King, 2016)
- Poor judgment and decision making (Moritz, Kother, Hartmann, & Lincoln, 2015)

Taking time to appreciate and build on your personal interests is another way to develop your intellectual wellness. Do you enjoy art, reading, or pottery? These activities support brain development by finding creative outlets for you to think critically. They also allow you to take time for yourself, away from your daily stress.

## Social Wellness

The ability to form and maintain positive relationships comprises a person's **social wellness**. People are social beings, and the ability to form healthy relationships with others has a positive impact on health and wellness. People who have a good social support network—family and friends who can provide comfort during times of stress—have

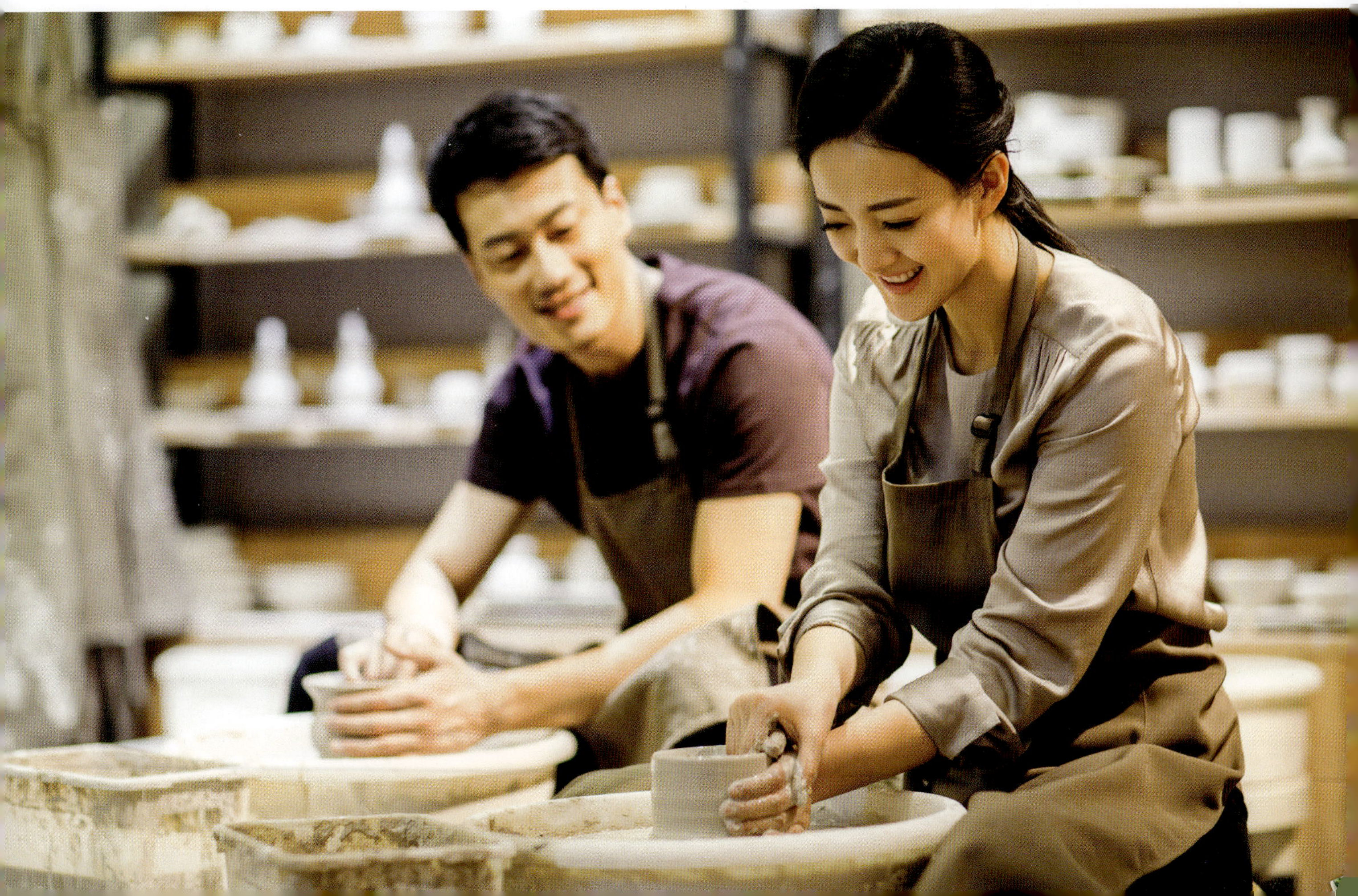

**Simply knowing you have someone there for you can provide a sense of comfort.**

better stress management skills and tend to have better mental and emotional health (Mayo Clinic, 2020). On the other hand, being physically and emotionally separated from others can lead to isolation and loneliness, which can lead to increased stress and poorer health outcomes (Mayo Clinic, 2020).

## Spiritual Wellness

**Spiritual wellness** can be defined as having a purpose and meaning in life or feeling a sense of connectedness with a higher power or the universe. Although it means different things to different people, many would agree that humans are spiritual people. A feeling of a connection can make you feel less alone, and a sense of purpose can help put things in perspective and allow you to focus on what's important—both of which can enhance your stress management skills (Mayo Clinic, 2021).

Spiritual health has been linked to many health benefits. People who express high levels of spiritual health have lower levels of depression, adapt better to stress, have healthier lifestyles, and require less medical care (Akbari & Hossaini, 2018). On the other hand, those without a clear purpose in life sometimes struggle with a lack of motivation or desire to deal with life's challenges—for these reasons, those who identify as having a high religious involvement are likely to live longer than those who do not (Cornah, 2006). Learning about other religions or spiritual practices can help bring better clarity about your own beliefs and values, which can serve as a framework to help guide your decisions to better align with your personal goals.

## Environmental Wellness

As described previously, the physical environment one lives in can contribute to wellness—in this case, our **environmental wellness**. This includes our immediate personal space and branches out to include larger areas, such as our community, country, and so on. Consider your own physical space: How would you describe it? Does it evoke feelings of peace and harmony? Does it evoke feelings of stress and chaos? Because our immediate surroundings are generally under our control, there are small and relatively easy things we can

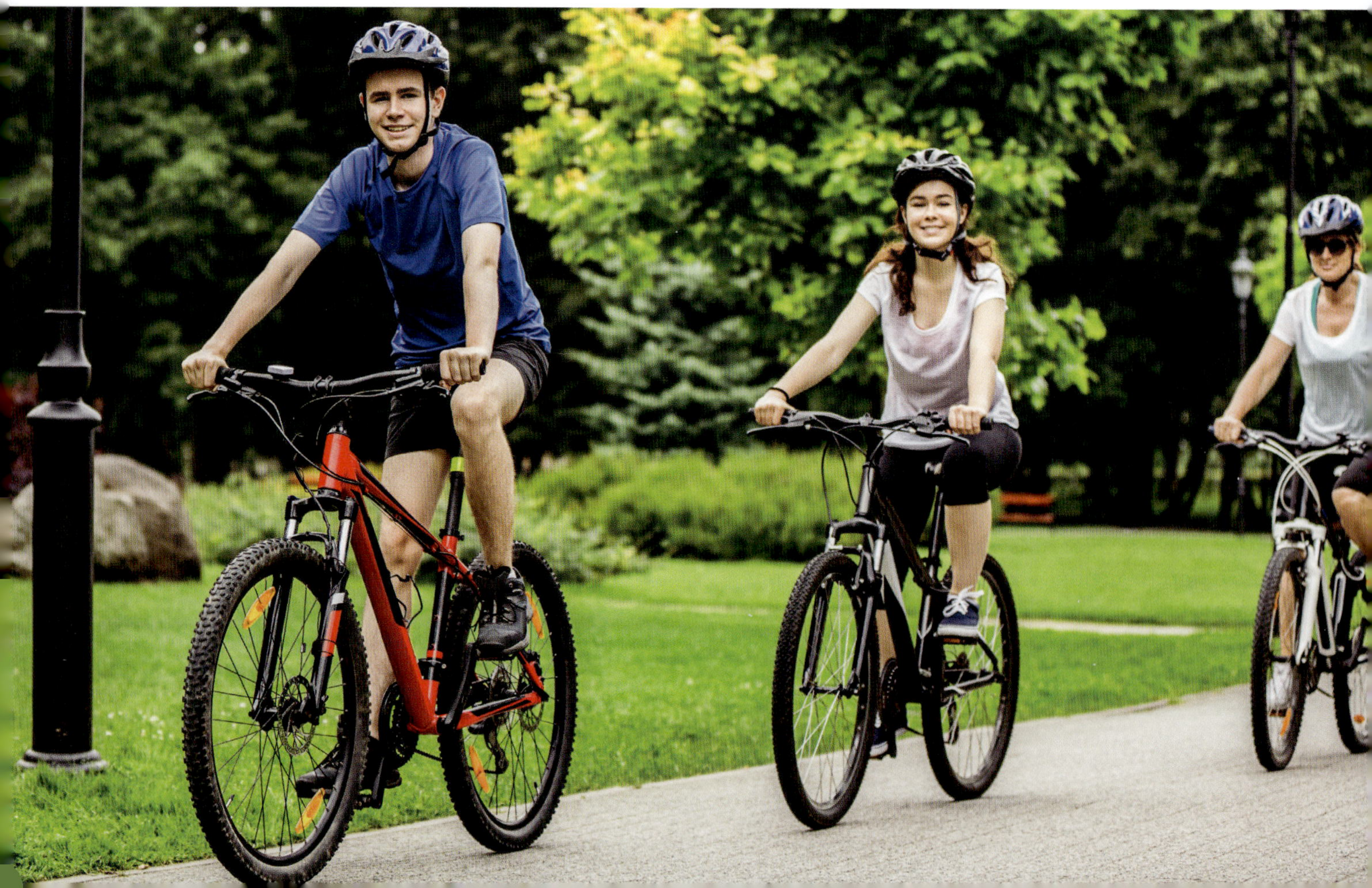

do to create a more tranquil environment, such as adding a plant or pictures or clearing out clutter. However, as one moves away from their immediate space, it is more difficult (and requires the effort of more people) to improve the larger area.

Health and living conditions go hand in hand. Poor housing conditions can lead to poor health outcomes, with people living in more deprived neighborhoods experiencing higher mortality rates and higher levels of stress (Lenthe et al., 2005). Information about where we live can provide evidence of our levels of wellness. Consider walking down the block in a neighborhood and making a determination about the wellness and stress levels of the people who live there. For example, are the houses in good shape or disrepair? What does the area around the houses look like? Are there well-maintained parks or evidence of poverty? Other environmental factors that affect our health, happiness, and stress include noise and light.

Consider the following and how they would impact your own levels of wellness:

- Living with the noise of a big city compared to the quiet of a rural area
- Living in a brightly lit area (e.g., next to a large 24-hour gas station) as compared to a leafy residential neighborhood
- Living near parks and green spaces
- Living in areas with high levels of crime
- Living in an area with a high unemployment rate

## Mind–Body Connection

The mind–body connection describes the influence the mind has on the body and vice versa. There is a strong relationship among our thoughts, subjective experiences, mood, and physiological responses (e.g., heart rate, blood pressure, perspiration) (Uzan, 2021). For example, many studies have shown the connection between poorly managed stress and hypertension, insomnia, digestive disorders, mental health issues, and diabetes (Witzel, Turner, & Hooker, 2021). Furthermore, stress, anger, helplessness, and hopelessness increase a person's susceptibility to disease and disorder (Pawar, 2020). Although dying of a broken heart is not possible, a condition called Takotsubo cardiomyopathy, known as *broken heart syndrome*, is believed to be caused by a surge of stress hormones entering the bloodstream and temporarily damaging the heart muscle (Zvonarev, 2019). Acute stress may also increase the risk of true coronary syndrome, resulting in cardiovascular death. For example, on the day of the 1994 Northridge earthquake, a 6.7 earthquake centered in southern California, a 260 percent increase in cardiovascular deaths was observed (Levine, 2019).

Mind–body practices can help promote a sense of control, enhance optimism, and help you cope with life's challenges, which can help reduce the risk of other health conditions (Dossett, Fricchione, & Benson, 2020). Using mind–body therapies can help with conditions from substance abuse to depression. The following list highlights some examples of mind–body therapies; these will be discussed in more depth in chapter 10.

- Meditation
- Yoga
- Mindfulness
- Art therapy
- Movement therapy

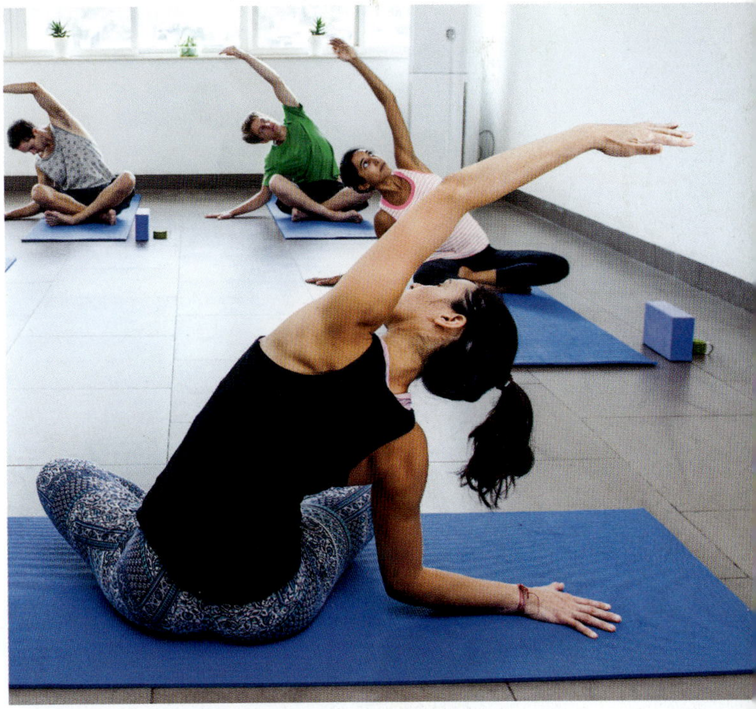

## Proactive Ways to Manage Stress

Advice for improving one's health is often grounded in a deficit approach, which begins with identifying weak areas needing improvement. This puts the journey toward better health in a negative light, which tends to diminish self-esteem and be counterproductive. On the other hand, a strengths-based approach identifies resources and assets afforded by an individual's personality and environment (figure 1.4).

This approach is often used in the helping professions (e.g., counselors, social workers, community health workers) to help clients bring about positive change. A strengths-based approach identifies your personal strengths and then uses them to support behavior changes. For example, let's say you wanted to improve your fitness, and your identified strengths are that you are very organized and love creating schedules. The strengths-based approach would have you create your own weekly physical activity schedule. Now let's say that instead of being organized, your strength is being social; you enjoy being around other people. In this example, you might improve fitness by signing up for a group activity class. In these ways, you are utilizing your strengths to best achieve your goals.

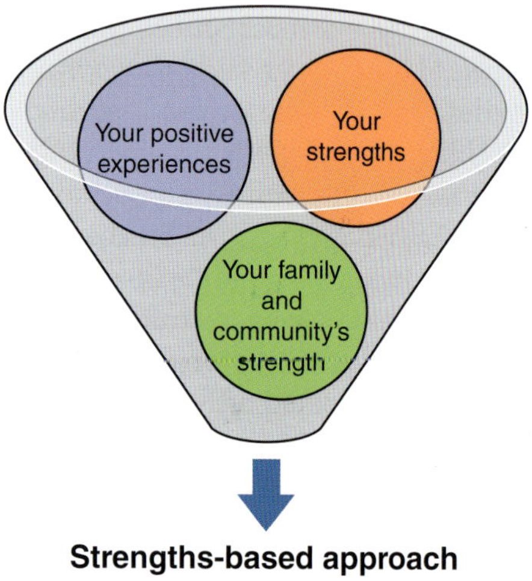


**Figure 1.4** Strengths-based approach to health and wellness.

**By focusing on your strengths, you can utilize your skills to improve your health.**

## Summary

This chapter explored definitions of health and wellness. In the context of stress management, behaviors that move you toward optimal levels of health also help with stress management. You cannot effectively manage stress levels if you engage in behaviors that do not support health and wellness. The next chapter will expand on the definition of stress and how it connects to your overall wellness. You will also learn about the stress response cycle and connect the changes that occur during a stressful event to your overall wellness.

## ONLINE RESOURCES

Visit HK*Propel* to access audio supplements, worksheets, and vocabulary flash cards for this chapter.

## DISCUSSION QUESTIONS

1. How does stress impact all areas of wellness? Explain how managing stress can help move a person toward optimal wellness.
2. Analyze your wellness using the six dimensions. Discuss ways to improve your own wellness.
3. What is the mind–body connection? Think back on your own life experiences and describe a time when your mental health impacted another aspect of your wellness. Describe the situation that led to the event and how it affected other aspects of your wellness.
4. What are the benefits of using a strengths-based approach to wellness? Why do you think this approach is supported by mental health professionals?

# 2

# Understanding Stress

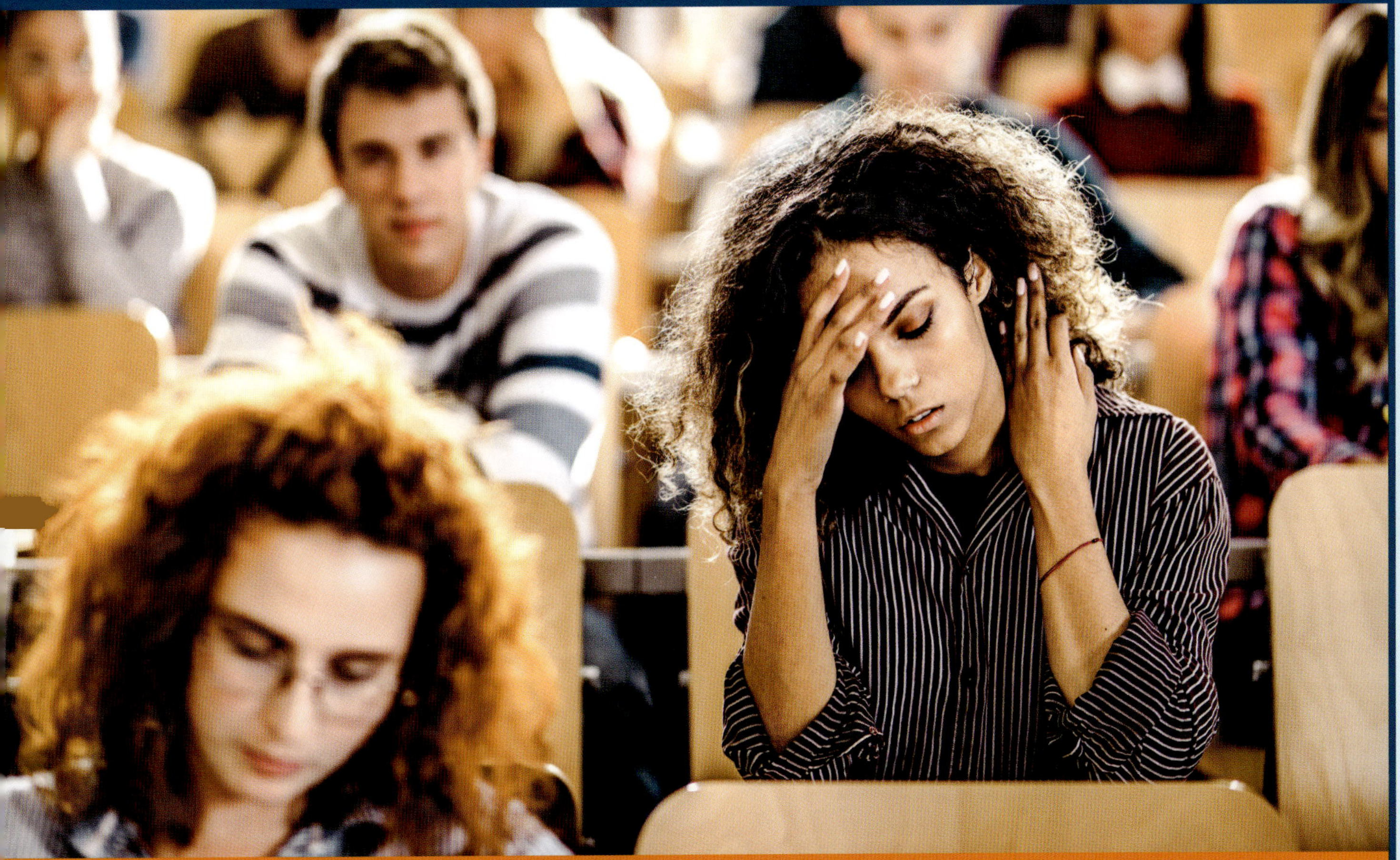

## LEARNING OBJECTIVES

After reading this chapter, you will be able to do the following:

- Explain the physiological responses to stress
- Identify the hormones involved in stress and their roles in the stress response stages
- Distinguish between eustress, distress, acute stress, chronic stress, trauma, and posttraumatic stress
- Evaluate factors that contribute to an individual's optimal stress level and stress reactivity
- Discuss the types of societal stressors and their impact

# KEY TERMS

- acute stress
- adrenaline
- adverse childhood experiences (ACEs)
- alarm stage
- autonomic nervous system (ANS)
- biopsychosocial (BPS) model of challenge and threat
- chronic stress
- cortisol
- distress
- eustress
- exhaustion stage
- fight-or-flight response
- freeze response
- general adaptation syndrome
- homeostasis
- internalized racism
- nomophobia
- parasympathetic nervous system (PNS)
- posttraumatic stress disorder (PTSD)
- resistance stage
- stress
- stressors
- stress reactivity
- sympathetic nervous system (SNS)
- technostress
- trauma

When was the last time you felt really stressed? What caused your stress? Was it too many assignments due in one week? Was it a fight with a friend? Was it not enough time in the day to get everything done? The source of stress is different for everyone, but learning to manage it can make the difference between living well and struggling. This chapter will help you understand the physical effects of stress to better understand the importance of managing stress.

## Stress and Stressors

**Stress** is defined as the body's response to events or thoughts that cause physical or emotional strain. One of the main functions of the body is to maintain a consistent internal environment while adjusting to a changing external environment, called **homeostasis** (Billman, 2020). This includes regulating blood pressure and blood pH (osmoregulation), blood sugar and breathing rate (chemical regulation), and body temperature (thermoregulation); if any of these systems falls out of homeostasis, it can disrupt the entire body and lead to disease or even death.

**Stressors** can be anything that disrupts the body's homeostasis. A stressor can be as simple as a loud noise or meeting a new person or as serious as experiencing extreme poverty, abuse, or violence. Stressors can be external, such as death of a loved one, a natural disaster, or work. They can also be internal, such as not meeting a goal you set for yourself, performing poorly on an exam, or feeling angry. There are different types of stress. Stress can be acute (short term) or chronic (long term). It can arise from something positive (eustress) or from something disturbing (distress). All of these types of stress disrupt the body's functioning. Consider your body temperature, which on average is around 98.6 degrees. This temperature remains constant whether it is hot or cold outside. When you are exposed to extreme heat (a stressor), your body temperature rises (stress), and your body sweats to cool off. When you are cold, your body shivers to produce heat. In this way, your body adapts to maintain its internal temperature (homeostasis). If stress is effectively managed, the body will return to homeostasis.

When you encounter high levels of stress, you diminish your body's ability to manage the stress. If your body's adaptation to cold starts failing, for example, your body would not be able to manage its internal temperature, which would put you in danger. If hypothermia continues for a long period of time, the blood vessels to the extremities constrict as the body diverts blood to maintain functioning of the main internal organs. This is when frostbite can occur. If the exposure continues, breathing and heart rate decrease, which ultimately can result in unconsciousness and death. Chronic stress similarly damages the body's ability to return to homeostasis, leaving you susceptible to disease. This will be discussed further in chapter 3.

Stress is a part of life experienced by all people. When our early human ancestors experienced stress, it likely occurred while hunting for food or while being hunted. In either case, the adaptations needed in the body were the same: When encountering danger, the body needs to temporarily increase its energy to run quicker (either toward prey or away from a predator). In the modern world, most of our stressors do not present a physical danger, but the body still undergoes the same physical stress responses as those of our ancestors.

## Stress Response Stages

In the 1930s, researcher Hans Selye coined the term **general adaptation syndrome** to describe the nonspecific signs of bodily damage associated with stress. While conducting research with cow ovarian extract in the hope of discovering and identifying female sex hormones, Selye discovered deterioration of the thymus gland and ulcers in the stomach lining of his research rats. He then began to give the same injections in specific organs, then expanded his experiment and injected other noxious agents into the rats, both with similar results. He found that he was able to reproduce reliable changes in all the species of test rats by injecting agents into them. He then placed the rats in physically stressful situations (e.g., cold roof, continuous running on a treadmill) and again found similar results. In all his experiences, the rats experienced adrenal hyperactivity, lymphatic atrophy, and peptic ulcers (Tan & Yip, 2018). He used the term *stress* to describe noxious agents that caused the changes in his test animals (Viner, 1999).

The general adaptation syndrome describes a series of changes that occur when a stressor is

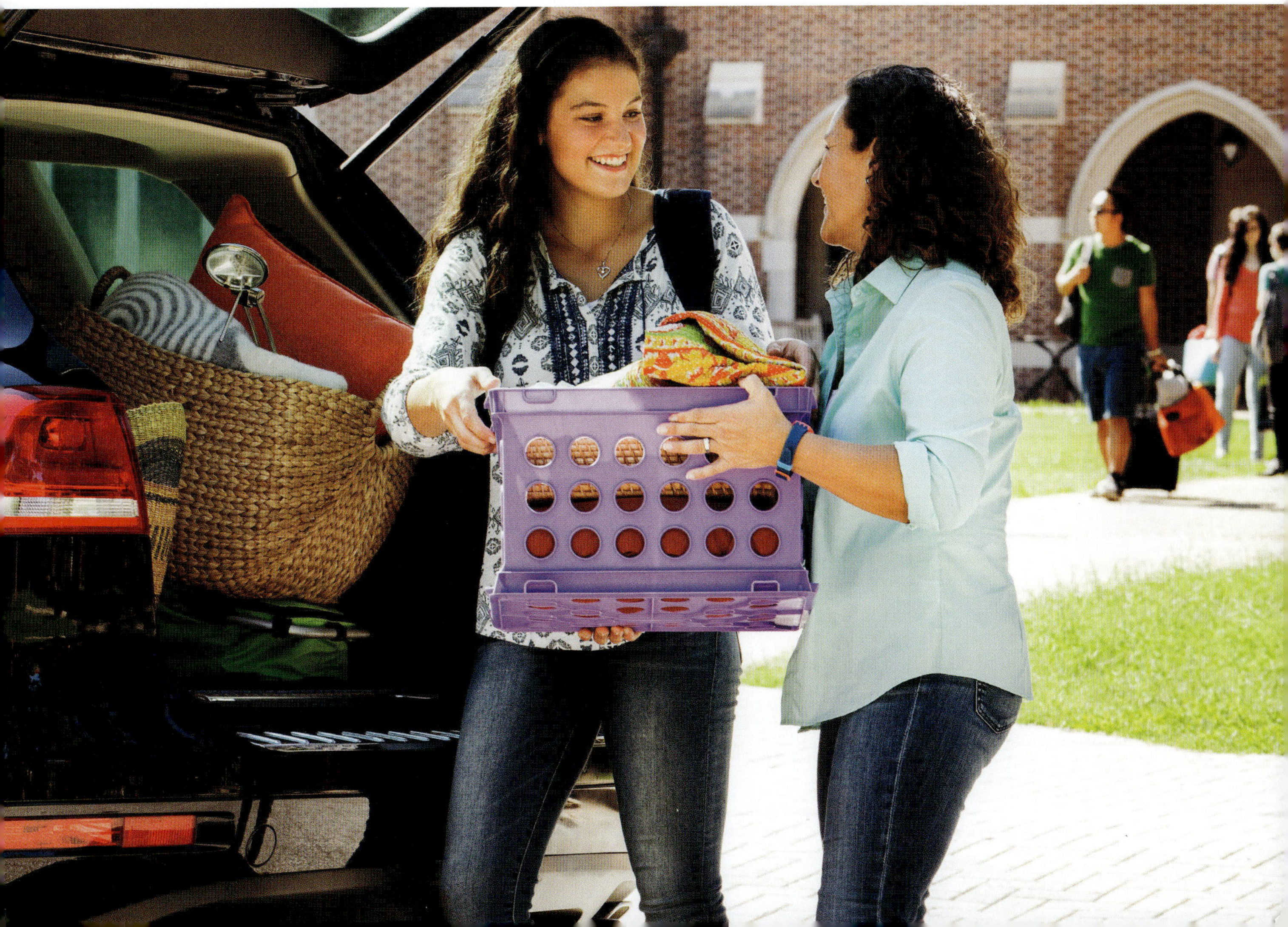

encountered, which follow a three-stage pattern that is common in both animals and humans (figure 2.1):

1. Alarm
2. Resistance
3. Exhaustion

The **alarm stage** is the body's initial reaction to stress. Walter Cannon (1915), a Harvard physiologist, first coined the phrase **fight-or-flight response** to describe the series of physiological changes that occur when a person encounters stress (figure 2.2). These changes are adaptations that evolved from our ancestors, who required an increase in energy to either hunt for food (fight) or run from becoming food (flight). In either case, the physical responses are the same. Have you ever been home at night and become frightened? After that initial fright, it might seem that every small sound of a branch hitting the window or creak in the floor has now become amplified. Your heart is racing and you feel tense all over. This is caused by the fight-or-flight response.

The fight-or-flight response is governed by the **autonomic nervous system**, which is responsible for managing the automatic functions in the body, including respiration, heart rate, blood pressure, and digestion. It is divided into two sections, the sympathetic nervous system and parasympathetic nervous system. The **sympathetic nervous system** is responsible for the initial response to stress (see figure 2.3). If your body perceives a threat, the sympathetic nervous system springs into action, producing physiological changes to improve the chances of a successful fight or flight. These changes make it possible for you to exert more physical strength and stamina—much like

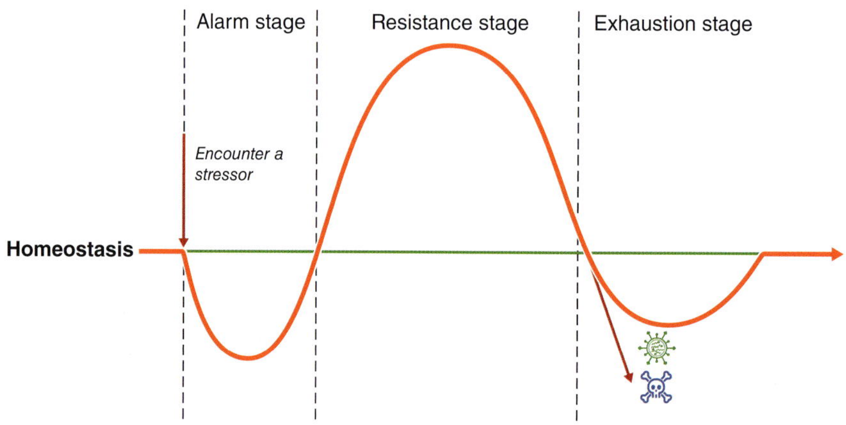


**Figure 2.1** General adaptation syndrome.

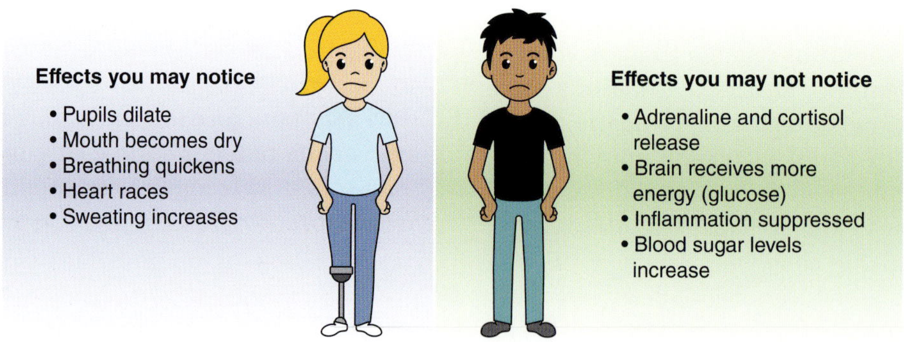
Effects you may notice
• Pupils dilate
• Mouth becomes dry
• Breathing quickens
• Heart races
• Sweating increases
Effects you may not notice
• Adrenaline and cortisol release
• Brain receives more energy (glucose)
• Inflammation suppressed
• Blood sugar levels increase

**Figure 2.2** Physiological changes during the fight-or-flight response.

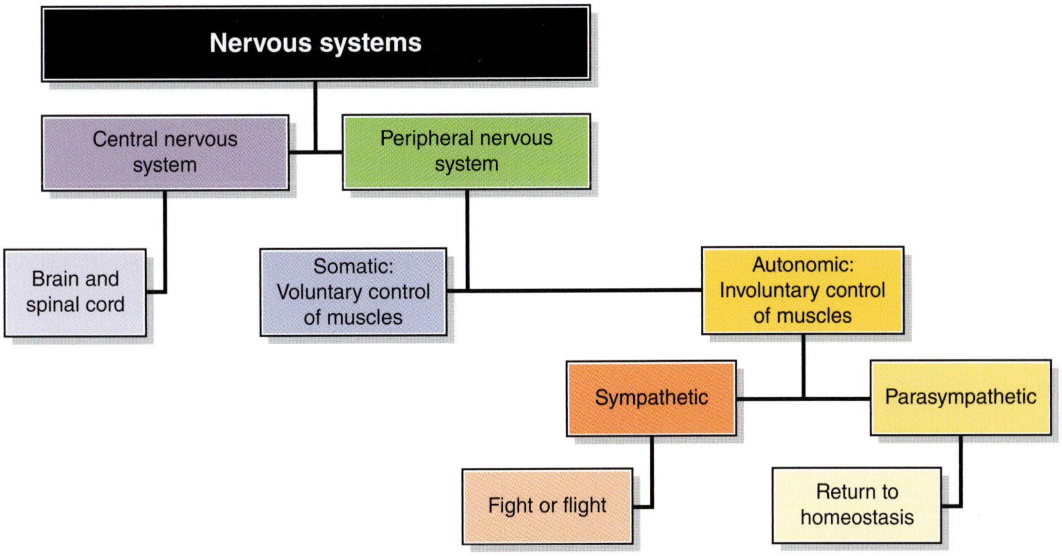


**Figure 2.3** The nervous system branches and roles.

a superhero! It also results in smaller changes such as dilated pupils to allow in more light and relaxed airway muscles to promote greater oxygen delivery.

The **parasympathetic nervous system** works to relax the body, performs necessary body functions when the body is at rest (e.g., digestion), and supports your body's efforts to return to homeostasis. When you encounter a stressor, your sympathetic nervous system is revved up and creates physical changes in your body to help you deal with the stress (e.g., increases heart rate). This alerts your parasympathetic nervous system into action to counteract the changes brought on by the sympathetic nervous system (e.g., decreases heart rate). Thus, these two systems work in opposition.

During the alarm stage, an area of the brain called the hypothalamus activates a series of events that trigger the adrenal gland to release the stress hormones adrenaline and cortisol (discussed in more detail in chapter 3). Adrenaline and cortisol work to control the physical adaptations to stress.

> **If we think of the autonomic nervous system as a car, the sympathetic nervous system is the gas pedal, and the parasympathetic nervous system is the brake.**

**Adrenaline**, also known as epinephrine, causes the air passages to dilate, which allows the lungs to provide the muscles with more oxygen and energy. It also causes the blood vessels to direct greater circulation to the major muscle groups (heart and lungs) and stimulates the body to produce sugar to use for fuel. Adrenaline can reduce the body's ability to feel pain and has been shown to improve strength and performance; its effects may last for up to an hour (Russell & Lightman, 2019).

**Cortisol** is another hormone that is released during an encounter with a stressor. Most cells in the body contain cortisol receptors, which means that cortisol can affect most organ systems in the body (Burgess, 2017). Cortisol helps regulate metabolism, inflammation, and memory formation (Russell & Lightman, 2019). Cortisol also helps the body downplay nonessential functions so that it can focus on essential functions during a stress event. It works to increase sugar in the bloodstream, increase the brain's ability to use glucose, suppress inflammation, regulate blood pressure, control sleep and wake cycles, boost energy, and increase the body's ability to repair tissues (Russell & Lightman, 2019). Because cortisol increases the amount of glucose and lipids in the blood during the stress response, prolonged stress impacts the way the body is able to utilize glucose and insulin. This increases a person's risk for developing type II diabetes (Hackett & Steptoe, 2017).

In the early 2000s, a third adaptive stress response was identified. This **freeze response** mimics a frozen state, like a deer in headlights (Bracha, Ralston, Matsukawa, Williams, & Bracha, 2004). This response, also called *tonic immobility*, is more likely to occur when a situation is more dangerous or a person has experienced previous trauma (Moller, Sondergaard, & Helstrom, 2017). Considered your ancient defense system, it is activated through a combination of the sympathetic nervous system and the dorsal vagal complex, a primitive system in the brain that activates to shut down other body processes when you experience a life threat (Porges, 2022). In extreme cases, this combination can cause a person to become immobilized with fear. Those in this state describe being hyperaware of their surroundings but unable to move. Other symptoms associated with the freeze response include the inability to speak, tremors in the hands and feet, decreased sense of pain, and a decreased responsiveness to physical stimuli (Fuse, Forsyth, Marx, Gallup, & Weaver, 2007).

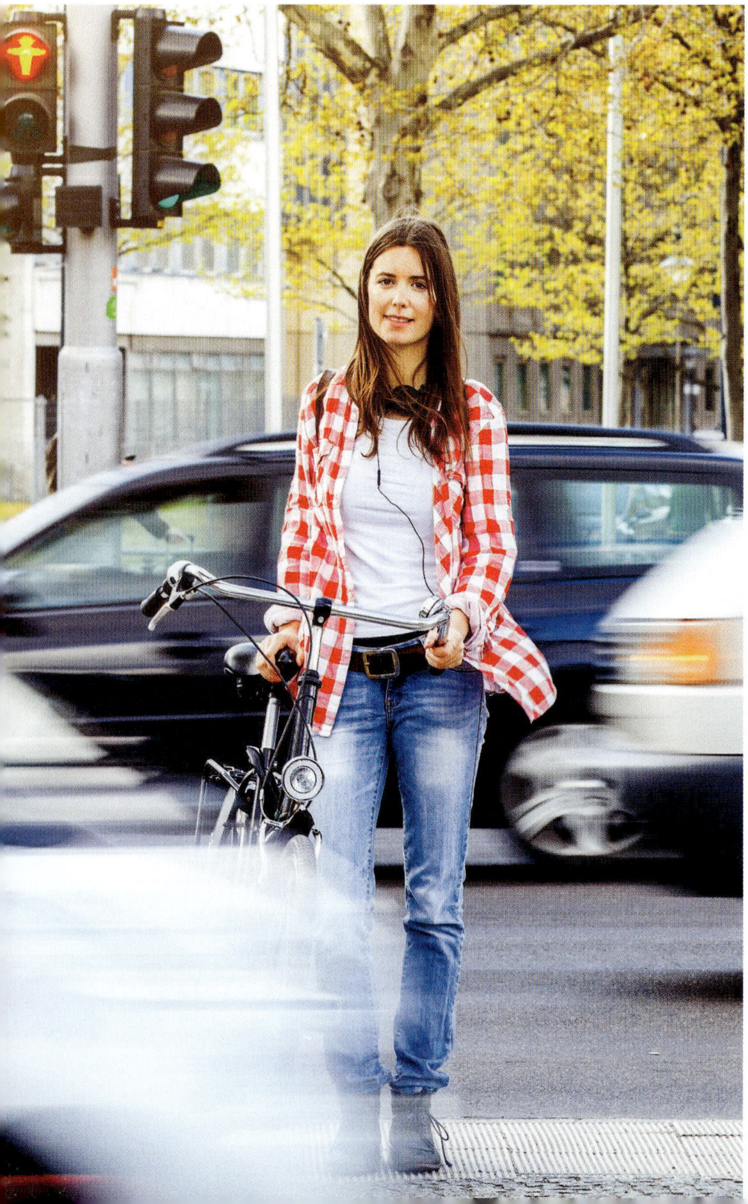

Freeze is triggered when fleeing or being aggressive is likely to be ineffective (Schmidt, Richey, Zvolensky, & Maner, 2008). This behavior is not exclusive to humans; animals have also used this response to escape predators. For example, opossums will flop on the ground and excrete a rotting scent to stop a predator from attacking. This behavior has also been witnessed in the Eastern hog-nosed snake, which will roll on its back, curl in a ball, and stick its tongue out to appear dead when under attack and may also defecate to help create a more realistic scene (Repp, 2020).

For humans, the freeze response is not a primary response like fight or flight. It is a secondary response that tends to occur in dangerous situations with feelings of intense fear and often includes being physically restrained (Fuse et al., 2007). A higher rate of freeze response has been shown among survivors of sexual assault, with almost half of all sexual assault survivors reporting some form of being frozen during their attack (Fuse et al., 2007).

In the **resistance stage** (sometimes referred to as the *adaptation stage*), the parasympathetic nervous system tries to counteract the changes associated with stress. If the stress ends, the body begins to decrease levels of cortisol and lower the heart rate and blood pressure to prestressor levels. If the stress continues, the body remains alert and stress hormones continue to be released. If the body spends too much time in the resistance stage, cortisol levels become too high and can be detrimental to your health, leading to sleep issues, weight gain, and other problems (see figure 2.4).

Regardless of how long a person is in the resistance stage, their energy becomes depleted and the ability to deal with additional stressors is diminished if they do not effectively manage the stress. Prolonged or chronic stress drains mental and physical resources, resulting in increased wear and tear on the body. During the **exhaustion stage**, your body's energy resources become depleted, and you may experience tiredness, depression, and anxiety. The immune system is significantly weakened, which may lead to a variety of other health issues.

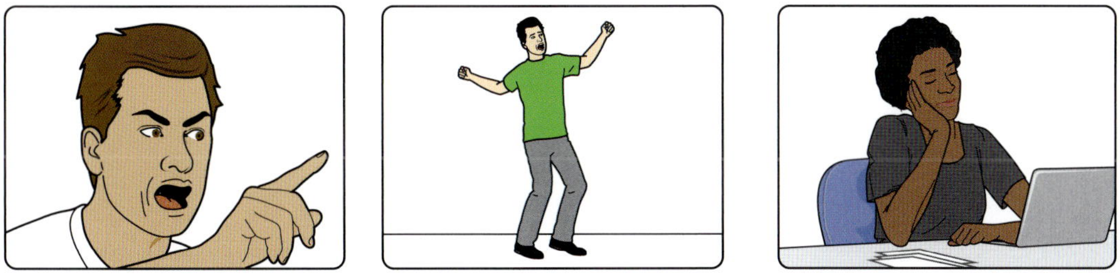


**Figure 2.4** Signs of being in the resistance stage.

However, effective stress management techniques can shorten the time the body stays in the resistance stage by activating the parasympathetic nervous system. This system works to restore normal breathing and heart rate, restore nonessential body functions that were placed on hold, and promote a sense of calm in the body. When you are able to manage your stress, your body is able to resume functioning at optimal levels.

How can you tell if your parasympathetic nervous system is working well? First, measure your resting heart rate. The average adult resting heart rate ranges from 60 to 100 beats per minute. Take a deep breath and hold it, noting how high your heart rate goes (an increase of about 20 beats per minute). Release your breath and measure how long it takes for your heart rate to return to the resting rate. If it is relatively quick, such as a one or two minutes, then your system is working well. If it takes a while to return to normal, that may indicate your parasympathetic nervous system is not working optimally (Garcia, Porto, Gomes da Cruz, & Molina, 2022). Don't worry—even if your parasympathetic nervous system is not working at optimal levels, you can practice stress management techniques to improve your body's functioning, including walks, meditation, yoga, and deep breathing. These will be further discussed in chapter 10.

## Types of Stress

When considering the different types of stress, you first think about the cause of stress, or stressor. Remember that stressors are anything that cause stress; they can be internal or external, vary from person to person, and range from mild to serious. The following sections will cover the different types of stress and their causes.

### Eustress and Distress

Although many people tend to think of stress as solely negative, stress is just the body's response to change and may be positive or negative (see table 2.1). **Eustress** is stress that is positive and can promote internal growth. Consider the following scenario: Aaliyah comes home from work and her partner asks, "How was your day?" Aaliyah responds, "It was such a stressful day." Aaliyah's partner tells her to sit on the couch while they bring her a cup of herbal tea to relax. Aaliyah's partner may have assumed that Aaliyah had a bad

**Table 2.1** Characteristics of Eustress and Distress

| Eustress | Distress |
|---|---|
| Not overwhelming | Overwhelming |
| Able to manage | Unable to manage |
| Increases motivation | Causes anxiety or concern |
| Improves performance | Decreases performance |
| Generally short term | Can be either short term or long term |

day. However, remember that stress can be positive or negative. In Aaliyah's case, it was positive: She had just received an important promotion, and it was her first week at her new job. She felt stressed because she was meeting new people, managing a new daily routine, and learning new skills, but she was managing the stress and finding the situation motivational.

Similarly, many college students report an increase in stress during the first few days of a new semester because they are learning a new schedule, going to new classes, and meeting new instructors and classmates. Although each new semester is ultimately helping you get closer to your goal of graduation, it may still be stressful as you adjust.

Generally, when people talk about stress in a negative light, they are really talking about **distress**, the type of stress that is uncomfortable and places additional burden on the body. Distress can be either acute, or short term, or chronic, which is considered long term. **Acute stress** only lasts a short time (seconds, minutes, or days). Imagine sitting at a stoplight in your car when suddenly—*bam*—you get hit from behind. Immediately, your heart starts to race, you can feel the blood pumping in your ears, your palms become sweaty, and you feel butterflies in your stomach. Thankfully, no one is hurt, and your car only has a small dent in the bumper. Once the police arrive and take down all the necessary information, you get to go home. As you drive home, you can feel yourself begin to relax a bit. Your heart rate begins to slow to normal, and you start listening to the radio again. This is an example of acute stress because it is short lived.

**Even though eustress is considered positive stress, your body still undergoes changes associated with stress.**

Another example of acute stress would be worrying about an upcoming exam. Even though your stress may last for days prior to the exam, it is still considered short-term stress. You know that once the exam has passed, your stress will go away. However, it can still be helpful to practice strategies (discussed in parts II and II of this text) to manage acute stress.

**Chronic stress**, on the other hand, can last for weeks, months, or years. Examples of chronic stressors include poverty, homelessness, housing insecurity, food insecurity, or being in a dysfunctional relationship. A common cause of stress for college students is the increasing burden of student loans. For some, these payments can be quite large, and if their postcollege income can't support that loan payment, the financial hardship can cause chronic stress for years to come. There are no quick and easy fixes for chronic stress; however, stress management techniques can help minimize the impact.

Chronic stress or the inability to manage stress may lead to excessive levels of cortisol in the body and increase the risk of certain health conditions, including the following (Mayo Clinic, 2019):

- Anxiety
- Depression
- Digestive problems
- Headaches
- Heart disease
- Sleep problems
- Weight gain
- Memory and concentration impairment

A cortisol test may be used to assess cortisol levels. Abnormal levels might result not just from problems with stress, but from disorders of the adrenal glands such as Cushing's syndrome (too much cortisol) or Addison's disease (too little cortisol).

## Traumatic Stress

**Trauma** is an emotional response to a disturbing event. Trauma can be further classified into three categories:

- Acute trauma: Results from a single event (physical attack, rape)
- Chronic trauma: Results from multiple disturbing events or a prolonged event (intimate partner violence, sexual abuse, bullying)
- Complex trauma: Results from a variety of disturbing events or experiences

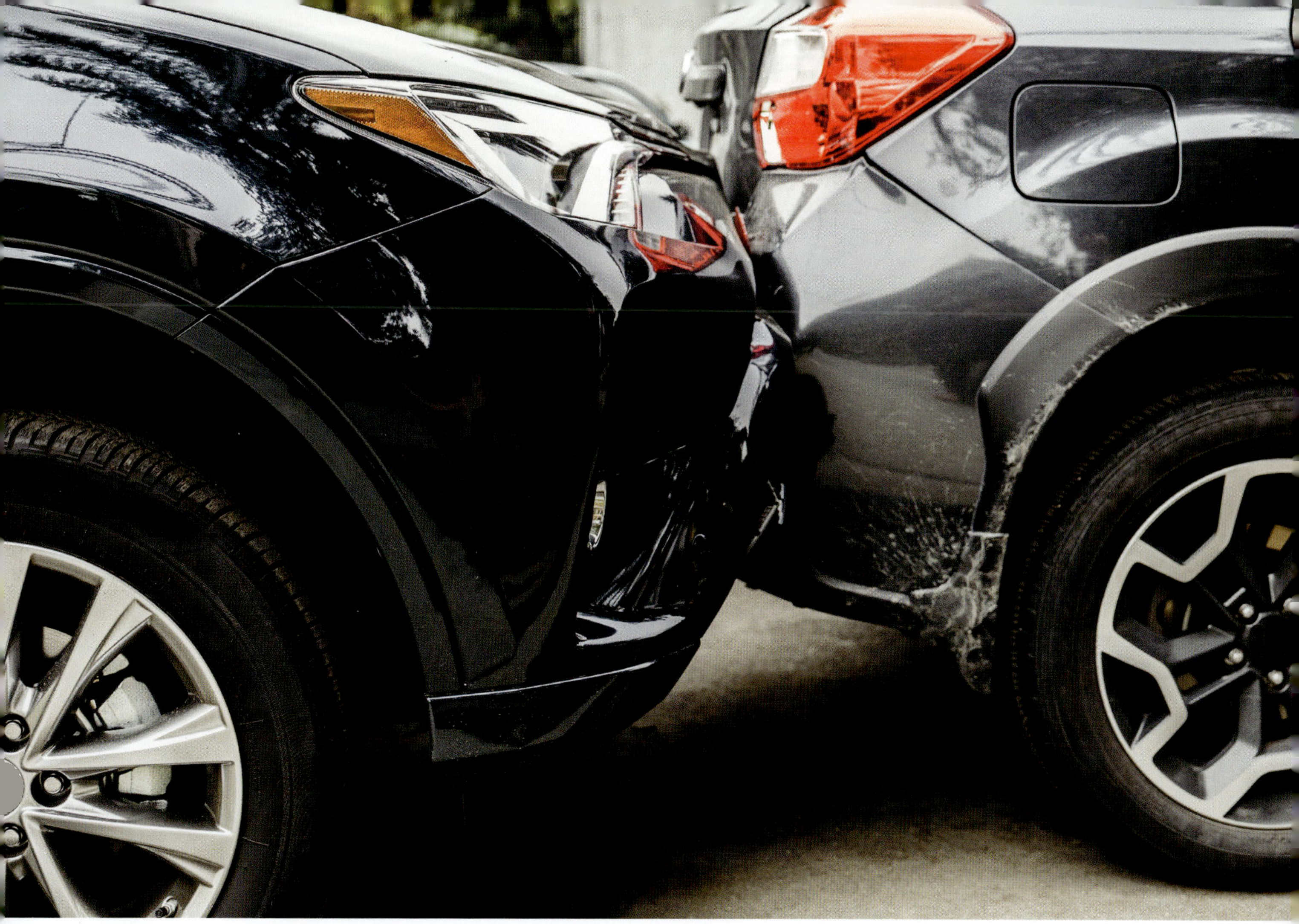

Trauma can occur at any age but has a particularly negative impact on children's developing brains. Depending on severity, traumatic events during childhood might be referred to as **adverse childhood experiences (ACEs)**; exposure to these events are common across all population groups in society (Yau et al., 2022). Experiencing ACEs during childhood and adolescence has a negative impact on brain development, especially the areas connected with cognitive functioning (Guinosso, Johnson, & Riley, 2016). Prolonged exposure to cortisol and adrenaline released as the body tries to regulate the stress response is associated with poorer early childhood brain development (Royce, 2021). Currently, over 60 percent of adults in the United States have experienced an adverse childhood event, with about 25 percent of adults having experienced three or more adverse events (Merrick, Ford, Ports, & Guinn, 2018).

Although ACEs occur among all subgroups of a population, they tend to be more common among those who identify as Black, Hispanic, or multiracial; those with less than a high school education; those with an annual income of $15,000 or less; those who are unemployed or unable to work; and those who identify as a sexual minority (Merrick et al., 2018). This is particularly concerning because the threat of ACEs is higher among those groups that often have fewer resources, making it less likely those impacted will be able to seek help to deal with the trauma. Furthermore, as the number of ACEs increase, health risks also increase, creating an additional burden for these low-resource groups. For example, homeless youth who have experienced an ACE are at greater risk for developing a substance use disorder later in life (Moss et al., 2020).

There are many different treatment options for people who have experienced ACEs. In recent years, more medical students and those in helping professions have been educated in trauma-informed care (Pletcher, O'Connor, Swift-Taylor, &

DallaPiazza, 2019). Trauma-informed care uses a strengths-based approach, which focuses on initial screening for trauma, creating a safe environment, and engaging patients in the treatment process (Bendall, Eastwood, & Scanlan, 2020). Additionally, there are a variety of treatment options for those who have experienced ACEs. For example, cognitive behavioral therapy has been shown to improve mental health outcomes for people who have experienced ACEs (Macdonald et al., 2016). There is some evidence to suggest parent training can be effective in improving outcomes for those who have experienced ACEs (Ziviani, Feeney, Cuckelly, Meredith, & Hunt, 2012). Finally, research suggests that engaging in programs to build resilience may be beneficial for young people with ACEs (Norris & Norris, 2021).

## Posttraumatic Stress Disorder

**Posttraumatic stress disorder (PTSD)** is a psychiatric disorder that develops in people who have experienced or witnessed traumatic events or circumstances (American Psychiatric Association, 2020). An example of some the events that can lead to PTSD include the following:

- Natural disaster
- Serious accident or life-threatening event
- Physical or sexual assault
- Childhood or domestic abuse
- Witnessing death
- War and conflict
- Torture
- Prolonged exposure to traumatic experiences

PTSD develops in about one in three people who experience a traumatic event (National Health Service, 2018). PTSD doesn't occur immediately and can take months to several years to develop after a traumatic event (Mayo Clinic, n.d.). It is not clear why some people develop PTSD and others do not. Most researchers agree that it depends on a variety of factors that include the severity of trauma experienced, previous history of mental illness, family history of mental illness, personality, and how the brain regulates chemicals and hormones (Mayo Clinic, n.d.). Women are more vulnerable to PTSD than men: One study found the risk for PTSD following a traumatic event for women versus men was twofold higher and that the duration of PTSD was also longer. This finding was attributed "to the greater effect of assaultive violence on women" (Breslau, 2002, p. 34).

Symptoms of PTSD can range greatly and include distressing memories of the traumatic event, flashbacks, nightmares, negative thoughts, feeling hopeless, memory problems, detachment, and feeling on guard. PTSD symptoms fall into four categories (American Psychiatric Association, 2020):

1. *Intrusion*. The person may have nightmares, flashbacks, and memories of the traumatic event. These experiences can be so realistic that the person feels as if they are reliving the event.
2. *Avoidance*. The person may try to avoid anything that reminds them of the trauma. This can include people, places, and objects. They may resist talking about what happened because mention of the trauma triggers distressing memories.
3. *Alterations in cognition and mood*. The person may not remember the traumatic event or have distorted beliefs about themselves as it relates to the traumatic event (e.g., "I am a bad person" or "it is all my fault"). They may be unable to experience any positive emotions, even during activities they previously enjoyed.
4. *Alterations in arousal and reactivity*. The person may act self-destructive and reckless or, conversely, become overly cautious and protective.

PTSD is treatable. The two major types of treatment are medications and trauma-focused psychotherapy. Trauma-focused psychotherapies address the memory of the traumatic event and provide the patient with different mechanisms and tools for dealing with the intrusive memory. Types of trauma-focused psychotherapies include the following (United States Department of Veterans Affairs, n.d.):

- *Prolonged exposure*. This teaches a person how to gain control by facing negative feelings.

- *Cognitive processing therapy*. This teaches a person how to reframe negative thoughts about a trauma.
- *Eye movement desensitization and reprocessing*. This teaches a person how to process and make sense of the trauma by recalling a memory from the traumatic event while paying attention to a back-and-forth movement or sound.

Treatment for PTSD is often short term and does not require a lifetime of attending treatment sessions. It is important to work with a mental health care professional to find the best treatment option. The sooner one obtains treatment, the closer one is to recovery.

**Because each person is different, treatment that works for one may not work for another. Some people may need to try several different approaches before finding one that works.**

## Optimal Levels of Stress

When people talk about stress, they usually speak of it like an unwanted visitor. A stress-free life may sound good on paper, but in actuality, it would not be very healthy. In the early 1900s, researchers Robert M. Yerkes and John D. Dodson discovered that too much stress can decrease task performance in mice, but so did too little stress. At optimal levels of stress, mice were better able to learn and perform tasks of moderate difficulty (Yerkes & Dodson, 1908). For easy tasks, the relationship between stress and learning was linear: The more stress placed on the mouse, the harder it was for the mouse to learn the task. However, for moderately difficult tasks, too little and too much stress both made it harder for the mouse to learn; the mouse was better able to learn the moderate tasks when there were optimal levels of stress.

> Stress should be a powerful driving force, not an obstacle.
>
> **Bill Phillips**

Similarly, humans require optimal levels of stress to be motivated. For more challenging tasks, the Yerkes-Dodson law states that a moderate level of arousal (i.e., stress) improves performance (Chaby, Sheriff, Hirrlinger, & Braithwaite, 2015). Figure 2.5 provides a visual representation of the Yerkes-Dodson law.

Without stress, boredom sets in and motivation to perform at an optimal level decreases. However, high stakes can improve focus—for example, the looming stress of a highly weighted midterm exam might push you to study harder. On the other hand, if the stakes are too high and the stress is not managed, it can impede performance. When people fail to perform at a level that would be expected under these circumstances, it is known as pressure-induced performance error, or more commonly as "choking under pressure." Choking under pressure occurs when cognitive resources are shifted toward stress and away from the task at hand (Sattizahn, Moser, & Beilock, 2016).

The amount of stress you need to improve performance depends on a few factors, including skill level, personality, confidence, and task complexity. For example, learning a new skill takes time and practice. Under these conditions, adding pressure and stress will most likely slow you down. If, on the other hand, you have more experience and a higher skill level, you may need additional stress to find the motivation to continue improving (Ciria et al., 2021). Personality also plays a role in

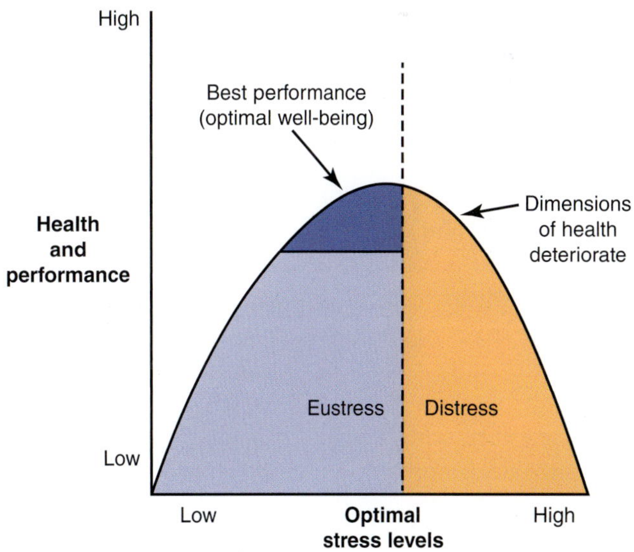


**Figure 2.5** Yerkes–Dodson law. The left side of the curve represents eustress, whereas the right side of the curve represents distress. Finding the optimal level of stress leads to higher levels of health and performance.

Reprinted by permission from N.E. Tummers, *Stress Management: A Wellness Approach* (Champaign, IL: Human Kinetics, 2013), 7.

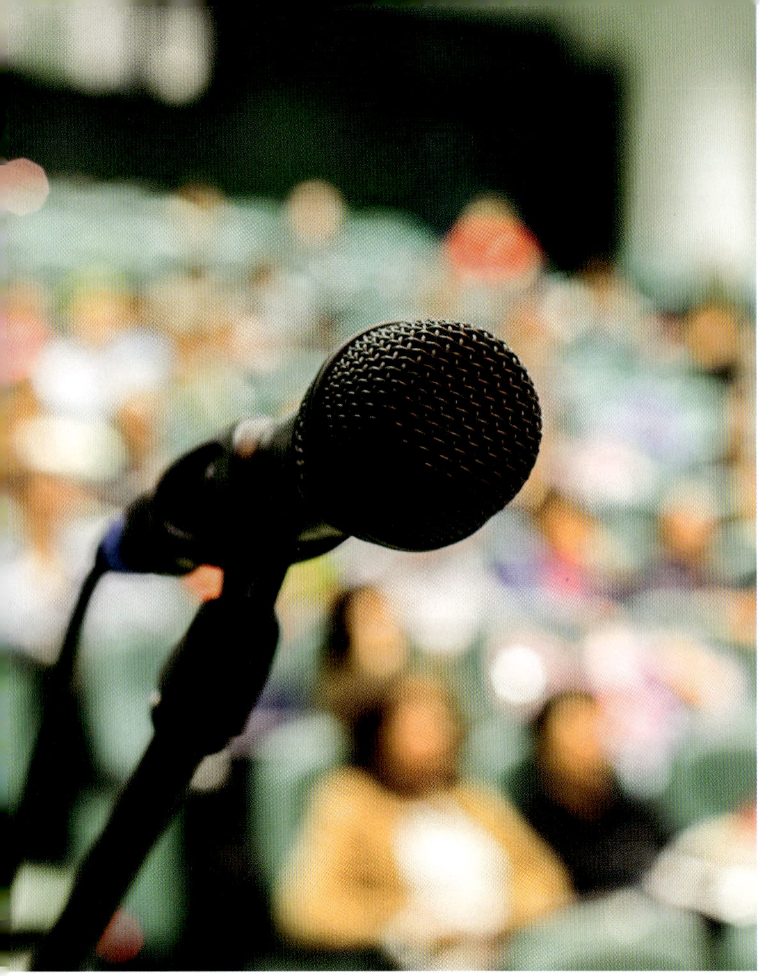

what levels of arousal are needed for peak performance. Some people enjoy working under greater amounts of pressure, whereas others feel overwhelmed and begin to underperform. You must consider your own susceptibility to stress and how you can best manage it (Sattizahn et al., 2016).

Related to personality is your level of confidence on a task. If you have a lot of confidence, then you may perform better under pressure, whereas if you lack self-confidence, then any pressure to perform may slow you down. Lastly, the complexity of a task plays a role in how much outside stress you may need for additional motivation. Consider a simple task you have been doing for a while. You may find yourself getting bored quite easily, which will slow down your performance. Although you may not be able to change the task to increase levels of arousal or stress, you may be able to offer yourself an incentive to complete the task in a particular amount of time. Consider assembly workers, whose tasks remain the same every day for years on end. Businesses use incentives and goals as a way to introduce stress and arousal to encourage peak performance. On the other hand, for more complex tasks, you may not need additional arousal for motivation if the task itself is difficult enough.

## Stress Reactivity

Two people can experience the same stressor but have very different perceptions of it. What accounts for those individual differences? **Stress reactivity** refers to the individual capacity to respond to stress—high levels of stress reactivity mean you have a strong reaction to stress, whereas low levels of stress reactivity mean you generally have lower reactions to stress. Different characteristics can shape a person's stress response. For example, studies have shown that stressful perinatal experiences (those occurring a few weeks before and after birth) may cause an individual to become more reactive to stress (Russell et al., 2018). Other factors that may increase stress reactivity in an individual include experiencing chronic stress (especially at a young age) and having a traumatic brain injury (Russell & Lightman, 2019). People with higher levels of stress reactivity are at higher risk of chronic conditions associated with stress such as hypertension and heart disease (Russell & Lightman, 2019).

Having an awareness of your own stress reactivity, particularly if it is high, can help you better manage your own levels of stress. Additionally, it may be helpful to have a toolbox of stress management techniques you can use when you encounter stressful situations. Having a high stress reactivity doesn't mean you are doomed to be stressed out—it just means you need to be mindful about how you deal with stress.

The **biopsychosocial (BPS) model of challenge and threat** is a framework used to describe how a stress is perceived and how you respond to your perception of that stress (Uphill, Rossato, Swain, & O'Driscoll, 2019). This framework posits there are two ways your body responds to a stressor: as a threat or a challenge. In the threat response, you perceive the stress as relevant but do not perceive that you have sufficient resources to deal with the stress. This results in less efficient cardiovascular output and an impaired decision-making ability (Gu, Ocampo, Algoe, & Oveis, 2022). On the other hand, when the stress is personally relevant and you feel you have the

## Same Day, Different Experiences

Devin and Reilly have been roommates since their freshman year of college. It is now their junior year, and each is handling the first day of the new semester very differently. Devin looks forward to receiving the syllabi for his classes, reading what will be expected of him for the semester, and meeting his teachers and classmates. Although the first day is a little stressful, he enjoys it. Reilly, on the other hand, has always hated the first day of class and gets himself worked into a frenzy worrying about who his teachers will be and what type of work will be expected of him. He more often than not misses the first day of class with a stomachache or headache. Although Devin and Reilly are experiencing similar situations, how they perceive them is very different.

It may seem odd to have such a different response to the same event. However, Reilly had an experience during his first day in high school that shaped how he views the first day of class. On Reilly's first day of high school, he was nervous but excited. When Reilly got to school, he realized he had forgotten his schedule. He attempted to remain calm and go to the office to obtain another copy but couldn't find his way to the front office. He asked some upperclassmen for directions, but they just laughed at him and walked away. As the minutes passed, he began to feel more panicked. He knew the bell was going to ring soon and he would be in trouble if he was caught in the hallway. By the time the bell rang, he was experiencing a racing heartbeat, sweaty palms, and shortness of breath. Although Reilly finally found a hall monitor to help him find the front office, that experience shaped how he has handled the first day of classes from that day forward.

resources needed to handle it, you perceive the stress as a challenge, which brings a certain level of pleasure or enjoyment. This results in more efficient cardiovascular output and improved cognitive and motor performance (Gu et al., 2022). The challenge response is useful in dealing with stressors that are work and performance related.

### Upbringing

How you were raised impacts your ability to manage stress. For example, having a caring and attentive mother can help you better manage stress levels as an adult. A study conducted on rats showed that those who experienced maternal deprivation showed much higher patterns of stress as adults compared to those who had a present mother; those who experienced mothering in a normal range showed more resilient patterns of stress and lower stress reactivity (Buchanan & Lovallo, 2019). A study on humans confirmed these results, showing children raised by sensitive and supportive mothers to have a stronger ability to delay gratification, stronger impulse control, and better working memory—all traits used to manage stress (Kok et al., 2022).

Levels of parental stress may also impact stress among offspring. Children raised in households with higher levels of stress are more likely to report symptoms of depression (Ren et al., 2022). Children raised in poverty have more risk factors, including psychological and physical stressors, family disruption, unresponsive parenting, and community violence, which increase levels of stress reactivity and conditions associated with stress (Sripada, Swain, Evans, Welsh, & Liberzon, 2014).

### Genetics

In recent years, some studies on genes have shown that they play a role in stress reactivity. Earlier in the chapter, you learned about how cortisol is increased during a stressful event. Gene alterations can impact the levels of cortisol in the body (Ising & Holsboer, 2006). One such gene alteration leads to decreased functioning of the cortisol receptors, which signal the brain to stop releasing cortisol when the levels become sufficient. The gene alterations lead to decreased recognition that there is enough cortisol in the body, which leads to prolonged cortisol release during a stressful event, resulting in higher levels of cortisol in the body (Turecki & Meaney, 2017).

### Sex Differences

Stress reactivity may differ by sex based on the type of stressor experienced. Women generally show

Research Spotlight

## Signs of Using Alcohol for Stress Relief

Although it's common for alcohol intake to increase in times of stress (Steckler, Kalin, & Reul, 2005), needing a drink every day is not a well-adapted approach to dealing with stress. Even though alcohol and other drugs may decrease the physical symptoms of stress in the now, these are not long-term solutions. Alcohol may make you feel better initially because it is a depressant (meaning it relaxes the body), but if you do not learn healthier behaviors to manage stress, it can ultimately make matters worse. The effect of alcohol only temporarily brings relief—once the alcohol wears off, so does the relief. An excess of alcohol consumption can lead to gut issues and excess weight gain, two additional stressors to add to the initial stress. Eventually, prolonged alcohol use stimulates the release of stress hormones, placing you at an even higher stress reactivity level (Anthenelli, 2012).

Answer each question to tell if you are using alcohol to deal with stress.

- Have your drinking habits significantly changed recently?
- Do you need alcohol after a stressful day to calm down?
- Do you have a difficult time unwinding after a long day without alcohol?
- Do you have a family history of substance use disorder?
- Do you use alcohol to reduce social anxiety?

If you answered yes to two or more questions, you may be using alcohol to deal with stress in an unhealthy manner. Consider talking to your doctor or a professional on campus.

higher reactivity to stressors that involve social rejection, whereas men show higher reactivity to stressors that involve a lack of achievement (Stroud, Salovey, & Epel, 2002). These differences may arise during puberty, after the sex hormones have had an impact on brain development.

Women may have another stress response adaptation that is separate from fight or flight. Cortisol is still involved in this process, but it is influenced by the release of oxytocin, a hormone responsible in part for romantic attachments and mother–infant bonding. In stressful situations, women are more likely to seek the help and support of others. If children are involved, women will go tend or nurture their children. This tend-and-befriend response is a stress response theory developed by Shelley E. Taylor that draws on the attachment caregiving system (Levy, Hlay, Johnson, & Witmer, 2019; Taylor et al., 2000). Because women have historically been positioned as caregivers, if women were to fight or run when faced with a stressor, they would leave their offspring and others vulnerable to the threat. Thus, the need to form strong attachments and social connections may have been another adaptation to help survive during times of stress (Levy et al., 2019; Taylor et al., 2000). Next time you are stressed, are you more likely to seek solace alone or seek the support of friends?

### Personal Health Choices

How you choose to deal with stress can affect your stress reactivity. Some behaviors, such as eating a nutritious diet, regularly exercising, and practicing meditation, can help decrease stress reactivity. These behaviors help train your parasympathetic nervous system to recover quickly after being deployed, making it more effective in counteracting the effects of stress. In chapter 1, you learned about the different components of wellness and their relationship with stress. In the following chapters, you will learn more about the ways each aspect of wellness influences stress and vice versa. In part III of this textbook, you will learn techniques to manage and avoid stress. These fall under personal health choices—those that move you either toward optimal wellness or away from it.

## Societal Stress

Even as the world rapidly changes, stress remains a constant. The world, your environment, and society all affect how you experience stress. Societal stress can be seen as a special type of stressor, one that is experienced and shared by a group of people in similar circumstances. For example, if you were to talk to your classmates about what stresses them out, many of them would share similar stressors, such as upcoming exams, papers, and academic strains. Recent events have had a particularly great impact on stress, not only for individuals but for society as a whole.

**People in similar circumstances share similar stressors.**

### COVID-19

At the end of 2019, an outbreak of COVID-19 occurred in China, which spread to the rest of the world and continued to pandemic levels over the next few months. In the early stages of the pandemic, almost 10 percent of the general population in mainland China reported experiencing moderate to severe stress (Wang et al., 2020). Between March and April 2020, as the virus rapidly spread worldwide, there was a matching rise in acute stress levels (Holman, Thompson, Garfin, & Silver, 2020). As many schools shifted to online learning, businesses closed or encouraged employees to work from home, and social distance precautions were set into place, many people began to experience boredom—one of the strongest factors for those experiencing stress during the pandemic lockdowns (Yan, Gan, Ding, Wu, & Duan, 2021).

One study found increased levels of depression, anxiety, and traumatic stress among the general population during the initial stages of COVID-19, with higher levels of anxiety more common among females who had children in the household and those who felt at personal risk of infection (Shevlin et al., 2020). Surprisingly, males and the oldest age group—two subgroups associated with higher COVID-19 mortality rates—showed lower levels of anxiety and depression during COVID-19 compared to the other subgroups, though the reason why is unclear (Shevlin et al., 2020).

Another study found that rates of posttraumatic stress in the general population may have increased because of COVID-19 (Cooke, Eirich, Racine, & Madigan, 2020). Not surprisingly, those who experienced higher levels of stress also experienced higher levels of emotional distress (depression, fear, compulsion-anxiety, and hypochondria). Additionally, these stressors were higher among those who were exposed to media that largely focused on the pandemic. Many news networks spoke about the dangers of the disease, especially during the initial stages of the pandemic, often excluding positive data (e.g., survivors, recovery odds) in favor of negative (e.g., infection and death rates). One study found that those who watched more television news programs during the COVID-19 pandemic experienced higher levels of PTSD than those who watched fewer news programs (Solomon, Ginzburg, Ohry, & Mikulincer, 2021).

It is not surprising, therefore, that Americans are suffering from higher levels of stress. In a recent survey, 77 percent of Americans say the future of our nation is a significant source of stress. This is the highest recorded level (American Psychological Association, 2020).

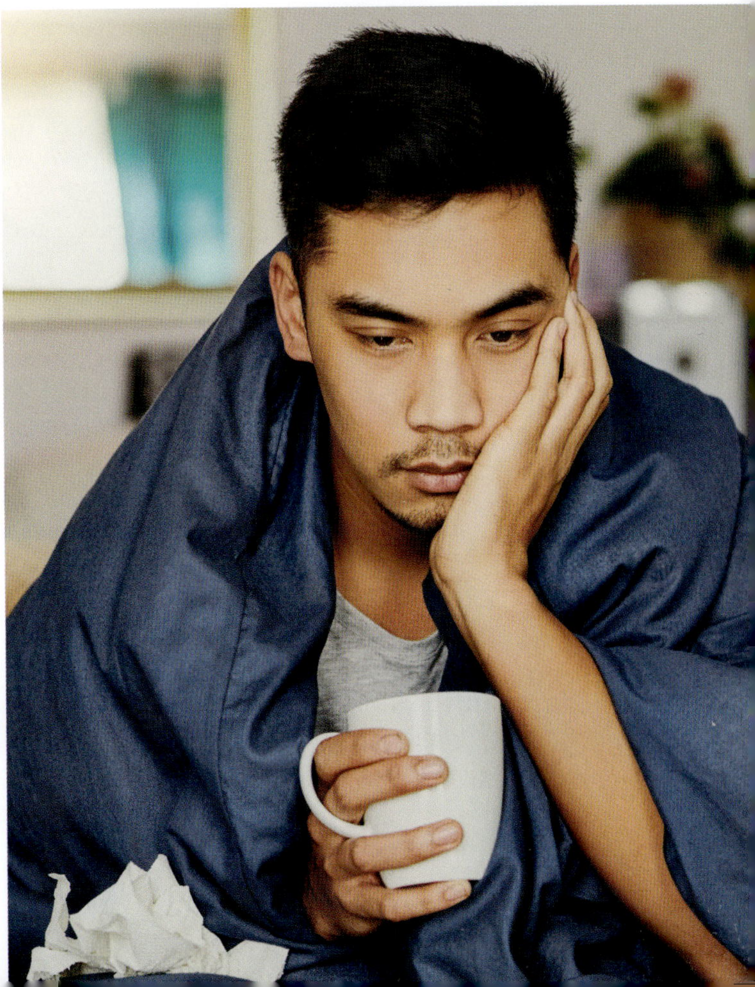

## Racism

Cultural racism can be measured by looking at levels of negative stereotypes in a population. Those from disadvantaged racial and ethnic groups face higher levels of negative racial stereotyping at all ages, leading to discrimination (intentional and unintentional) and resulting in higher levels of stress among the members of those groups.

One such experience was shared by Dr. Roberto E. Montenegro in a 2016 article in the *Journal of the American Medical Association*. Dr. Montenegro and his wife were invited to an upscale restaurant to celebrate the completion of his doctoral dissertation with several other faculty members. While waiting in line for the valet at the end of dinner, a woman exited her vehicle, walked by several couples, and handed Dr. Montenegro her keys without saying a word. He quickly handed the keys to the valet. A few minutes later another couple arrived and also approached him, although the woman realized her mistake and apologized before she gave him her keys. This type of behavior, though certainly not intentional, still leaves a negative impact on the person. Dr. Montenegro recalls feeling embarrassed, angry, and hurt, his heart racing and his face becoming flushed—all signs of stress.

Inequities such as discrimination, institutional racism, and civil unrest create higher rates of stress for minorities, and over the past decade racism and discrimination have been on the rise in the United States (Pew Research Center, 2019). In a survey on stress in America conducted by the American Psychological Association (2020), 48 percent of Black Americans reported that discrimination is a significant source of stress, and 59 percent of all Americans saw police violence toward minorities as a significant source of stress. Almost 65 percent of American Jews have reported experiencing some form of discrimination—a 20 percent increase since 2016 (Pew Research Center, 2019). In 2017 a "Unite the Right" rally in Charlottesville, Virginia, saw protestors chanting "Jews will not replace us"; in 2018, a gunman murdered 11 people in the Tree of Life Synagogue in Pittsburgh, Pennsylvania (Wright, Volodarsky, Hecht, & Saxe, 2021). There has also been an increase of anti-Semitism on college campuses (AMCHA Initiative, 2018); such behavior can lead to an increase in anxiety and stress among Jewish people.

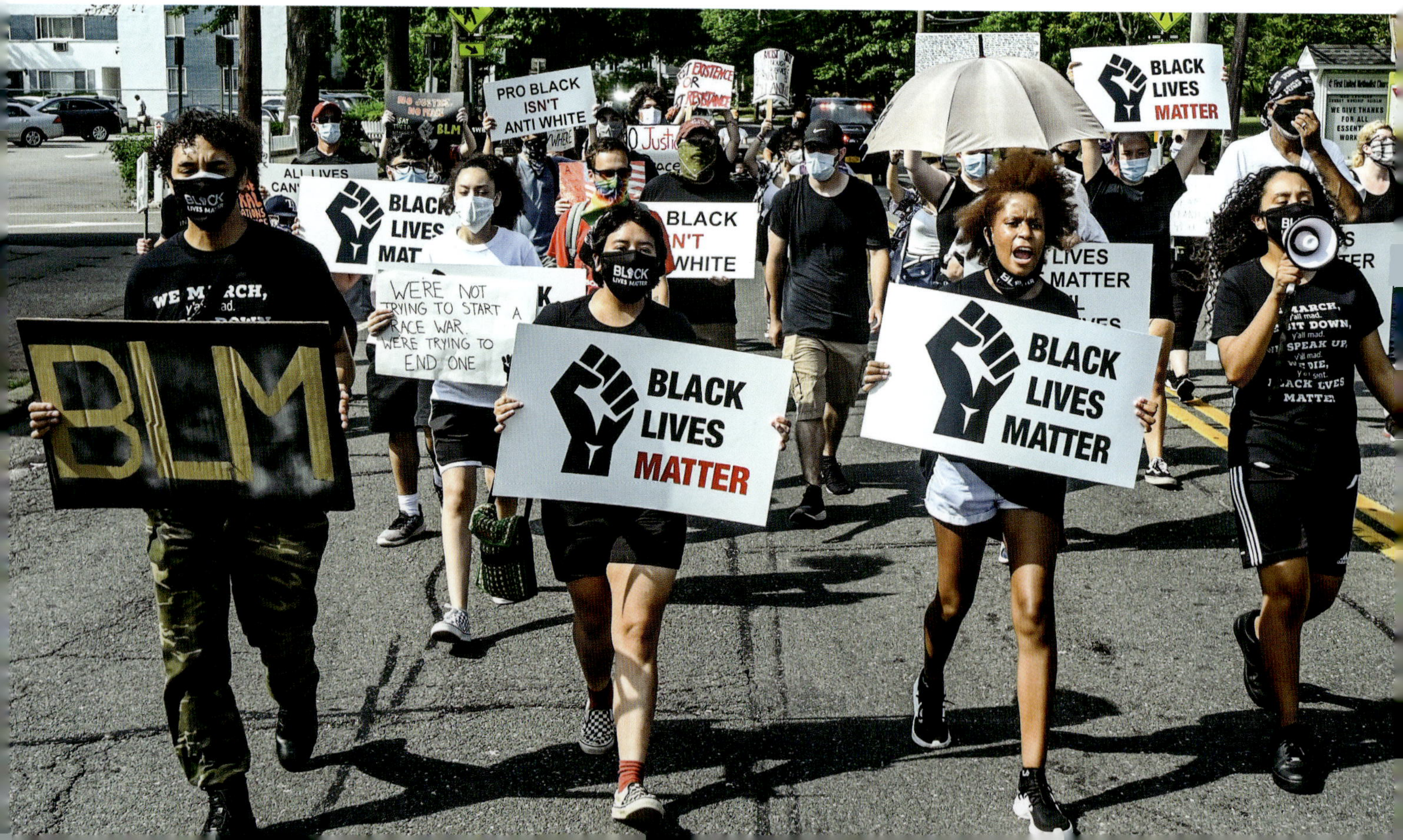
PRO BLACK ISN'T ANTI WHITE
BLACK LIVES MATTER
WERE NOT TRYING TO START A RACE WAR WERE TRYING TO END ONE
BLM
BLACK LIVES MATTER
BLACK LIVES MATTER

The United States saw a particular increase in racism against Asian American and Pacific Islander (AAPI) people during the COVID-19 pandemic. Not surprisingly, those who experienced anti-Asian racism reported higher levels of stress, depression, and anxiety, and many Asian Americans reported being more fearful of anti-Asian hate than the virus itself (Saw, Yellow Horse, & Russell, 2021). Those aged 60 and older were particularly fearful of this increased racism, with almost all of them (98 percent) reporting a belief that the United States has become more dangerous for Asian Americans (Stop the Hate & AARP, 2022).

A unique stressor occurs when negative stereotypes of minority populations are internalized within members of those populations, known as **internalized racism** (Potapchuk, Leiderman, Bivens, & Major, 2005). Black Americans who have high levels of internalized racism experience higher levels of anxiety and distress compared to those who do not internalize racism (Sosoo, Bernard, & Neblett Jr., 2020). These higher levels of internalized racism are also associated with higher levels of stress and poorer mental health (Mouzon & McLean, 2017), as well as lower self-esteem, lower self-worth, and increased anxiety (Williams, 2018). Consider Dr. Montenegro's story: If he experienced that same situation when he was younger, he might have started to believe he could only grow up to be a valet or have a similar job that did not require an advanced education, and it would have changed his entire life plan.

## Technology

In modern times, we have access to technology at our fingertips. Being connected to technology at all times has its benefits, but excessive use—defined as having a high amount of cognitive, emotional, and behavioral involvement with technology—can induce stress (Hefner, Knop, Schmitt, & Vorderer, 2019). Studies suggest that problematic smartphone use is higher among people who have elevated levels of stress (Chiu, 2014). Although smartphones can provide a sense of connection with others, they can also block connections: Excessive phone use reduces the number of face-to-face interactions with other people (Bhattacharya, Basher, Srivastava, & Singh, 2019) and is associated with higher levels of loneliness, which may be attributed to this decrease in meaningful face-to-face interactions and increase in superficial connections (Mahapatra, 2019).

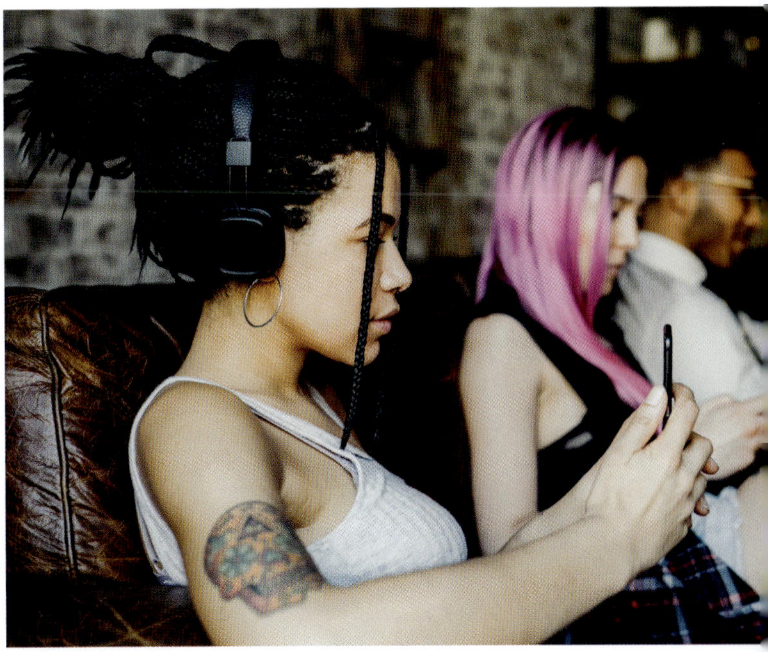

Have you ever left the house without your phone? How did it make you feel? Chances are, you were a little stressed about leaving it behind. **Nomophobia** (literally "no mobile phone phobia") is a psychological condition describing an intense level of fear some people feel when they are separated from their phone (Bhattacharya, Basher, Srivastava, & Singh, 2019). In a recent study on the impact of being separated from a mobile phone, participants who were separated from their mobile devices experienced higher levels of stress, which led them to seek out their mobile device and intentionally move to be physically closer to it (Konok, Pogány, & Miklosi, 2017). People who suffer from nomophobia prefer to connect with people virtually and avoid face-to-face social situations. They tend to keep their phones near them 24/7 and even check their phones throughout the night, causing interrupted sleep in addition to increased stress.

**Technostress** is a term coined in the 1980s that refers to the inability to cope with new technologies in a healthy manner (Brod, 1984). As the pressure to use more technology increases, so do the effects of technostress. There are different types of technostress:

- *Techno-overload.* This stress arises when users are confronted with too many streams of information at one time.
- *Techno-uncertainty.* This results from feelings of inability or uncertainty when using a new form of technology. Because each new piece of technology or update requires additional knowledge and practice to learn in a relatively short amount of time, this can bring about stress.
- *Techno-insecurity.* This describes the fear associated with losing one's place to technology or to another person who has more experience with technology.
- *Techno-complexity.* This describes the stress that occurs when users find the technology difficult to understand or feel incompetent with the new technology (Bondanini, Giorgi, Ariza-Montes, & Vega-Munoz, 2020).

It may seem hard to understand how one could get stressed from learning to use new technology. It is likely that every time an updated version of an electronic device or a new game comes out, you and your friends can't wait to get your hands on it. For younger people, new technology represents fun, status, or just a better way to connect with others. However, for older people, the thrill is often gone. Imagine you are studying for a final exam that covers an entire textbook. During the final two weeks of class, the teacher introduces another—albeit shorter—text to be covered on the exam. Although it may be interesting, not as long, or even better than the previous book, the

## Fear of Missing Out

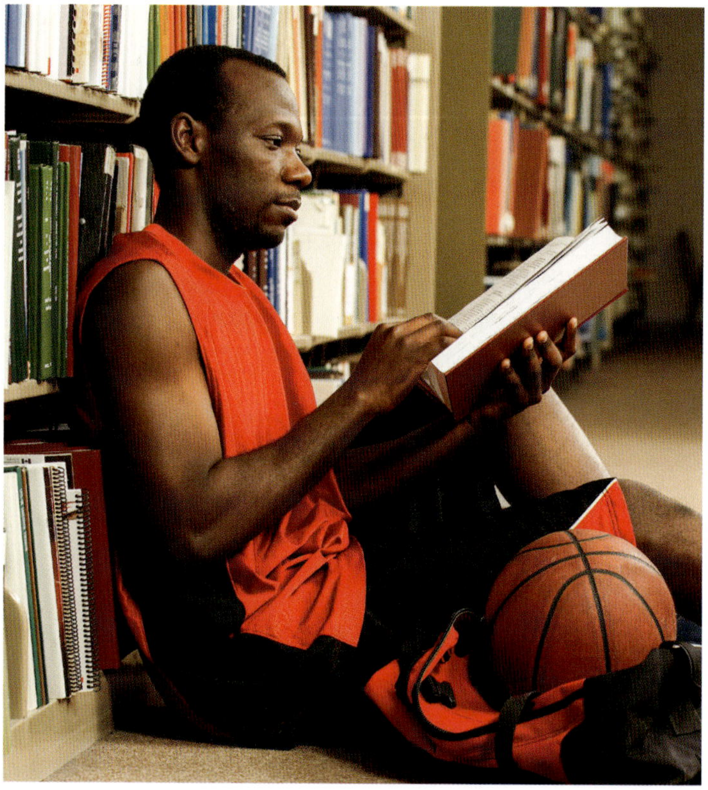

It is a Thursday night, and Ramal has an important exam tomorrow morning. He is a little nervous about the test and is planning to study after dinner. As he is preparing dinner, he gets a text from his friends. They are all going to the bar to see a local band and want Ramal to join them.

Ramal feels conflicted. He knows he should stay home, but he really wants to join his friends and have fun. As he is weighing his options, he sees his textbook at the edge of the table. That is enough to prompt him to tell his friends he will not be able to join them. After dinner Ramal opens his book and notes and begins to review them. He notices he is having trouble focusing because he keeps thinking about his friends. What are they doing? How much fun are they having? What is he missing out on? These concerns have a name: the fear of missing out (FOMO).

The fear of missing out refers to the perception that one is missing out on an activity that will not repeat itself. The fear of missing out is increasing as more people are constantly connected to social media and technology. The more a person is connected to those platforms, the higher likelihood of them developing FOMO at some point in their life (Tandon, Dhir, Almugren, AlNemer, & Mantymaki, 2021).

fact that you must read it quickly to prepare for the upcoming final may cause you stress. This is often how older people feel when introduced to new technology.

There are tools available to help users deal with technostress. One is to provide technical support for new and existing technology. It may also be beneficial to create smaller communities where users can share their experiences and challenges and collaboratively discuss ways to overcome those challenges. When a new technology is being considered for a project, it may be helpful to involve the stakeholders in the decision-making process; those who feel they are part of the final decision are more likely to engage with the new technology (Bondanini, Giorgi, Ariza-Montes, & Vega-Munoz, 2020).

## Climate Change

Climate change is another world phenomenon that impacts mental health and stress (figure 2.6). First, climate change may be responsible for causing or at least contributing to extreme climatic events, defined by the scientific community as events that are rare or outside of normal range (Cianconi, Betrò, & Janiri, 2020). Second, when natural disasters hit, many people in the affected area experience stress and serious mental health consequences. However, it is not only disasters themselves that increase stress levels: Worrying about climate change may also increase stress and impact mental health (Weir, 2016). Considering some of the dire climate predictions, it is hard not to worry about the future, but how these predictions will unfold are yet to be seen.

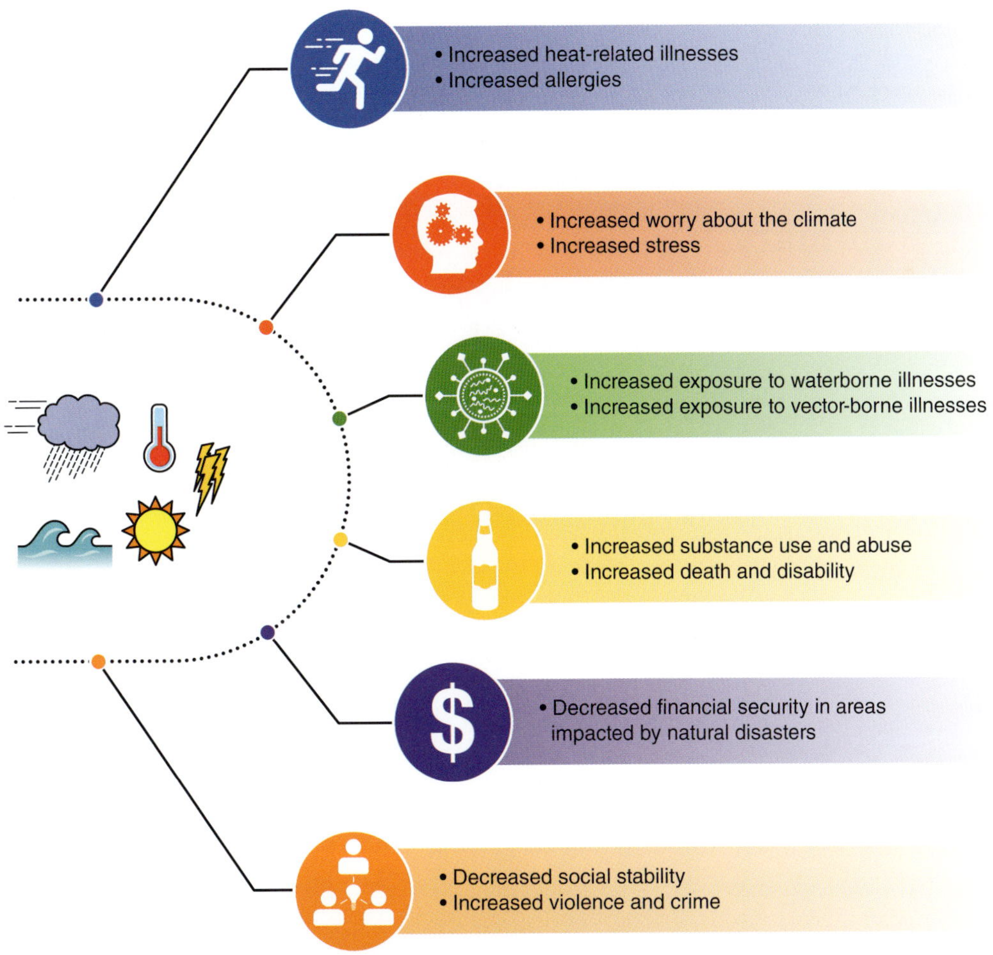


**Figure 2.6** How climate change impacts wellness.

Case Study

## Coping With Stress in College

Hannah, a freshman soccer player, is excited to be starting her college career. However, she feels a lot of pressure from her family and coach to perform well. She needs to maintain a 3.0 GPA and attend all practices and games to maintain her full-ride scholarship. Hannah is also the first one in her family to attend college, and her parents are constantly telling her how proud they are. She feels that her classes are very difficult and the soccer practices are exhausting. When she gets home after practice, she usually just eats dinner and watches television.

Hannah's first game is coming up and her coach told her she is not performing well in two of her classes, which puts her at risk for being ineligible. To make matters worse, her counselor also told her if her GPA drops, she is in danger of losing her scholarship. Hannah tells her counselor she is feeling overwhelmed and is having a difficult time concentrating on her work.

Her counselor asks her about her high school experience with managing sports and academics. Hannah shares that she used to create a weekly schedule to make sure she would have enough time to study. After discussing this option more, Hannah concludes she needs to resume her weekly scheduling to better manage her schoolwork. She leaves the meeting with her counselor feeling optimistic and motivated.

### Discussion Questions

1. How did Hannah's high school experience help prepare her for college?
2. What do you think would have happened if Hannah continued down the path she was on?
3. When is the last time you felt overwhelmed?
4. What are techniques you use to cope with those feelings?

## Summary

This chapter presented information about stress and how it impacts the body. When the body encounters stress, it goes through a three-stage process called general adaptation syndrome. These stages are alarm, resistance, and exhaustion. Stress can be identified as eustress (positive) or distress (negative). It can also be acute or chronic, depending on how long it lasts. Avoiding all stress is not possible nor healthy; each person has an optimal level of stress that improves motivation and performance, known as the Yerkes-Dodson law. Each person responds to stress differently, depending on factors such as upbringing, genetics, sex, and personal health choices. Although reactions to stress are individual, societal stresses that those are shared among a group of people in common circumstances.

## ONLINE RESOURCES

Visit HK*Propel* to access audio supplements, worksheets, and vocabulary flash cards for this chapter.

## DISCUSSION QUESTIONS

1. Compare and contrast *distress*, *eustress*, and *posttraumatic stress*. In what ways are they similar? In what ways are they different?
2. Explain how technology impacts stress levels. Describe a time in your life when technology caused distress. Describe a time when technology caused eustress.
3. Stress is not always negative. Describe a time in your life when you encountered eustress or positive stress. How were you able to grow and learn from that experience?
4. Imagining a life without stress may sound nice, but in reality, it would be detrimental. What is the impact of having too little stress? What is meant by optimal levels of stress?

# 3

# Stress and the Body

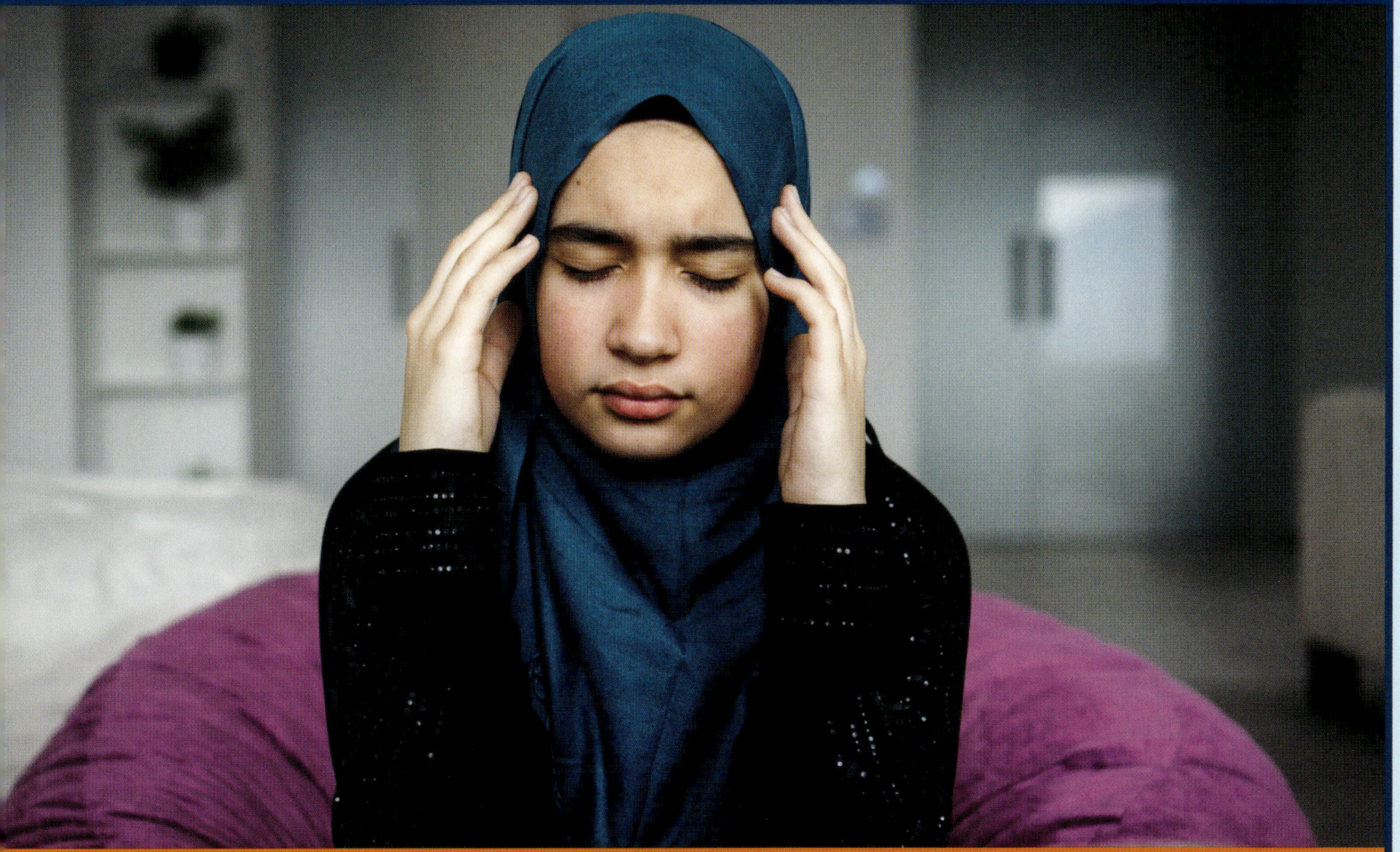

**LEARNING OBJECTIVES**

After reading this chapter, you will be able to do the following:

- Summarize the effects stress has on the body systems
- Discuss how chronic stress can increase your risk for acute and chronic illnesses
- Describe how chronic stress can produce physical symptoms of discomfort
- Justify the importance of effectively managing your stress to improve body functioning

# KEY TERMS

- cardiovascular system
- central nervous system
- endocrine system
- enteric nervous system
- glucocorticoids
- hypertension
- hyperventilation
- hypothalamus-pituitary-adrenal axis (HPA axis)
- immune system
- integumentary system
- musculoskeletal system
- perception
- peripheral nervous system
- renal system
- reproductive system
- respiratory system
- reticular activating system (RAS)
- sarcopenia

To begin to understand the role of stress, it is important to understand the body and its different systems. Information about the outside world—sights, sounds, smells, tastes, body position, and more—comes in through your senses. When you encounter a stressor, it starts with the senses receiving the information and relaying that information to the brain. The brain then triggers a series of changes, starting with the release of **glucocorticoids**, which begins the physical response to stress. From there, the body moves glucose into the bloodstream, increases heart rate and blood pressure, and decreases digestion to ensure that the alarm response is focused on essential functions. All body systems are connected in their response to both acute and chronic stress.

## Nervous System

The nervous system is the command center of the body. It has two parts: The **central nervous system**, which consists of your brain and spinal cord, and **peripheral nervous system**, which contains the nerves that branch out from the spinal cord to the rest of the body (figure 3.1).

All information received in the body goes to the brain for interpretation. Whether physical or psychological, the brain is responsible for creating a **perception** of the information. The stress you feel is a result of your perception: Whether an event is perceived as stressful depends on your expectations, previous experiences, and personality (see chapter 2). The brain has three main areas: the cerebrum, cerebellum, and brain stem (figure 3.2). The cerebrum, which is covered by

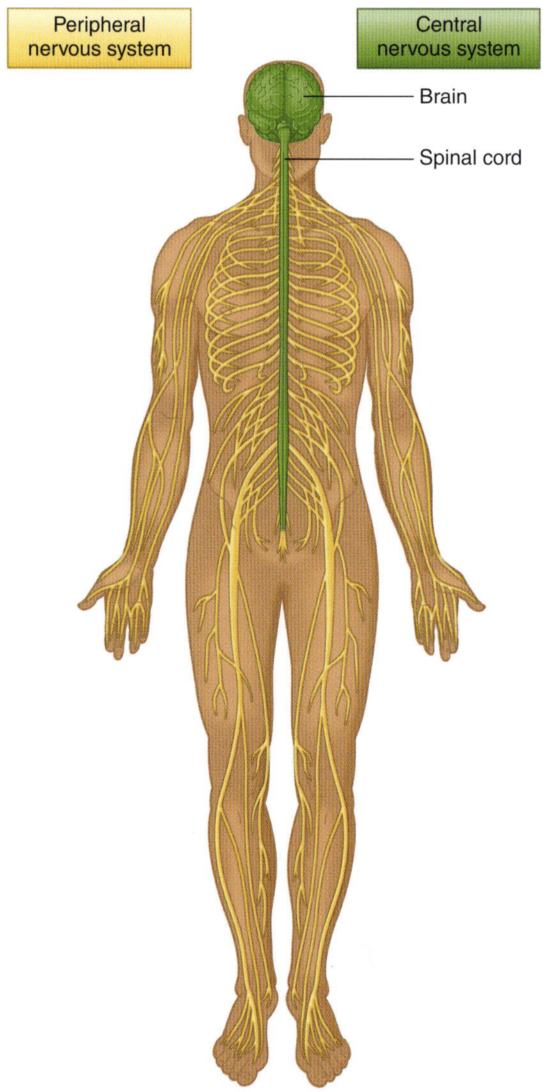


**Figure 3.1** Your body's nervous system.

the cerebral cortex, is the largest part of the brain and has two hemispheres and four lobes, each of which is responsible for different behaviors (known as brain lateralization). The left hemisphere controls the right side of the body and is responsible for language, logic, and math. The right hemisphere controls the left side of the body and is responsible for creativity, intuition, art, and music. The two halves communicate through a bundle of fibers called the corpus callosum. The cerebellum works to maintain balance and posture and coordinates voluntary muscle control. The brain stem, consisting of the midbrain, pons, and medulla oblongata, connects the cerebrum and cerebellum to the spinal cord. It is also responsible for regulating automatic and homeostatic functions like breathing, heart rate, digestion, and wake and sleep cycles. Deeper in the brain is the diencephalon, which includes the hypothalamus.

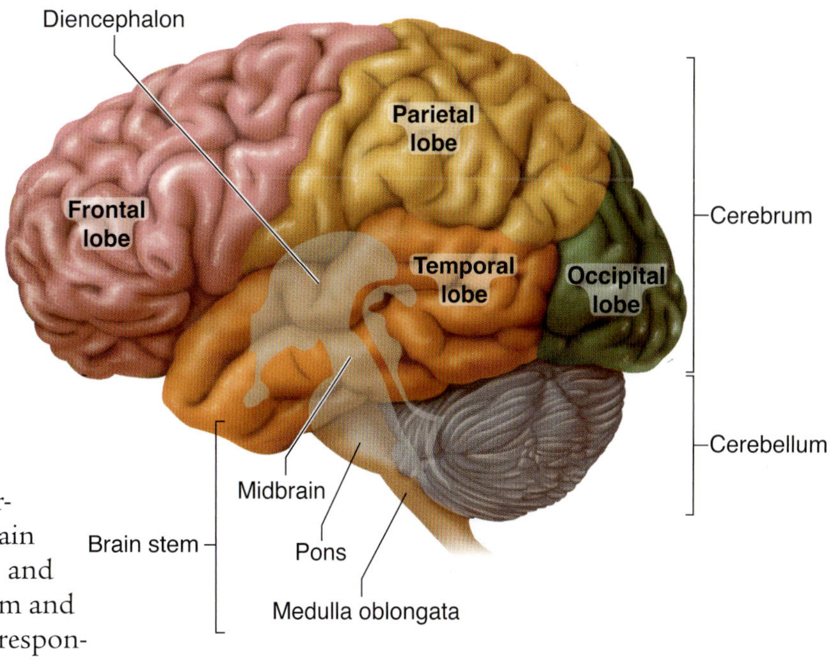


**Figure 3.2** The different parts of the brain.

## Brain Systems and Stress

Your brain acts as a regulator for stress. It identifies and tags stressors and begins a series of physical responses to manage those stressors (general adaptation syndrome, discussed in the previous chapter). The limbic system is a set of structures in the brain that includes the hypothalamus, thalamus, amygdala, and hippocampus. It links conscious and unconscious functions and also plays a role in memory and learning. The amygdala and hippocampus work together to regulate emotions (Torrico & Abdijadid, 2019). The amygdala creates emotional memories, which tend to elicit a heightened physical response. For example, if you have ever touched something very hot, you probably took your hand away from the heat source before you even felt the pain. Your amygdala creates a fear-based memory of being burned so that when you are near a similar heat source, you will remember fear and stay away from getting burned again.

### Stress and Fear

While on a bike ride with her friend, Pilar lost control going down a steep hill and fell. She didn't require any medical care but was pretty scraped up. She refused to get back on her bike to ride home but instead walked her bike all the way back. The next day her friend invited her on another bike ride. Pilar agreed, but as she neared her bike, she began to feel nervous. Her palms got sweaty, and her heart rate increased. Her amygdala created an effective fear-based memory to help Pilar remember the danger of riding her bike. Her body responded by activating the stress response because of the emotional attachment to riding a bike—in this case, fear.

When you were young and fell off a bike, you may have heard a parent tell you to get right back on. They were trying to reduce the chances of creating a fear-based memory so you wouldn't be scared to ride the bike again. On the other hand, this fear can also serve as a protective factor. For example, it was once a common punishment for teenagers caught smoking cigarettes to be forced to smoke the whole pack, which would cause them to be sick. This was an attempt to invoke a fear and disgust association with cigarettes in order to remove the temptation to smoke.

Emotions tend to be reactional and not proactive, and it can be difficult to overcome emotions that are tied to an event. You can, however, be proactive in your thinking and use imagery and positive self-talk (discussed in chapters 5 and 6 of this textbook) to help overcome and manage your emotions.

When you receive information about the world, it filters through the **reticular activating system (RAS)**, a bundle of nerves in the brain stem responsible for processing and filtering information. When functioning properly, it helps tune out background noise in a class so you can focus on the teacher. It also can help you hear your name being called in a crowd of people or allow a mother to hear her child call out "mom" in a room full of kids. When the RAS is not aroused, you may find it difficult to focus and concentrate. When the RAS is overstimulated, you may feel restless, hyperactive, and easily startled. People with ADD or ADHD are thought to have an understimulated RAS. Stimulants are used to treat these disorders by allowing the RAS to properly filter information.

The stress response begins with the **hypothalamus-pituitary-adrenal axis (HPA axis)** activation, triggered by signals from the limbic system and amygdala. Once a stressor filters through the RAS, it gets sent to the hypothalamus. The hypothalamus responds by activating the sympathetic nervous system, releasing a hormone called corticotropin-releasing hormone (CRH) into the bloodstream (figure 3.3). The CRH travels to the pituitary gland and signals the gland to release adrenocorticotropic hormone (ACTH) into the bloodstream. ACTH travels all the way to the adrenal glands (located near the kidneys), activating them to release the hormone cortisol into the bloodstream and creating the fight-or-flight response.

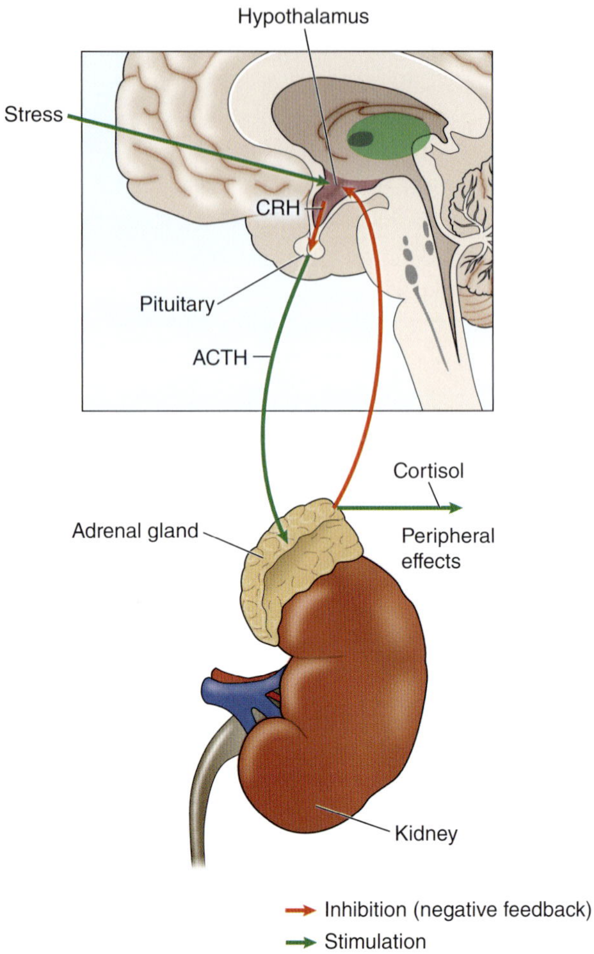


**Figure 3.3** HPA axis activation.

When under normal amounts of stress, the system works as it should and remains healthy. When you encounter too much stress, the body continues to send out CRH and ACTH, which tell the adrenal gland to continue to secrete adrenaline and cortisol. This can have detrimental health effects, as previously described in chapter 2. Repeated exposure to stress may also impact memory and cognition and result in mood disorders, such as depression (Chrousos, 2009).

## Learning and Memory

Many people feel stress when under pressure, such as when they are taking exams. However, too much stress can impact your ability to learn and perform well. Think of the game Simon: The game consists of four buttons that each light up a different color, and you have to copy the order of the lights. To start, the game moves slowly, but as the game progresses, the lights go faster, creating anxiety to keep up. Although simple, the act of keeping the correct order of lights becomes more difficult as the sequence becomes quicker, creating a sense of running out of time. The increased stress or anticipation that occurs during this game makes it more difficult for your brain to learn.

New information is coded in your brain in two ways. If the new information is related to prior knowledge, it is processed via the medial prefrontal cortex. If the new information is not related to prior knowledge, it is processed through the hippocampus. However, your ability to learn new information and retrieve prior information is disrupted when you are under stress (Vogel, Kluen, Ferandez, & Schwabe, 2018). Remember, when stressed, your body releases cortisol, which—among other functions—reduces the functioning of processes that do not contribute to the fight-or-flight response. The release of cortisol reaches its peak levels 20 to 30 minutes after the onset of stress (Vogel & Schwabe, 2016). After peaking, it can take over an hour for cortisol levels to return to normal levels. During this time your hippocampus and medial prefrontal cortex functioning is altered, particularly as it relates to memory recall. This explains why, for example, you may have performed more poorly than you expected on a high-stakes exam you felt prepared for: When you are under stress, your brain has a difficult time retrieving information.

**The more stressed you feel during an exam, the more you are inhibiting your brain to recall learning.**

## Endocrine System

The **endocrine system** (figure 3.4) is responsible for making and releasing hormones, which control mood, growth, development, metabolism, and reproduction. Table 3.1 presents the glands in the endocrine system and their roles. The endocrine system is also responsible for the fight-or-flight response.

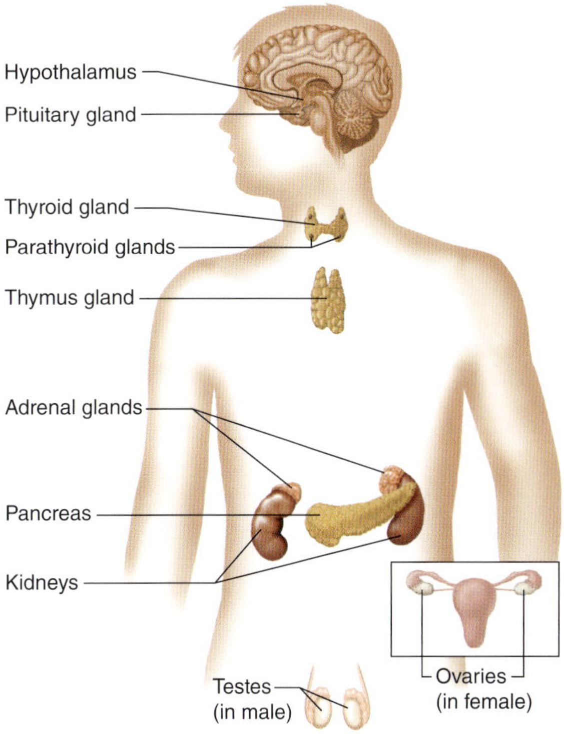


**Figure 3.4** Main components of the endocrine system.

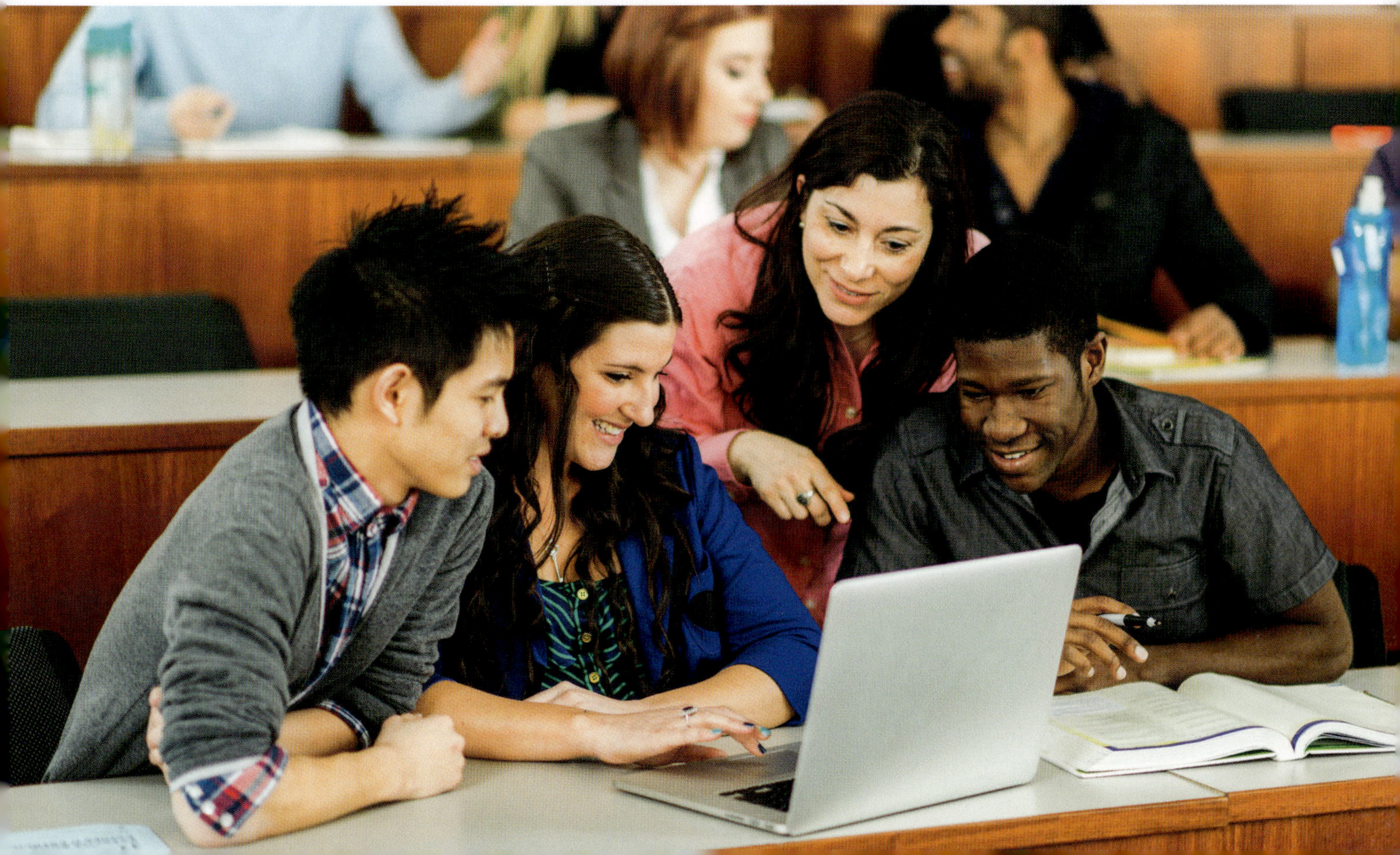

**Table 3.1** Glands of the Endocrine System and Their Roles

| Gland | Role |
|---|---|
| Hypothalamus | Connects endocrine system to the nervous system |
| Pituitary gland | Tells other glands in the body what hormones to produce and release; considered the master gland |
| Pineal gland | Produces melatonin to help your body fall and stay asleep |
| Thyroid gland | Controls growth and metabolism |
| Parathyroid | Plays a role in bone health |
| Thymus | Makes white blood cells and regulates immune system development |
| Adrenals | Control fight-or-flight hormones |
| Pancreas | Creates hormones responsible for digestion and blood sugar. |
| Ovaries | Produce hormones to help develop puberty, regulate menstrual cycle, and support pregnancy in biological females |
| Testes | Produce hormones to help develop puberty and produce sperm in biological males |

Research Spotlight

## Marie Antoinette Syndrome

Can extreme stress (like being captured during the French Revolution) really turn your hair gray overnight? Although waking up to a full head of white or gray hair is best left to the realm of fiction, it does seem that stress can contribute to gray hair. Noradrenaline released during stress depletes melanocyte stem cells, a skin cell responsible for giving hair its pigment. Too much stress, therefore, eventually depletes pigment and causes the hair to come out gray (Zhang et al., 2020).

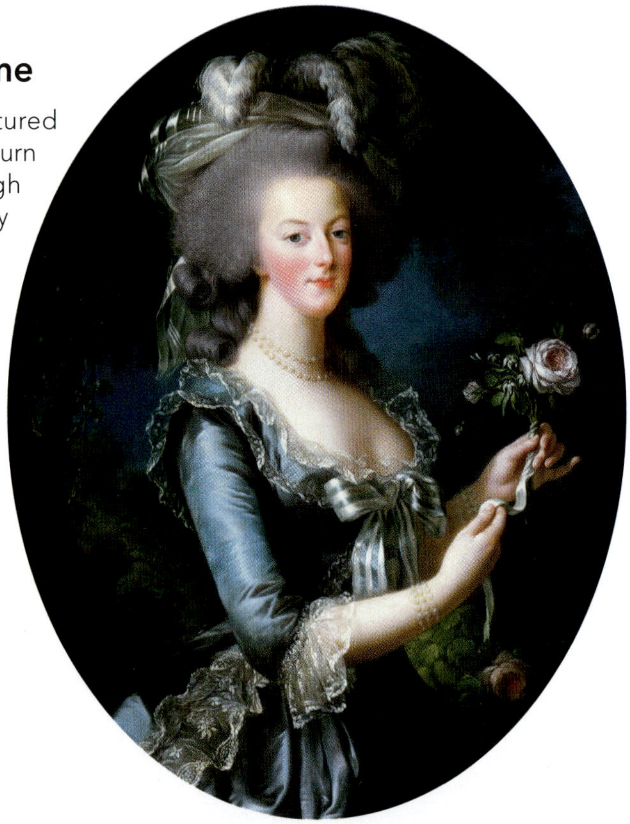

Any type of stress elicits a response from the endocrine system. However, psychological stressors have the potential to elicit even stronger responses from the endocrine system, particularly if the stress involves uncertainty and unpredictability (Henley, Kaye, & Lightman, 2011). Chronic stress can have damaging and lasting effects on the endocrine system. For example, Graves' disease is an autoimmune disorder that results in the overproduction of thyroid hormones (also known as hyperthyroidism); stress has been shown to be linked to the development of Graves' disease (Vita et al., 2016).

## Reproductive System

Because the endocrine system is closely related to the **reproductive system**, the hormones involved in reproductive functioning are also affected by stress. Because sex is generally not considered a primary physical function, energy is diverted to other systems necessary for the stress response, reducing the normal functioning of the reproductive system and contributing to causes of infertility in both males and females.

Chronic stress reduces the testosterone levels in biological males (Jaurez-Rojas, Vigueras-Villasenor, Casillas, & Retana-Marquez, 2017), which has been associated with diminished libido (sex drive) and normal sperm cell production. Chronic stress can also impact the production of healthy sperm cells by influencing the degeneration of seminiferous tubules (where immature sperm mature) (Jaurez-Rojas et al., 2017). Moreover, chronic exposure to stress can lead to functional damage of the testes (Shen et al., 2020). These alterations all contribute to infertility in males.

Biological females also have testosterone, albeit in much smaller amounts compared to males. Lower amounts of testosterone in females can lead to decreased sexual drive, sexual satisfaction, and mood (Scott & Newson, 2020). Studies have found that when under stress, female rats will not seek out sex (Magarinos & Pfaff, 2015). Stress can also contribute to hypothalamic amenorrhea, or the ceasing of menstruation caused by the hypothalamus (Valsamakis, Chrousos, & Mastorakos, 2019). Finally, increased levels of cortisol can impair egg cell development, which, in turn, makes fertilization more difficult (Joseph & Whirledge, 2017).

Human bodies are uniquely designed, and when under stress, they go through changes that make it difficult for reproduction to take place. Sometimes the stress is caused by a delay in conception, which can then further reduce chances of getting pregnant. Regardless of the cause of stress, practicing stress management techniques, particularly mind–body programs, can improve the chances of getting pregnant (Rooney & Domar, 2018).

## Cardiovascular System

The **cardiovascular system** is a closed system consisting of the heart and blood vessels (figure 3.5). The heart is a muscle that circulates blood through the body via arteries, veins, and capillaries. During a stress response, the stress hormones adrenaline, noradrenaline, and cortisol increase heart rate. Additionally, the blood vessels dilate, increasing the amount of blood that's pumped through the body. Once the stress event has passed, the body resumes homeostasis.

Chronic stress places additional burdens on the cardiovascular system and increases the risk of cardiovascular disease (Yaribeygi, Panahi, Sahraei, Johnston, & Sahebkar, 2017). Imagine dribbling a basketball. Under normal conditions, it doesn't take a lot of effort and you can probably go for a long time before you become tired. Now imagine you have to dribble the ball as quickly as possible: If that stress is short lived, it will not take a lot of additional effort, and your heart rate and breathing will quickly return to normal. However, if you were to continue to dribble the ball as quickly as possible for as long as possible, you would eventually tire out. Your heart is similar. Under normal amounts of stress, your heart can handle the additional work. When stress is prolonged or chronic, however, the heart doesn't have an opportunity to rest and can become strained. This can contribute to an increased risk of heart attack (Yaribeygi et al., 2017).

Stress is also a risk factor for **hypertension**, or high blood pressure. Under normal resting conditions, a healthy blood pressure is considered to be anything below 120/80. Blood pressure above 140/90 is considered hypertension and is a risk factor for cardiovascular disease. High blood pressure can reduce the elasticity of the arteries,

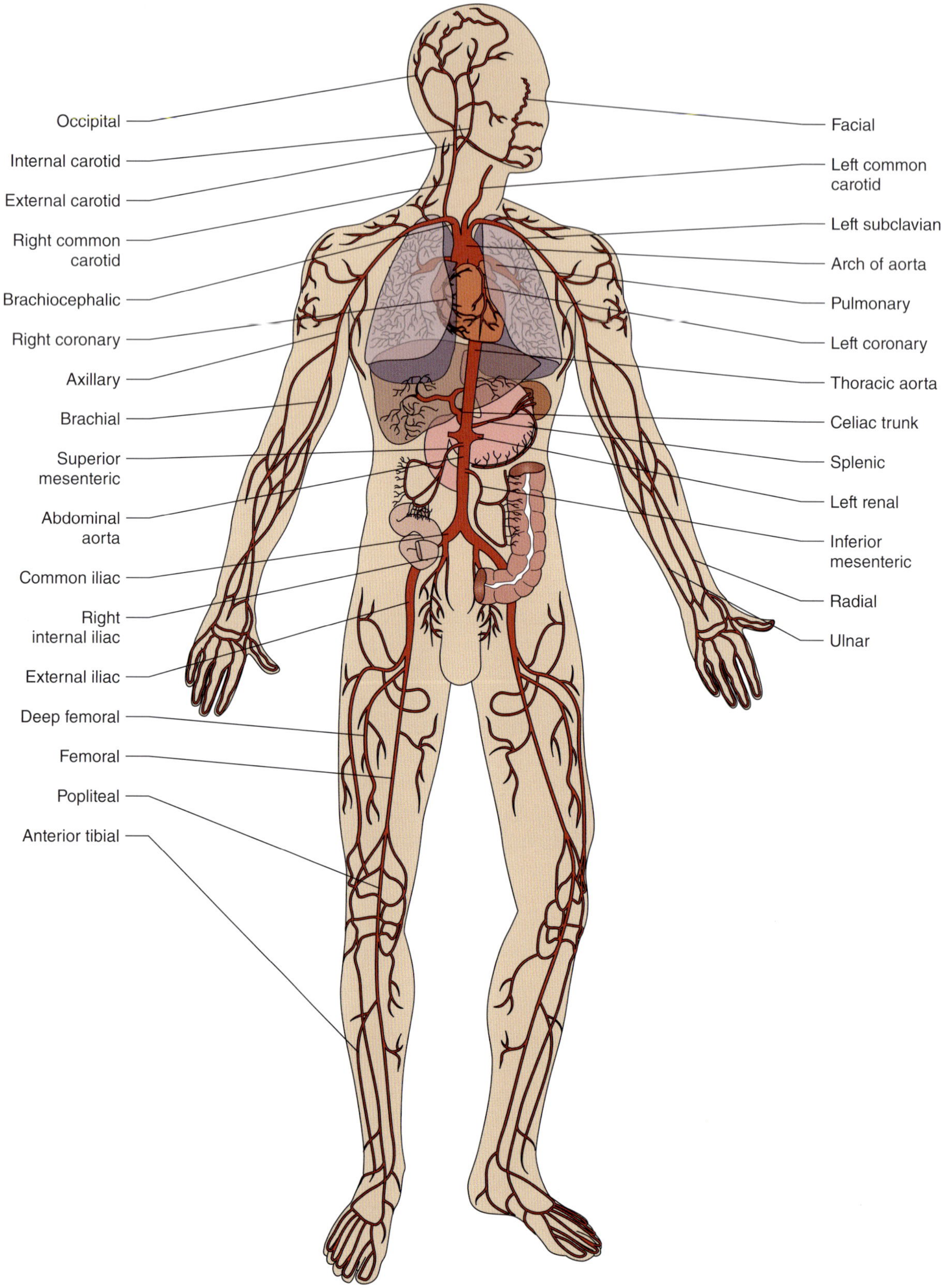


**Figure 3.5** The cardiovascular system supplies blood to your body.

decreasing the amount of blood that flows to the heart and increasing the risk of heart attacks and heart failure. Consider the previous example of dribbling a basketball: The blood pressure would be measured by the force of the basketball hitting the floor, and the harder and faster you dribble, the higher the force.

Stress can also contribute to inflammation of the circulatory system. Inflammation is your body's response to an injury or illness. Prolonged inflammation in the arteries may promote the growth of plaque or loosen plaque in your arteries and trigger blood clots, all of which can contribute to heart attacks (American Psychological Association, 2018). Inflammation has also been linked to increased cholesterol, another risk factor for cardiovascular disease.

## Enteric Nervous System

The **enteric nervous system** is part of the autonomic nervous system that regulates digestion. This system is sometimes referred to as the *second brain* because of the constant communication between the brain and the gut. The brain–gut axis describes this deep connection. For example, have you ever said you have a gut feeling about something? You may not be far off from the truth: The gut sends messages to the brain that can impact mood. In fact, 95 percent of the body's serotonin is found in the gut, not the brain (Abdel-Haq, Schlachetzki, Glass, & Mazmanian, 2019). More neurons also reside in the gut than in the entire spinal cord (Iliades, 2018).

**It is not surprising that stress, which forms in the brain, can impact the gut.**

How often have you heard the terms "butterflies in my stomach," "gut-wrenching," or "my stomach is tied in knots"? These are all terms that describe the physical effects stress has on the stomach. This phenomenon is not limited to adults: Almost 20 percent of children experience stomach pains that are not related to an illness (Newton et al., 2018).

Many believe an increased production of stomach acid is the cause of stress-induced stomachaches, but this is not correct. When the stomach acid used to break down food is present, the sphincter between the esophagus and stomach is closed, indicating digestion is functioning well (Rosen & Winters, 2020). During a stress response, digestion—a nonessential function—is slowed or stopped altogether, resulting in the production of less stomach acid. This causes the sphincter between the stomach and esophagus to remain open, allowing the little stomach acid that is present in the stomach to come up and irritate the esophagus. A similar misconception exists regarding ulcers: Though ulcers may be worsened by stress, they are caused by bacterial infection.

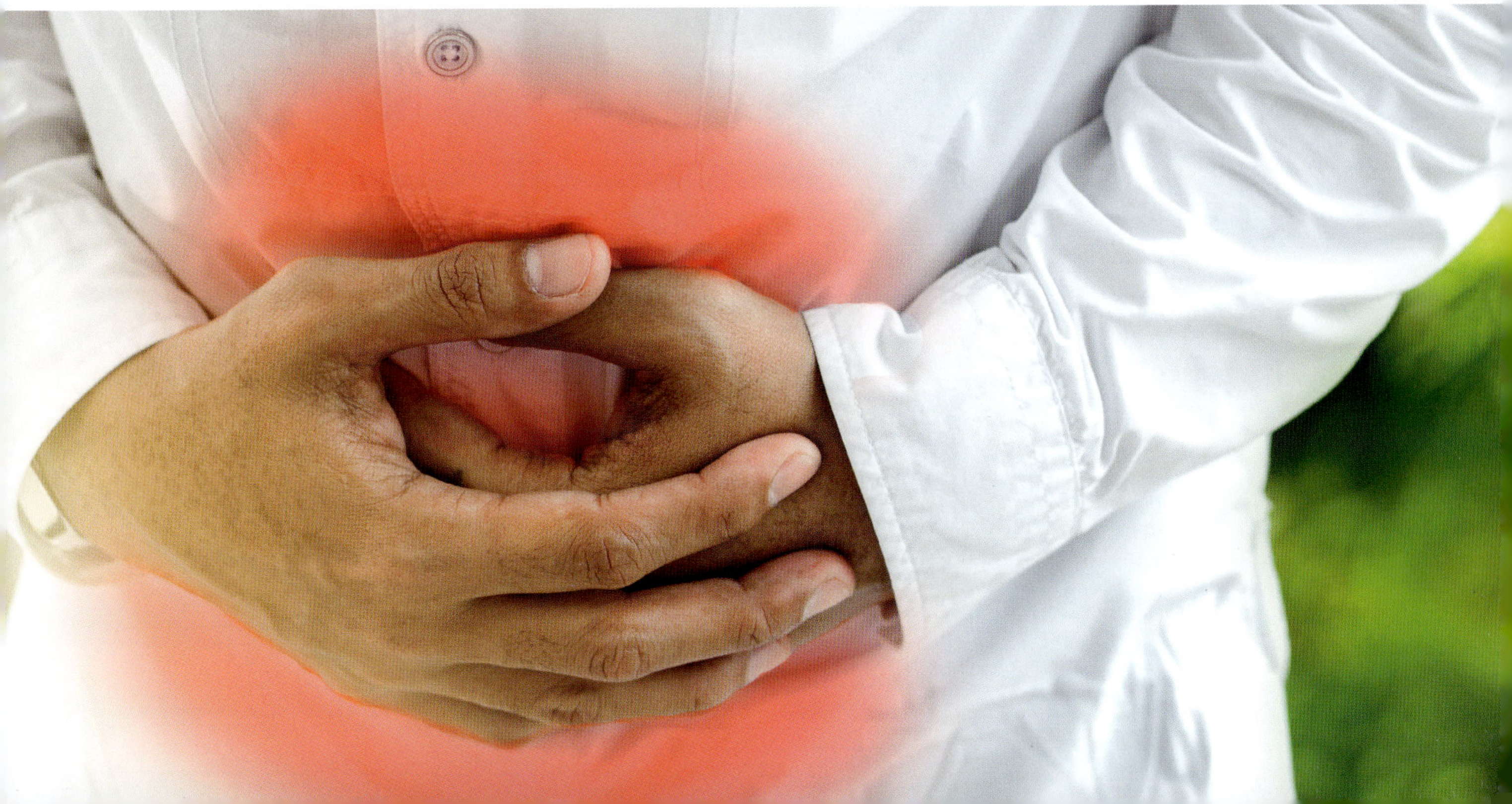

## Renal System

Stress can impact the **renal system**, which is responsible for creating urine, by affecting how quickly food passes through the body, which can cause quite a bit of discomfort. When you encounter stress, your body redirects blood and other resources to essential functions and away from your stomach; as such, the initial response to stress may be diarrhea. But the slowed rate of digestion from prolonged stress can result in constipation. These conditions are magnified for people who suffer from irritable bowel syndrome and similar conditions (Chan et al., 2019). Chronic stress has also been shown to have similar effects on the urinary system; initial exposure may cause frequent urination, followed by decreased urinary function and frequency and increased susceptibility to lower urinary tract infections with continued exposure (Gao & Rodriquez, 2022).

A leaky gut is a condition that occurs when the lining of the gut becomes more permeable and no longer works properly as a barrier. As such, bad bacteria and food particles are able to enter the gut, which can damage your health (Camilleri, 2019). Both chronic and acute stress release cortisol into the bloodstream, which weakens the gut barrier. Harmful bacteria and other food particles can then pass through the barrier, causing an inflammation response to fight off the bacteria (Madison & Kiecolt-Glaser, 2019), which further disrupts normal digestion.

## Musculoskeletal System

The **musculoskeletal system** includes the bones, muscles, tendons, cartilage, ligaments, and joints and works to provide the body's movement and stability. Muscle tension is part of the stress response—when under stress, you may feel tightness in your back or a stiff neck. This is because stress causes your muscles to contract as part of the fight-or-flight response. Muscle tension is also a short-term protective factor against injury and pain (American Psychological Association, 2018). When the stressor passes, the muscles will release the tension. However, under conditions of long-term stress, the chronic muscle tension can cause you to experience aches and pains.

**Think back to the last stressful day you had. What did you feel like at the end of the day? Were you sore? Did your back hurt? Did you experience a headache?**

### Stress Gains

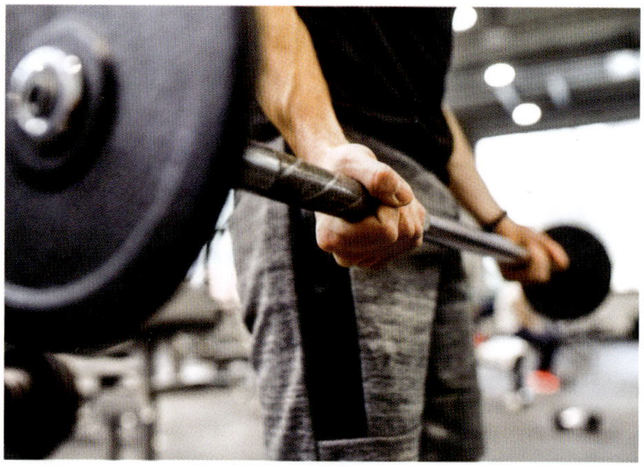

Henry is a college student who attends a gym and works with a weightlifting trainer. He has formed a nice workout routine and has been able to stick to his schedule. Recently, Henry lost his job to downsizing, and he is now worried how he will pay rent. Moreover, one of his professors asked to see him about his poor performance on the last exam. Since the stress has started, Henry has not seen the same benefits from weightlifting; in fact, he sees more fat development in his abdominal area. He knows he has not changed his diet or workout routine and can't figure out why his body is changing. The only difference is the amount of stress he feels. Henry is struggling because the chronic stress is affecting the availability of energy he needs to build muscle. He needs to better control his stress in order to reduce his cortisol levels and help him reduce the excess abdominal fat cells.

Chronic stress can also contribute to **sarcopenia**, or muscle loss. In low doses and for short periods of time, the stress hormone cortisol can improve muscle function. However, during chronic stress, cortisol is continually released in the body and inhibits skeletal muscle mitochondrial functioning (Stefanaki, Pervanidou, Boschiero, & Chrousos, 2018). Because the mitochondria is the cell's energy source, the energy available to the muscle cells is reduced. Think of it as a car: The mitochondria is the engine that allows the car to go. If the engine is not functioning properly, the car's functioning will be limited no matter how full the gas tank is. Similarly, even if you are eating right, muscular mitochondria that is inhibited by stress will not be able to convert the fuel to energy for muscle use.

Hyperplasia, or enlargement of tissue or an organ due to the increased reproduction rate of the cells, is one possible cause of the increase in fat around the abdominal region. Adipose tissue (fat) serves as stored energy in the body and contains precursor cells that can be triggered to convert to fat cells. Cortisol can signal these precursor cells to convert to fat cells at higher rates (Bahrami-Nejad et al., 2018). This is especially true if higher amounts of cortisol are released at night, which is more likely during conditions of chronic stress. Other studies show a relationship between obesity and stress. For example, one study found that stress significantly contributed to the development and maintenance of obesity (van der Valk, Savas, & van Rossum, 2018). This is even more true among individuals who have higher amounts of abdominal fat.

## Respiratory System

The **respiratory system** is responsible for supplying your body with oxygen and removing carbon dioxide. The main components of this system include the mouth, nose, trachea, bronchi, bronchioles, alveoli, and lungs. Air enters through the nose or mouth and travels through the trachea to the entryway of the lungs. The air travels through large branches in the lungs called bronchi, which divide further into bronchioles and end in tiny sacs called alveoli. The alveoli take in the oxygen through capillaries and transmit them to the heart to be distributed to the rest of the body.

**Take a minute and think about your breathing. Breathe deeply and think about how relaxed you feel.**

When you are relaxed, your muscles mainly work in the inhalation stage of breathing; the exhalation stage is primarily passive. However, when under stress, your body focuses its energy on essential functions and requires more oxygen (Seo, Kim, Kim, Lee, & Park, 2019). The sympathetic nervous system signals your lungs to breathe faster, placing muscular effort on both inhalation and exhalation. When this occurs for too long, it can exacerbate other conditions. For example, those who suffer from asthma or emphysema may find it more difficult to breathe when under stress (Vafaee, Shirzad, Shamsi, & Boskabady, 2022). This signal can also go in the other direction: If you start to breathe rapidly, your brain will assume you are under stress and signal the sympathetic nervous system to deploy the fight-or-flight response. This can encourage **hyperventilation** (rapid breathing that is brought on by stress) or panic attacks and increase feelings of anxiety for those who are prone to those experiences.

Think about the last time you saw a scary movie. Did you find yourself holding your breath? Did you gasp when you experienced a jump scare?

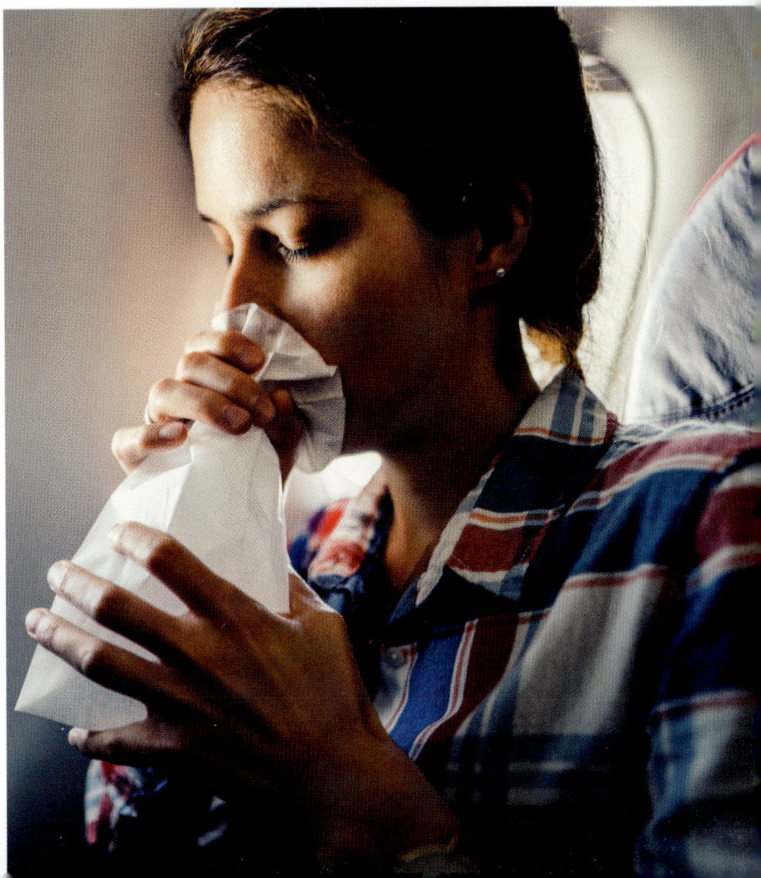

These are normal reactions to stress. Fear is a strong emotion that evokes the fight-or-flight response. Even watching a person take short, quick breaths can put you in a state of stress as you mimic the actor's breathing rate.

Learning controlled breathing techniques can stimulate the body to modulate the effects of stress. Whereas quick and shallow breathing can ignite the sympathetic nervous system into a stress reaction, deep and controlled breathing can signal the brain to switch off the fight-or-flight response and return to homeostasis (De Couck et al., 2019). More about controlled and rhythmic breathing will be presented later in this text.

## Immune System

The **immune system** includes the lymphatic system, spleen, bone marrow, white blood cells, antibodies, and thymus and is responsible for detecting and fighting infection in the body. When it recognizes antigens, or foreign substances, it triggers an attack. The immune system has two different attacking mechanisms: The innate immune system is generalized and used for all interactions with antigens. The adaptive immune system is more targeted and uses specific antibodies to attack specific antigens. The immune system stores information about previously encountered antigens so that when the body encounters the same antigen, the antibodies recognize it and are able to deal with them effectively. The purpose of a vaccine is for the immune system to create antibodies of the targeted disease to be able to fight it effectively.

Your body has been trained to respond to stress as if it is a physical threat. As a result, it prepares itself for a battle: During acute stress, the body increases immune cells and sends them to areas in the body most likely to be involved in an injury. However, most cases of modern stress do not involve a physical threat.

Chronic stress can decrease the functioning of the immune system, making you more susceptible to getting sick and less able to fight off diseases, infections, and injuries when they occur. The continued release of cortisol suppresses the proteins needed to make immune cells (B and T cells). Moreover, the immune system begins to ignore the cortisol's signals and stops responding to those signals. However, inflammation markers still continue to increase in response to chronic stress, which can also harm the body and place you at higher risk for other conditions such as cancer, cardiovascular disease, and obesity. For example, stress is believed to contribute to DNA damage, which results in malignant tumors. Stress, via glucocorticoids, may reactivate viral infections that contribute to cancer, such as the human papillomavirus (HPV). Glucocorticoids may also promote cancer tumor growth, advancing the cancer stage. (Eckerling et al., 2021). Another study found an association between psychosocial stress and cardiovascular disease, suggesting that stress can be a risk factor for chronic diseases (Dar et al., 2019).

> Worry affects the circulation, the heart, the glands, the whole nervous system.
>
> **Charles Horace Mayo**

## Integumentary System

The **integumentary system**, consisting of skin, hair, and nails, creates the physical boundary between the body's external and internal environment. The skin is the body's largest organ and contains two types of sweat glands: eccrine and apocrine glands. Eccrine glands cover most of your

### Post-Finals Week Crash

Many college students who are finishing up assignments while planning and studying for exams experience increased levels of stress as finals week approaches. Studies have shown decreased immune system functioning and greater susceptibility to illness (particularly upper respiratory tract infections) among students experiencing stress (Assaf, 2013; Turner et al., 2020). As you approach finals week, consider taking proactive approaches to manage your stress. It may help you from getting sick later.

Case Study

## The Immune System Versus the Wildebeest

Drob is an adult male caveman. His role is to help feed the family by going on weekly hunts and bringing back meat. While quietly sitting in the brush and sharpening his spear, he sees what looks to be a wildebeest in the distance coming his way. His heart starts racing as he plans his route of attack. Meanwhile, inside his body, his immune system is fast at work, producing more immune cells (neutrophils, eosinophils, lymphocytes, monocytes) and distributing them in the blood. These immune cells are also sent to the skin, gastrointestinal lining, and other frontline areas in the body in anticipation of an injury. The body also increases its inflammation markers, which are released before inflammation occurs.

Drob is now crouching down and waiting for the wildebeest to get closer. His muscles are tight with anticipation. At the right moment, Drob jumps up with the spear in hand and goes for the wildebeest. The wildebeest anticipates this move, deflects the spear, and scratches Drob with its horn before scurrying away. Thankfully, Drob's immune system was ready for this and quickly gets to work fighting off infection and beginning the healing process.

Drob is older now and is still hunting, though he is not as effective as he used to be. Sitting in the bush patiently waiting for his next animal, he sees something in the distance. His heart begins to race, and his immune system sends cells to their position. Drob coughs, and the animal runs away. His body begins to return to normal. A while later, Drob sees another animal, and his body again activates the stress response. Drob shifts his position a bit, which alerts the animal, and Drob misses another opportunity. Sometime later, Drob sees yet another animal, and his body again sets off the stress response. However, Drob is too slow. He misses, and he gets scratched. Unfortunately, under conditions of chronic stress, Drob's immune system has stopped responding, and his minor cut quickly becomes infected. Constant exposure to stress with no time to effectively manage it results in a weaker, less responsive immune system, which can place you at risk for infections, diseases, and illnesses.

### Discussion Questions

1. Why is it important to rest and recover after encountering stress?
2. What can occur when the body's immune response is reduced?
3. This case study highlights physical stress, but your immune system doesn't differentiate between a physical and emotional threat. Sometimes people are not aware that the stress they are experiencing is wearing down their body. How can you determine if stress is wearing you down?

body but are mostly concentrated in your palms, soles of your feet, forehead, cheeks, and armpits. The sweat released from these glands contains mostly water and is designed to cool your body, hydrate your skin, and balance your body fluids and electrolytes. Apocrine glands are larger and concentrated in areas of your body where you have a lot of hair follicles (armpits and genital regions). These secrete a thicker sweat that contains more lipids (fat) and proteins.

Think about the last time you had to give a presentation or went to a job interview. Were you nervous? Did you notice yourself sweating more? When under stress, the body produces and releases more sweat, specifically from the apocrine glands. The lipids and proteins contained in this sweat is believed to feed the bacteria located on the surface of your skin, which causes body odor (Swaney, Nelsen, Sandstrom, & Kalan, 2023). Many people say that the sweat produced under stress smells much different (and stronger) than regular sweat.

Stress can also impact how your skin looks. Flushing, a common symptom of stress, occurs when the blood vessels in the skin enlarge to

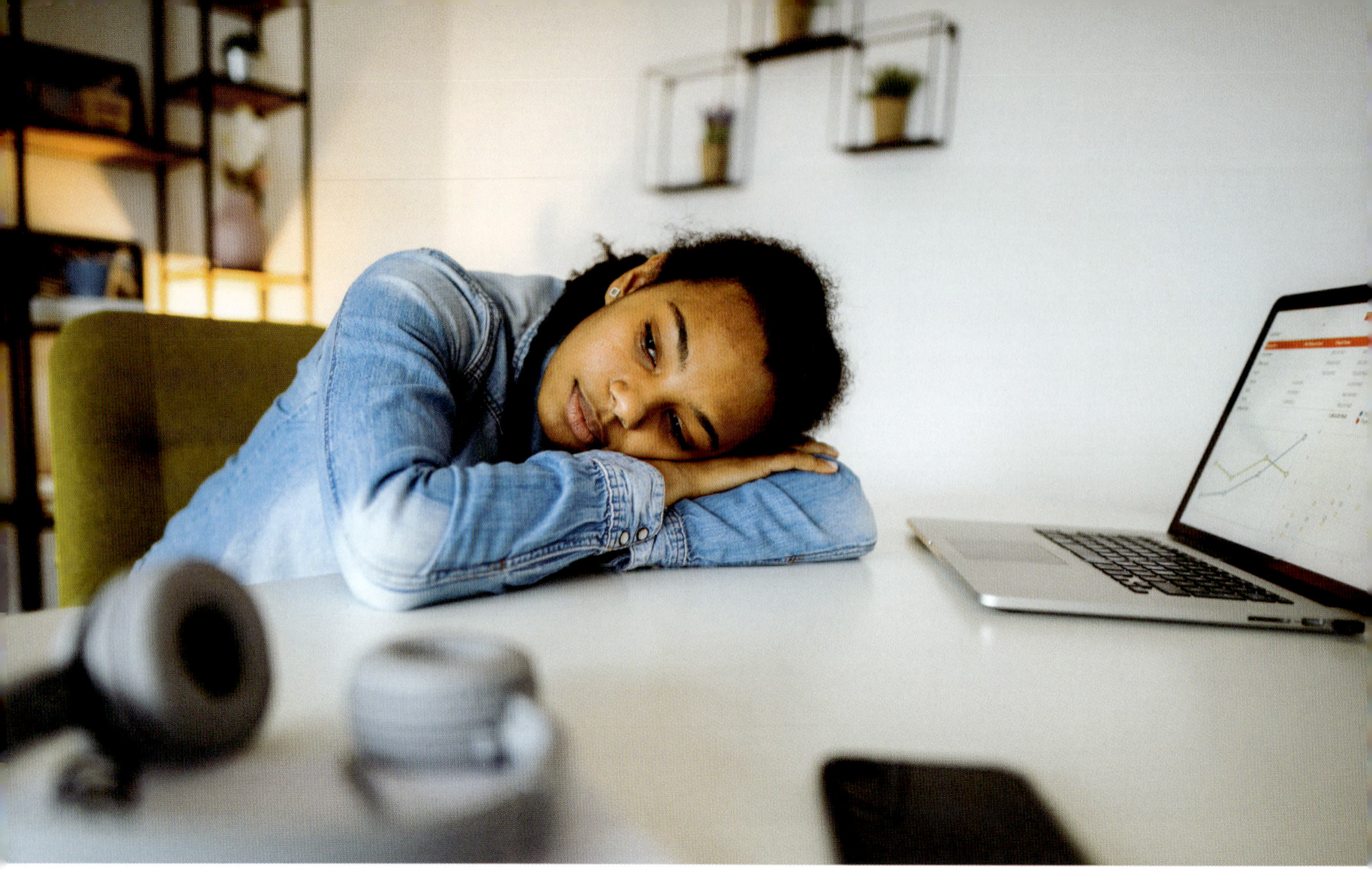

accommodate an increase in blood flow, which causes the skin to become reddened and feel warm. Higher levels of stress are also correlated with an increase in acne and its severity (Zari & Alrahmani, 2017). Cortisol sends a signal to the hypothalamus to release corticotrophin-releasing hormone (CRH), believed to stimulate additional oil release from sebaceous glands around the hair follicles in your skin and face (Chen, Zhang, Xu, Wan, & Wang, 2022). When these glands get clogged, it can lead to acne.

You might describe someone who looks older than they are as having "lived a hard life." Although stress doesn't cause premature aging, it does affect the condition of your skin. Stress can affect the integrity of the stratum corneum, or outer layer of your skin. Cortisol interferes with the skin's ability to store water and encourages your sweat glands to release more sweat. This combination of water loss and inability to store water results in very dry, itchy skin (Chen, Zhang, Xu, Wan, & Wang, 2022). Stress may also worsen the appearance of wrinkles by affecting the proteins in the stratum corneum, which reduces the elasticity in the skin, causing wrinkles to form (Chen et al., 2022). Dry skin can also enhance the appearance of wrinkles by making them more visible.

## Summary

Stress affects all body systems. When stress is acute and managed well, the body can deal with the stress and return to normal functioning. When stress is not managed well and becomes chronic, all body systems are at additional risk for both acute and chronic health conditions. Learning how to effectively manage stress can help your body function optimally. In the following chapters, you will learn how to better cope with stress to reduce this potential negative impact.

## ONLINE RESOURCES

Visit HK*Propel* to access audio supplements, worksheets, and vocabulary flash cards for this chapter.

## DISCUSSION QUESTIONS

1. Describe how stress impacts the major body systems. In your response, describe how stress reduces their functioning.
2. Reflect on your own physical symptoms of stress. Do you get headaches? Stomachaches? Describe your own symptoms of stress and explain why you experience those symptoms from a physiological perspective.
3. Think about some common phrases related to stress: "white as a ghost," "butterflies in my stomach," "tied in knots." How do these phrases relate to the physical changes occurring in the body?
4. Many students experience heightened levels of stress during exam week. Imagine you are put in charge of offering student activities to reduce stress prior to and during exam week. What types of activities would you plan? How would those activities reduce stress? How would you know if your program was successful?

PART II

# Managing Stress Using Dimensions of Wellness

# 4

# Physical Wellness

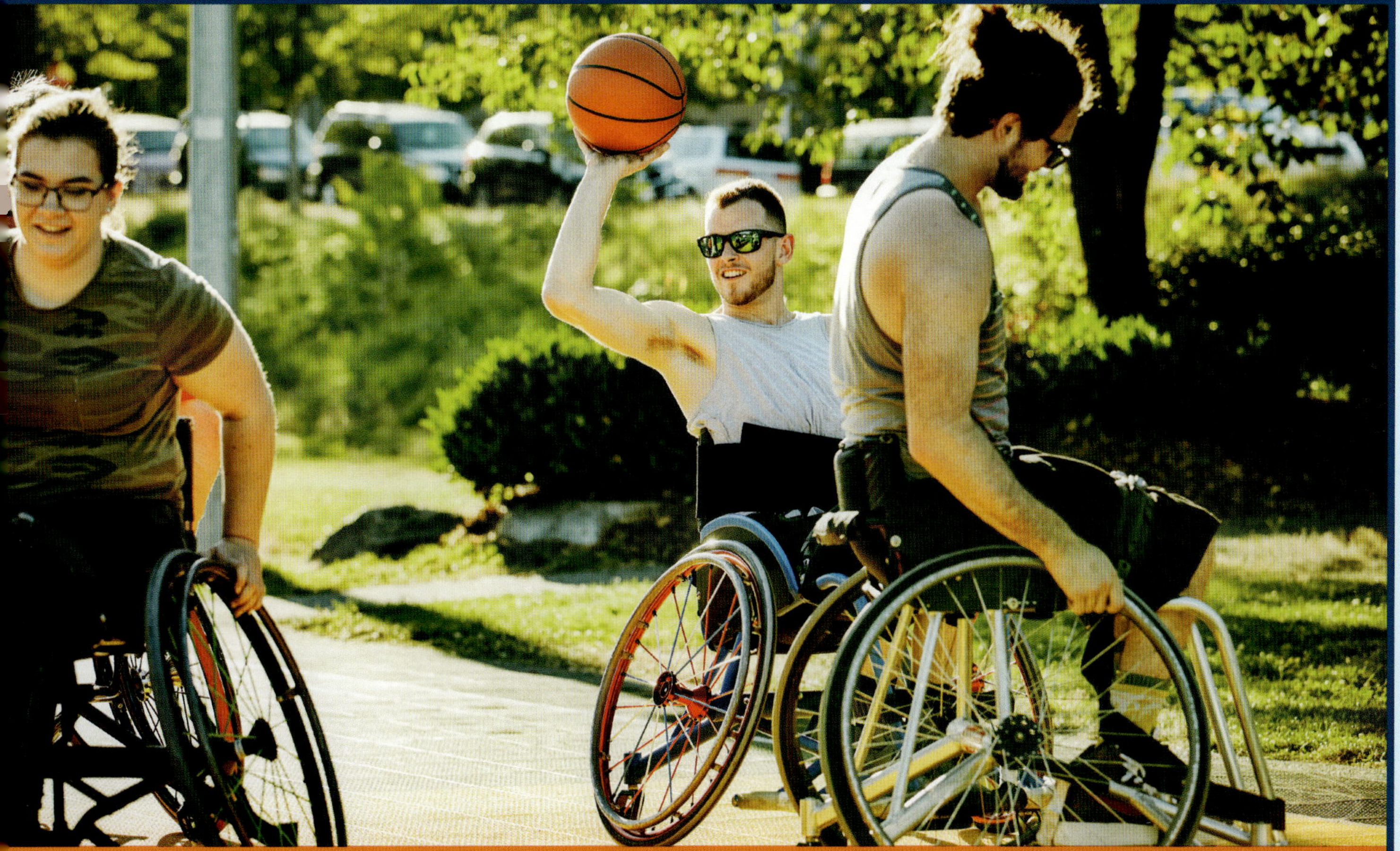

## LEARNING OBJECTIVES

After reading this chapter, you will be able to do the following:

- Explain the impact of stress on physical activity
- Discuss how physical activity can moderate stress
- Examine the relationship between nutrition and stress
- List strategies to help you practice healthy eating habits
- Evaluate the importance of sleep and its impact on stress
- List strategies for improved sleep hygiene
- Identify ways to induce the relaxation response

# KEY TERMS

cortisol awakening response (CAR)
dietary patterns
emotional hunger
exercise
hyperpalatable foods
immersion
incubation
insight
leisure physical activities
microbiota
morbidity
mortality
nutrient-dense foods
obesity
obesogenic diet
physical fitness
prebiotic
probiotic
psychobiotic diet
relaxation response
rest
sleep
sleep hygiene
stress eating
stress modulation effect

When you hear the term *physical wellness*, what comes to mind? Do you think about exercise or a healthy diet? Recall the definition of wellness from chapter 1: It embodies the decisions you make each day and how those can help or hurt your health. For example, although diabetes cannot be cured, a person with this condition can still achieve optimal wellness by making good decisions that help manage their blood sugar. Most people view physical wellness solely in terms of diet and exercise, but it also includes components of sleep, rest, and safety.

This chapter will discuss ways you can achieve optimal wellness, which is highly linked with lowered stress. For example, think about the last time you engaged in physical activity. How did you feel during the activity? How did you feel after? Stress was probably the last thing on your mind because physical activity is a great way to clear your mind and reduce stress. This chapter will highlight the relationships between stress and physical activity, nutrition, sleep, and decision making. Finally, you will learn some physical activities and relaxation techniques that can help you cope with stress.

## Physical Activity

Physical activity is defined as any movement that results in energy expenditure. **Leisure physical activities** are those not associated with essential activities of daily living and include sports, fitness classes, and walking or running. Leisure physical activities also include all forms of **exercise**, defined as a planned and structured activity with the goal of improving or maintaining physical fitness (such as yoga or weightlifting). Children tend to naturally engage in physical activity, but as we age, it often becomes necessary to make time to exercise.

**Physical fitness** is a set of health- and skill-related attributes that enable you to be active. The health-related components include cardiorespiratory endurance, muscular endurance and power, strength, and flexibility. The skill-related components include reaction time, balance, agility, and speed. Good physical fitness allows you to do the things you need to do every day without strain and has shown to decrease **morbidity** (i.e., chronic health conditions) and **mortality** (i.e., death).

**Physical fitness is the ability to perform tasks of daily living such as walking up stairs, carrying in groceries, and lifting heavy items.**

Physical activity has also been associated with the following health benefits (U.S. Department of Health and Human Services, 2018):

- Reduction in all causes of death
- Reduced risk for coronary heart disease, stroke, cancer, diabetes, and obesity
- Reduced risk for hypertension and high cholesterol

- Ability to engage in activities needed for daily living
- Improved brain health and cognition
- Reduction in falls and injuries

Being physically fit allows you "to carry out daily tasks with vigor and alertness, without undue fatigue, and with ample energy to enjoy leisure-time pursuits and respond to emergencies" (U.S. Department of Health and Human Services, 2018). The following classifications can help you determine your current fitness level and identify what is needed to move to the next level, if necessary:

- Inactive: No moderate- or vigorous-intensity physical activity
- Insufficiently active: Some moderate-intensity activity but less than 150 minutes of moderate-intensity or 75 minutes of vigorous-intensity activity per week
- Active: Between 150 and 300 minutes of moderate-intensity activity per week; this level meets the key guidelines for adults
- Highly active: More than 300 minutes of moderate-intensity activity per week; this level exceeds the key guidelines for adults

The health benefits of exercise increase with each level. Additionally, any length of physical activity, whether taking the stairs or parking farther away from an entrance, has health benefits (U.S. Department of Health and Human Services, 2018).

## Impact of Stress on Physical Activity

Think about a stressful time in the semester, perhaps when a large research paper is due or during final exams. During these times of heightened stress, do you think about going for a run or taking a class at the gym? Probably not. Stress has been shown to have a negative impact on physical activity (Stults-Kolehmainen & Sinha, 2014), with people under higher levels of stress more likely to be physically inactive than those experiencing lower levels of stress (Yoon, Park, & Park, 2019). Higher levels of stress have been associated with lower levels of all health-promoting behaviors (Tucker, Weymillerr, Cutshall, Rhudy, & Lohse, 2012) and can even predict negative health behaviors such as physical inactivity, poor nutrition, and drug and alcohol use (Dar et al., 2019; Schultchen et al., 2019; Weidner, Boughal, Connor, Pieper, & Mendell, 1997).

High-stress populations have been studied to examine the impact that stress has on physical activity behaviors. For example, military spouses experience higher levels of stress during their spouse's deployment, with stress level increasing and physical activity decreasing with the length of deployment (Padden, Connors, & Agazio, 2011). First-time mothers also tend to experience high stress during the first year, leading to lower levels of physical activity and higher levels of body mass index (Vernon, Young-Hyman, & Looney, 2010). Caring for a spouse with a chronic disease has been shown to be similarly stressful (Liu, Heffernan, & Tan, 2020), with higher levels of stress and lower levels of physical activity reported as the spouse begins to take on the role of caregiver (Connell, 1994; Doyle et al., 2021). Finally, certain subpopulations of college students—for example, first-generation students (House, Neal, & Kolb, 2019), those from historically marginalized backgrounds (Martinez, Lewis, & Marquez, 2019), and students from lower-income families (Moore et al., 2021)—tend to experience higher levels of stress. Among these groups, those who identify with having higher stress have also shown to have lower levels of physical activity (Bennett et al., 2006).

People who deal with high levels of stress tend to have lower levels of overall physical health and functioning (Cheng, Kawachi, Coakley, Schwartz, & Colditz, 2000). With low levels of physical health, performing the necessary functions of daily living becomes difficult and the desire and ability to engage in physical activity also declines. Of course, not engaging in any activity or exercise reduces the body's ability to function, and it increasingly becomes more difficult to perform daily functions. The relationship becomes cyclical, with increased levels of stress promoting a more sedentary lifestyle (figure 4.1).

As you read this section, did you envision the times when you felt stressed and didn't want to do anything? Even though it can be difficult to put the stress aside and engage in physical activity, going to the fitness center may be the best thing you do. The next section will focus on the positive impact physical activity has on stress.

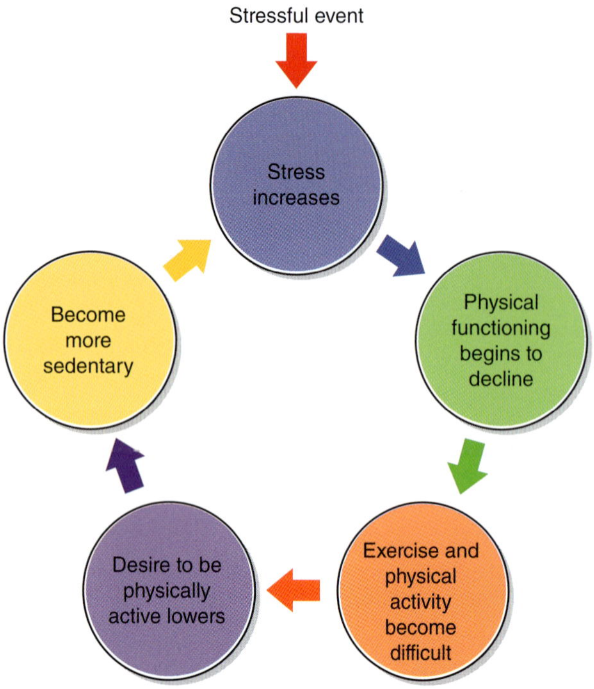


**Figure 4.1** Stress can negatively impact physical activity.

## Impact of Physical Activity on Stress

Physical activity offers many benefits that have been shown to improve health, including a **stress modulation effect**, or the ability to control and manage stress levels.

The transition from high school to college is difficult for many. Some feel that students in this phase are still in the late stages of adolescence rather than adulthood as they navigate their own perspectives and work toward independence (Sawyer, Azzopardi, Wickremarathne, & Patton, 2018). Reasons for increased stress levels during this time include lack of sleep, lack of time, and increased academic and family pressures. College students report more stress related to academic performance, learning efficacy, and pressure to succeed, especially in the first years of college (Beiter et al., 2015; Liu, Ping, & Gao, 2019). Financial stress tends to be high: As many as 75 percent of college students experience moderate to high financial distress while in college (American College Health Association, 2020). Reasons cited include the increasing cost of college, the cost of living, student loan uncertainty, and the inability to work as many hours as desired during the semester (Moore et al., 2021).

**College is a time associated with high levels of stress.**

Engaging in any form of physical activity during your college years can reduce feelings of stress. College students who engage in physical activity have responded that they experience lower levels of stress, feel more confident at handling stress, and forget their stressors during the physical activity (Sharp & Barney, 2016). Furthermore, those students who engaged in physical activity reported that engaging in physical activity provided opportunities to release stress in a healthy manner. Those students also admitted that they would feel more irritable if they were not engaged in physical activity. Not only did physical activity reduce their stress levels, but it also helped improve their overall mood.

Too much stress can cause academic performance to decline by making it difficult to focus on studying and performing at a peak level. Because engaging in physical activity lowers stress, it can also increase your academic success. One study showed that students who were physically active had lower levels of cortisol (stress hormone) and increased levels of serotonin (hormone related to happiness and well-being), increasing their likelihood of academic success and greater cognitive functioning compared to those students who were less physically active (Ahghadir, Gabr, & Iqbal, 2020).

Any type of physical activity can modulate stress. People who engage in leisure physical activities experience lower rates of perceived stress compared to people who do not (Herbert, Meixner, Wiebking, & Gilg, 2020). Unfortunately, stress can reduce the desire to exercise (Stults-Kolehmainen & Sinha, 2014). When people say they do not have time to engage in leisure physical activity, they may mean they do not have the motivation—a symptom of stress. However, the research is clear that exercise may be exactly what they need.

Here are some ideas on how to fit leisure physical activity into your routine:

- *Use the fitness center.* Many colleges have fitness centers on their campuses. These are often free, included in student fees, or

Case Study

## Stressed and Sick

Alex is a college junior under a lot of stress. He has two midterm papers due and two midterm exams the same week, and he has been burning the candle at both ends. Just as Alex is ready to have this week over with, he begins to feel a cold coming on. Alex thinks that he can't get sick now—this is the worst timing!

Is it a coincidence that Alex is getting sick during a stressful time? Recall from chapter 3 that high levels of stress can make you more susceptible to getting sick. Furthermore, those with higher levels of stress may experience longer and more severe levels of illness (Fleshner, 2005).

However, engaging in physical activity can lower stress and reduce the likelihood of getting sick. A study conducted on adolescent girls found that those who reported high levels of exercise and high levels of stress had lower levels of disease incidence compared to those who had lower levels of exercise and high levels of stress (Brown & Siegal, 1988). More recently, a study conducted on cancer patients found that including exercise in treatment protocols resulted in lower stress and illness (Sung et al., 2019). These findings suggest that physical activity helps modulate stress and its impact on the immune system.

### Discussion Questions

1. How can getting sick during a stressful event make it worse? Has this happened to you?
2. What are some physical activities you enjoy? How could you incorporate those activities into your weekly routine?
3. What would you tell someone who tells you they don't have time for physical activity because they have too much work to do?

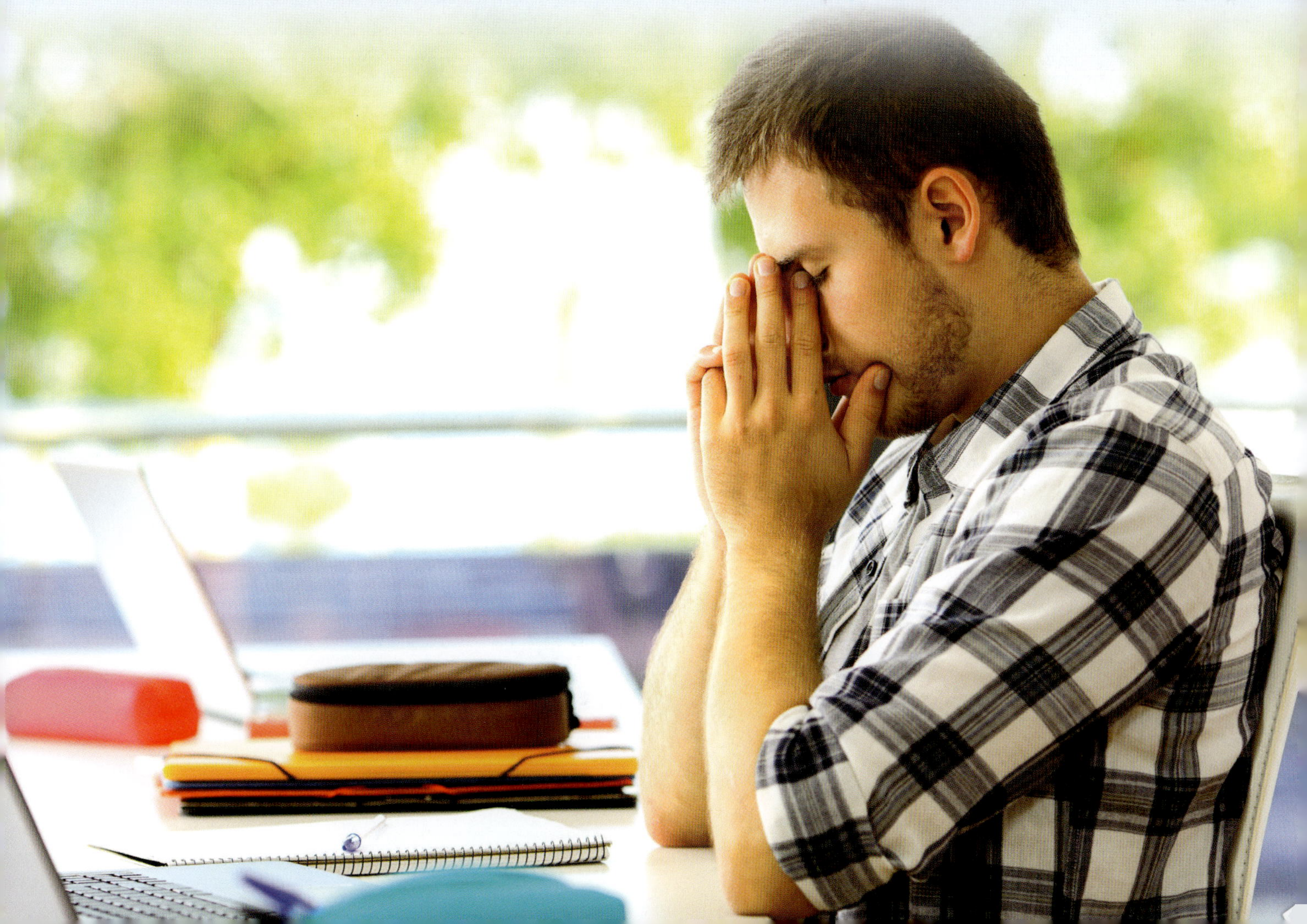

offered at a low cost. Use the fitness center right before or after class while you are on campus.

- *Partner with a friend.* Ask a friend to join you. When you schedule an activity with a friend, it is harder to blow it off. You can take a class, pick up a sport during open gym, or just meet at the fitness center to work out.
- *Take a class.* Find a class you are interested in taking at your school's fitness center or through your park district or local community center. Many offer low-cost classes that can be easy to fit in your schedule.
- *Find an app.* There are many apps (some free) that can help guide you through an exercise routine. There are also apps to help you with motivation.
- *Set time in your schedule.* Give yourself 15 to 30 minutes to engage in leisure physical activity. When you plan for something and write it down, you are more likely to do it.
- *Do something you enjoy.* Treat the activity as a true leisure and get excited about doing it.

When you were in grade school, physical education was likely a requirement. Additionally, many colleges require students to engage in a physical activity class as a requirement for graduation. Some companies also offer incentives to their employees who engage in exercise. Even if a physical activity routine is required or otherwise obligatory, the positive impact of that activity is still seen as a modulating effect on stress (Greenwood et al., 2013).

However, there are times when excessive exercise can be hurtful. Exercise addiction, or compulsive exercise, is defined as engaging in physical exercise in a rigid manner, refusing to stop or reduce the physical exercise despite the negative effects, and experiencing distress when the physical exercise has stopped. Men tend to be more at risk, as are bodybuilders, runners, and triathletes. It has also been associated with those who have an eating disorder (e.g., anorexia) and those with body dysmorphia or body dissatisfaction (Colledge & Meyer, 2022). Exercise addiction has been associated with an increased risk of suicide among individuals with disordered eating (Smith et al., 2013). Many with this ailment have developed a tolerance to exercise that allows them to work through the pain, ignoring the body's signals that something is wrong (Berczik et al., 2012). This places them at higher risk for overuse injuries.

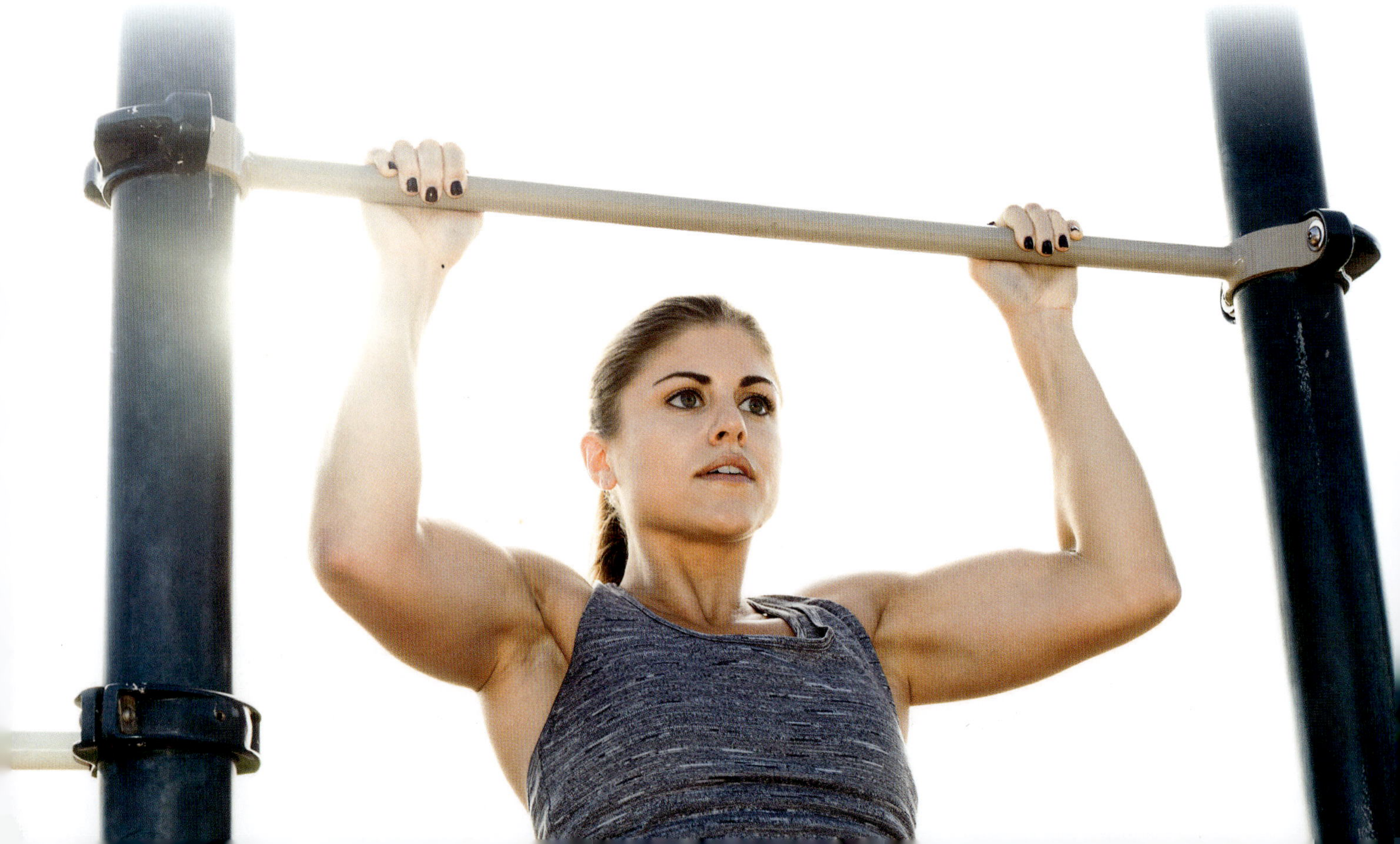

Research Spotlight

## Endorphins

Have you ever heard of the term *runner's high*? It is a feeling of euphoria that follows a lengthy and strenuous exercise routine as a result of **endorphins**. These chemicals are made in the hypothalamus and pituitary glands to help relieve stress and pain.

Endorphins come from the words *endogenous*, which means "within the body," and *morphine*, which is an opiate pain reliever. Endorphins act on the opioid receptors on the brain to reduce pain and boost feelings of pleasure. As you may have expected, endorphins are part of the brain's reward circuit. If the reward circuit is activated, it brings you pleasure, thus making you want to repeat the behavior. Endorphins have also been found to reduce feelings of stress and may explain why exercise is such a great stress modulator (Amir, Brown, & Amit, 1980; Pilozzi, Carro, & Huang, 2020).

Exercise isn't the only way to increase endorphins in the body. Other ways include the following:

- *Giving.* Donating and volunteering have been shown to activate endorphins in the brain (Mani & Mishra, 2021).
- *Yoga and meditation.* Some of the stress-relieving effects of yoga and meditation may be caused by the release of endorphins during the practice (Permana, Lindayani, Hendra, & Juniarni, 2020; Romero-Ramos, Gonzalez Suarez, & Ramos, 2022).
- *Spicy foods.* Recent research suggests eating spicy foods may prompt an increase in endorphins (Bosland, 2016).
- *Dark chocolate.* Eating dark chocolate can lead to an increase in endorphins (Magrone, Russo, & Jirillo, 2017).
- *Laughing.* Laughing increases endorphins and has a general positive impact on the body (Zhao et al., 2019).

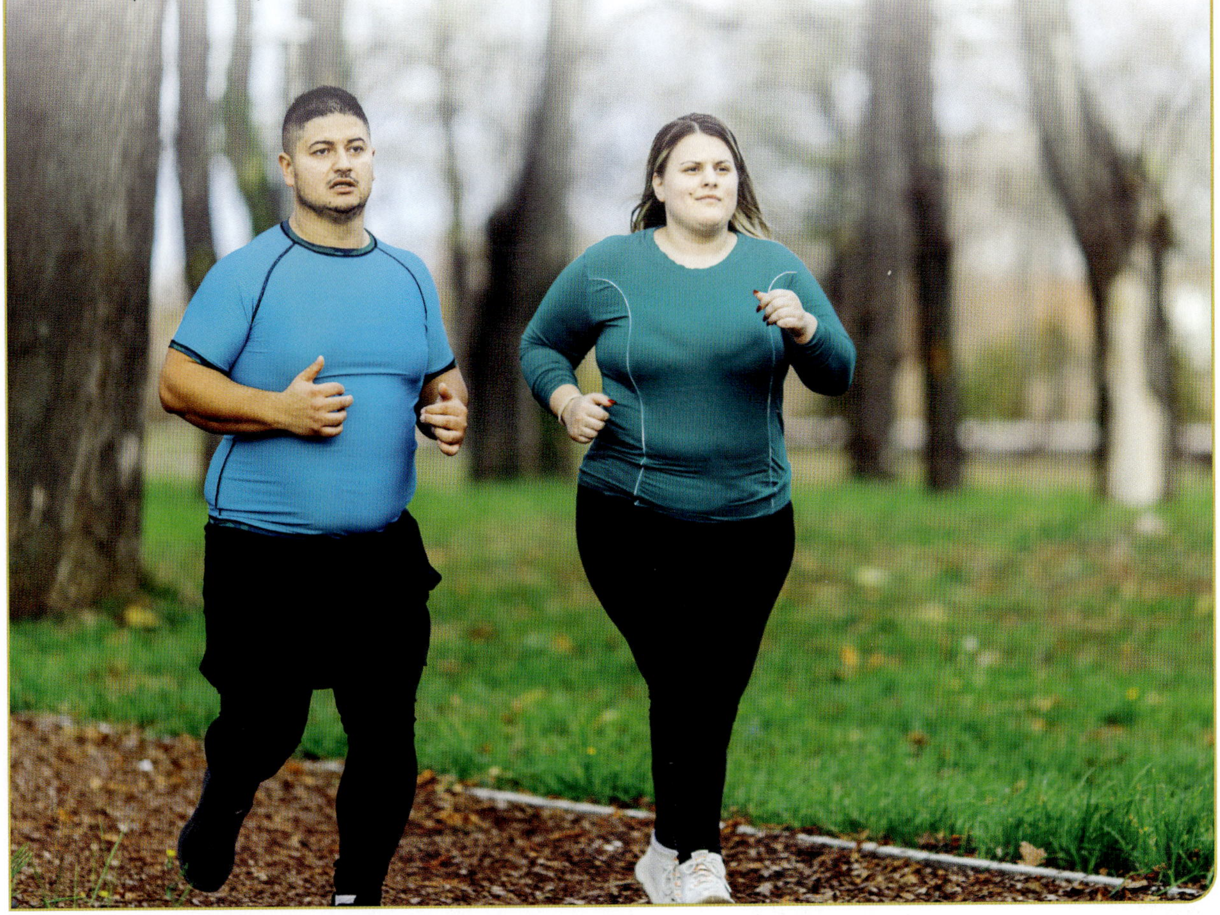

## Healthy Eating

**Dietary patterns** reflect a person's general eating habits and how those habits influence health. Each person's dietary pattern is different; however, there are some agreed-on guidelines for a healthy diet (U.S. Department of Agriculture and U.S. Department of Health and Human Services, December 2020). Although a healthy diet should be started early in life, it is never too late to start to receive the health benefits. Experts agree that a healthy diet should focus on **nutrient-dense foods**, or foods that provide vitamins, minerals, and other health-promoting components while remaining low in sugar and fat.

Unhealthy eating patterns such as the overconsumption of fat-dense foods, sugary beverages, and prepared meals have been linked to obesity, type 2 diabetes, and cardiovascular disease. These conditions are chronic, require lifelong management, and can lead to death. Healthy People 2030, a framework developed by the Office of Disease Prevention and Health Promotion to identify public health priorities and improve the health of people living in the United States, aims to reduce the proportion of children, adolescents, and adults with obesity (Office of Disease Prevention and Health Promotion, 2020). Currently, about two in five U.S. adults and one in five U.S. children have obesity, and more are overweight (Hales, Carroll, Fryar, & Ogden, 2017). In the United States, type 2 diabetes is the seventh leading cause of morbidity and mortality (Gonzalez-Zacarias, Mavarez-Martinez, Arias-Morales, Stoicea, & Rogers, 2016), and the prevalence of diet-related chronic diseases has risen since the COVID-19 pandemic (Ajabshir et al., 2021). As such, the need for an improved dietary pattern among Americans is great.

The U.S. Department of Agriculture and the U.S. Department of Health and Human Services have released the 2020-2025 Dietary Guidelines for Americans to help you make healthy choices. In this most recent edition, they recognize the importance of healthy dietary patterns over a lifetime, not just a focus on macro- and micronutrients.

The United States Department of Agriculture developed MyPlate to present healthy eating habits to Americans (figure 4.2). The MyPlate is a visual image of the food categories that should be consumed by meal on a daily basis. The plate is divided into four sections with a small outside section for dairy. The dietary recommendations include the following:

**A healthy diet should contain a variety of foods and vary day to day.**

- Make half the plate fruits and vegetables
- Use whole grains
- Vary the vegetables
- Vary the protein
- Move to low-fat or fat-free dairy
- Limit fat, sodium, and sugars

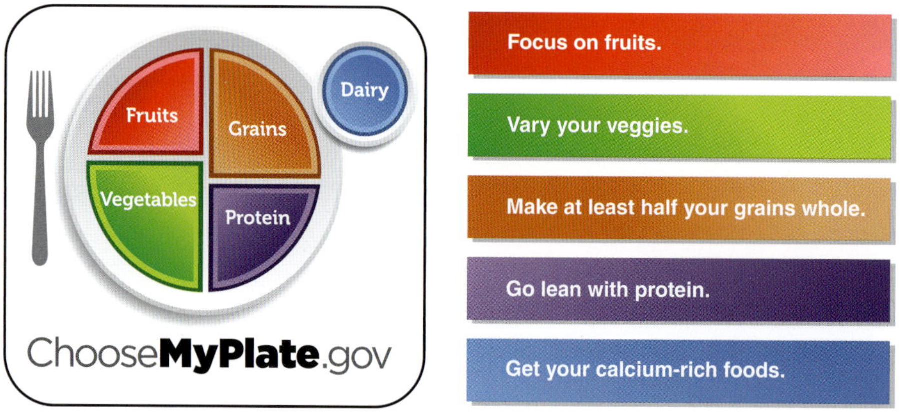


**Figure 4.2** Consider your typical dinner plate. How does it compare to MyPlate?
From U.S. Department of Agriculture. Available: www.choosemyplate.gov.

## Impact of Stress on Eating Patterns

Do you ever find yourself eating more when you are stressed? There are several ways stress impacts eating patterns. First, stress reduces cognitive processing, specifically executive processing and self-regulation. Second, increased cortisol can lead to an increased appetite. Stress can also increase addictive behaviors, including increased eating. Finally, the stigma associated with weight gain can lead to an increase in stress, which results in an increase in **stress eating** behavior.

> The doctor of the future will no longer treat the human frame with drugs, but rather will cure and prevent disease with nutrition.
>
> **Thomas A. Edison**

Exposure to chronic levels of stress can reduce the functioning of the prefrontal cortex, an area of the brain that helps with self-regulation and controlling impulsive behavior (Arnsten, 2009). In a study on rats, those that were exposed to high levels of stress were shown to have changes in their brain anatomy, physiology, and biochemistry in areas related to self-regulation (Murray & Hamoudi, 2016). In humans, there have been numerous studies that suggest chronic stress in childhood can reduce the ability for children to form and develop self-regulatory behaviors (Murray & Hamoudi, 2016). As the ability to self-regulate diminishes, unhealthy behaviors tend to increase, including unhealthy eating. The impact of stress on self-regulation cannot be understated: If you do not have the ability to self-regulate, you will have a difficult time improving dietary habits.

Although some people have a reduced appetite when stressed, this tends to be a symptom of short-term stress. When you experience persistent or chronic stress, cortisol levels remain elevated, leading to increased appetite and a likely increase in food intake (Chao, Jastreboff, White, Grilo, & Sinha, 2017). These combined factors can lead to an increased risk of **obesity**, a complex, treatment-resistant disease involving having excess body fat. Obesity has been related to intake of **hyperpalatable foods**, which are foods that are high in sugar and fat, have low nutrition value, and may also have addictive properties (Gearhardt, Grilo, DiLeone, Brownell, & Potenza, 2011).

Chronic stress may change the structure and functioning of a person's brain to make them more prone to addiction by increasing the sensitivity of the reward pathway in the brain (Volkow, Wang, Fowler, Tomasi, & Baler, 2012). As chronic stress increases, impulse control systems go down and reward pathway sensitivity increases, all of

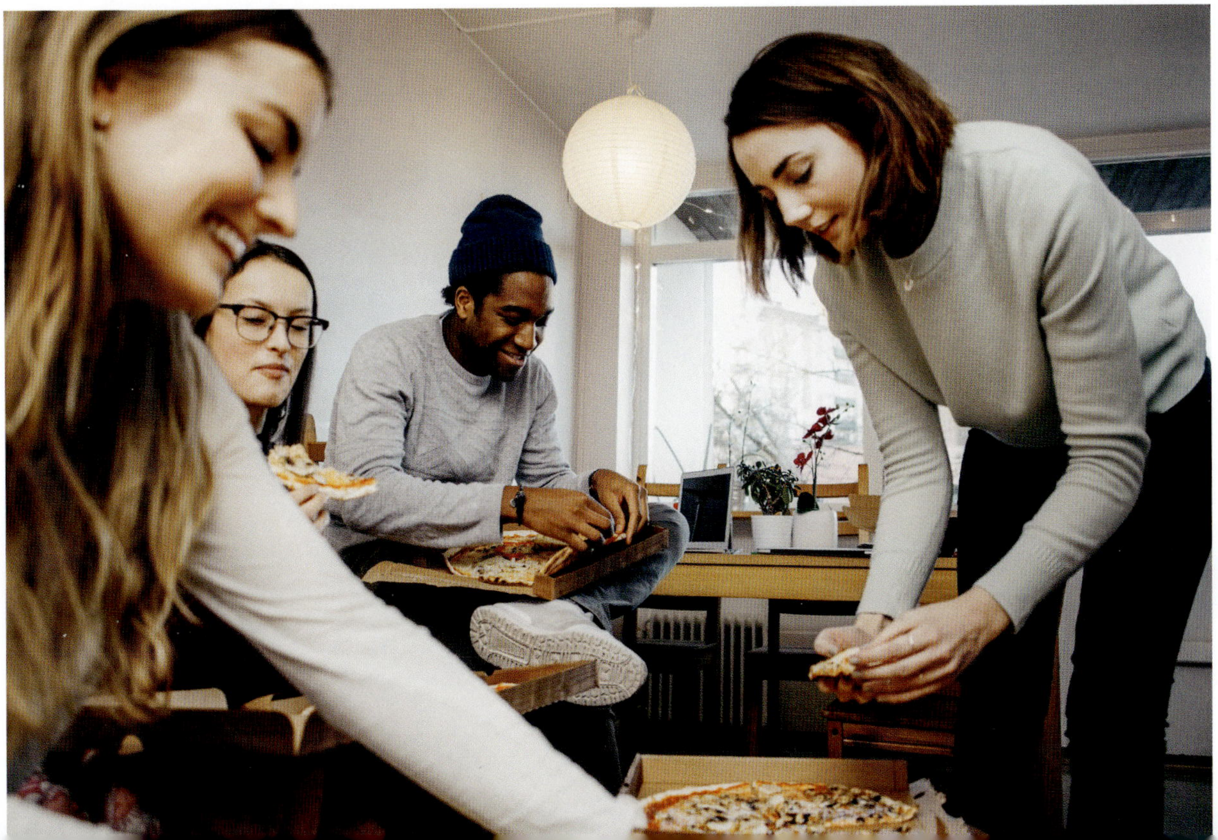

which increase the likelihood of engaging in addictive behaviors, including increased eating as well as alcohol, drugs, tobacco, gambling, or shopping.

With rates of obesity increasing in the United States, it is important to find ways to maintain a healthy diet and avoid stress eating. Keeping a food diary is one such strategy; the following tips can help you get started.

1. *Maintain a food diary*. Tracking food intake has been shown to help people make better decisions to improve their diet (Jimoh et al., 2018). Note your patterns of hunger, behavior, and feelings and emotions as you eat. This can help identify situations that trigger stress eating to help you avoid them in the future.
2. *Analyze your food diary*. It is common for people to eat for reasons other than physical hunger. Sometimes referred to as **emotional hunger**, this eating occurs in response to emotion (e.g., boredom, sadness, anger), not a physical need for food. Emotional hunger first starts in the brain and the body responds, whereas physical hunger begins in the stomach and moves up to the brain. Being able to recognize these patterns is the first step in being able to change them. See table 4.1 for ways to distinguish between physical and emotional hunger.
3. *Plan for success*. Now that you have identified your triggers for stress eating, make a plan to avoid them. For example, if you tend to eat as a result of boredom every night before bed, create a new bedtime routine so that eating does not become the focal point.

## Impact of Eating Patterns on Stress

The type of foods you eat can either reduce or magnify the impact of stress. For example, hyperpalatable foods may provide short-term relief of stress symptoms. In a study on rats, those that had access to hyperpalatable food showed a reduction in stress symptoms compared to those that did not (Pecoraro, Reyes, Gomez, Bhargava, & Dallman, 2004). The key to remember is that hyperpalatable foods are a temporary solution, not a long-term one. Using hyperpalatable foods to manage symptoms related to stress places you at higher risk of chronic illnesses, including obesity—and the stress will continue to return. Ultimately, people who consume **obesogenic diets**, or diets high in saturated fats and sugar, report higher levels of perceived stress compared those who do not. Obesogenic diets may also make you more sensitive to the negative effects of acute stress, which results in an impact on cognitive performance (Delgado, Dexpert, Sauvant, Cryan, & Capuron, 2021).

Diet may also serve as a protective factor against stress. Gut health—the balance and function of bacteria in the gastrointestinal tract—plays an important role in how well the body functions. It includes maintaining healthy **microbiota**, which are bacteria that work together to protect the intestine against harmful pathogens (Kamada, Seo, Chen,

**The desire to eat hyperpalatable foods when under stress is not a weakness or lack of self-control, but rather a behavior that has proven to provide short-term relief.**

**Table 4.1** Physical Versus Emotional Hunger

| Physical hunger | Emotional hunger |
|---|---|
| You recognize eating is necessary for life. | You feel guilty after eating. |
| The hunger occurs out of a biological need. | The hunger occurs out of an emotional need. |
| The hunger comes on slowly. | The hunger comes on quickly. |
| You can wait to eat. | You want to eat now. |
| You have eaten in the last 3 to 4 hours. | You have eaten within the last hour. |
| You are open to different foods. | You desire a specific food. |
| You stop when you feel full. | You have a limited response when you feel full. |

& Nunez, 2013). The gut microbiota have been shown to play a role in modulating the impact of stress and improving overall mood—people who have higher levels of specific microbiota such as *Bifidobacterium* and *Lactobacillus* in the gut exhibit less effects from stress (Cryan et al., 2018). As more research comes to light on the link between the gut and the body, it may be beneficial to follow a dietary pattern that improves gut health. This **psychobiotic diet** includes foods that are high in **probiotics** (healthy gut bacteria) and **prebiotics** (fiber-rich foods that feed the healthy gut bacteria) (Cheng, Liu, Wu, Wang, & Tsai, 2019).

**Consuming probiotics and maintaining gut health can help reduce your stress levels.**

In recent years, several studies have looked at the impact of psychobiotic diets on health, including stress. One study examined a group of healthy volunteers with relatively poor eating habits and found that participants who were placed on a psychobiotic diet rich in prebiotics felt less stress and scored lower on the perceived stress scale compared to those in the control group (Berding et al., 2020). In another study, participants who ate products with a variety of probiotics exhibited better working memory during an acute stressful event compared to those who didn't receive the probiotic (Cryan et al., 2018).

The psychobiotic food pyramid is shown in figure 4.3 to highlight the different levels of food and how much (or little) to eat at each level of this diet (Anderson, Cryan, & Dinan, 2017).

A good way to begin a psychobiotic diet is by reducing the consumption of level 4 foods. Overconsumption of sweets and red meat is common, and many people report feeling physically better within one to two weeks of reducing their intake of these foods (Anderson et al., 2017). Next, begin to add the level 1 and level 2 foods. These are foods that should be consumed more often. Most experts agree it is best to start small and make gradual adjustments to one's diet. This allows you to get used to small changes first and begin to incorporate them into lifestyle habits before moving on to the next change.

If you are not ready for a psychobiotic diet, there are other foods that may improve your health and stress levels. When there is too much or prolonged exposure to cortisol in the body, it can lead to an increase in blood pressure and inflammation. Foods that have anti-inflammatory properties may therefore help reduce cortisol levels; these include the following (Cleveland Clinic, 2021):

- Foods high in vitamin B (whole grains, meat, eggs and dairy, legumes, seeds and nuts, dark leafy vegetables, fruits)
- Foods high in omega-3 fatty acid (avocados, chia seeds, flaxseeds, fish, olive oil, walnuts)
- Magnesium-rich foods (avocados, bananas, broccoli, dark chocolate, pumpkin seeds, spinach)

It has also been shown that following the Mediterranean diet may also help you reduce cortisol and overall stress levels (Shively et al., 2020). One study conducted on university students found lower levels of stress and anxiety among students whose eating habits aligned with the Mediterranean diet (Trigueros et al., 2020). This diet places an emphasis on vegetables, fruits, whole grains, and beans and legumes, as well as low-fat dairy, nuts, and some fish and poultry (American Heart Association, 2020). Foods that should be limited include sugars, sodium, highly processed foods, refined carbohydrates, saturated fats, and processed meats. In additional to lowering cortisol

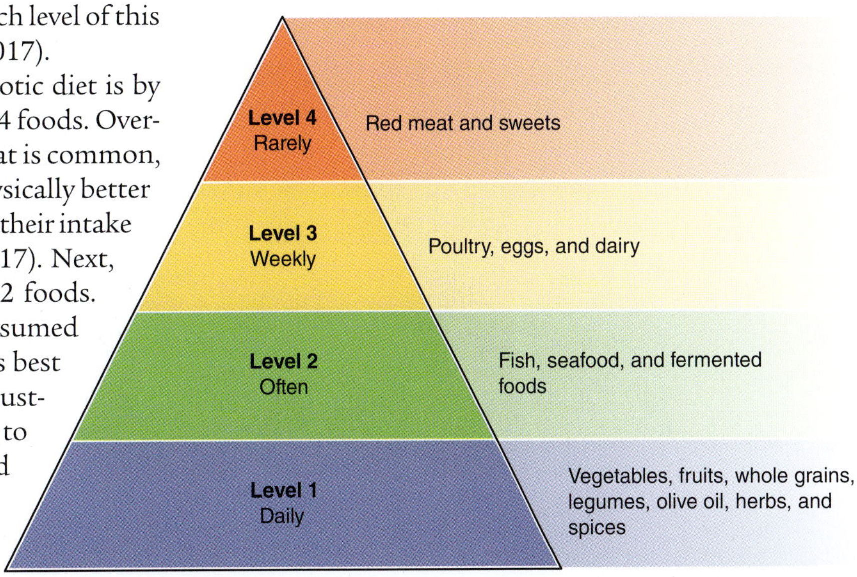


**Figure 4.3** Psychobiotic food pyramid.

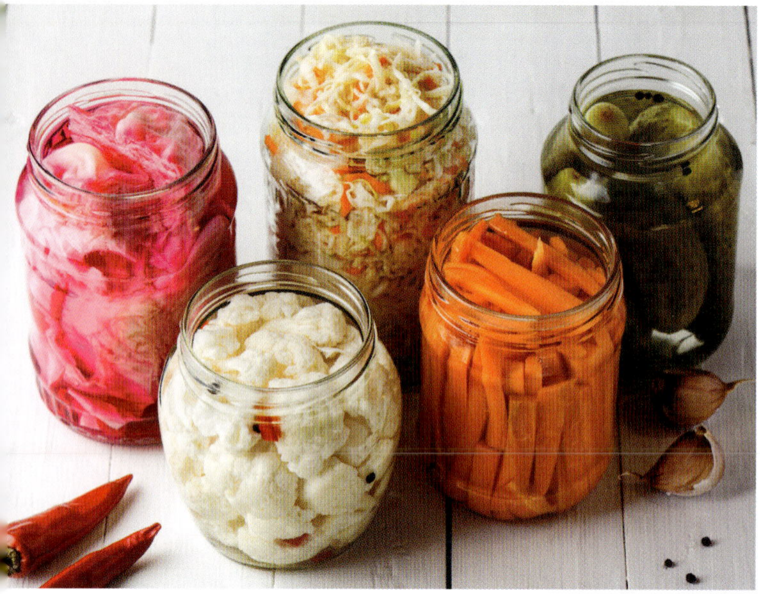

and stress levels, a Mediterranean diet may also reduce the risk of chronic health conditions such as heart disease and dementia.

Next time you feel stressed, try focusing on foods that do not contain high amounts of saturated fats and simple sugars. Try making small changes in your diet at first. If you can reduce the impact stress has on your life, these small dietary changes can make a big difference in your overall health and wellness.

## Rest, Relaxation, and Sleep

Your body is always working. Think about the last couple of days. How much time did you spend resting, relaxing, or sleeping? All of those are necessary to help restore your energy levels. When you allow time for yourself to rest, you feel better and are more energized. Rest, relaxation, and sleep promote optimal wellness just as much as what you eat and how much you move.

### Stress and Sleep

**Sleep** is a basic necessity for physical health and plays an important role in the consolidation of memory. Additionally, during sleep, toxins are removed from the brain and the rest of the body (Shuttleworth & Foster, 2020). Sleep is controlled by the brain and consists of five stages, as shown in figure 4.4 (Hasan, Heyat, Siddiqui, Azad, & Askhtar, 2015).

1. *Drowsy*. This stage is the shortest and lasts 5 to 10 minutes. The body begins to feel sleepy and moves into very light sleep. Some may experience light muscle jerks or muscle contractions during this stage.
2. *Sleep*. The brain waves become slower with bursts called sleep spindles.
3. *Moderate sleep*. Brain waves (delta waves) begin and are interspersed with smaller and faster waves.

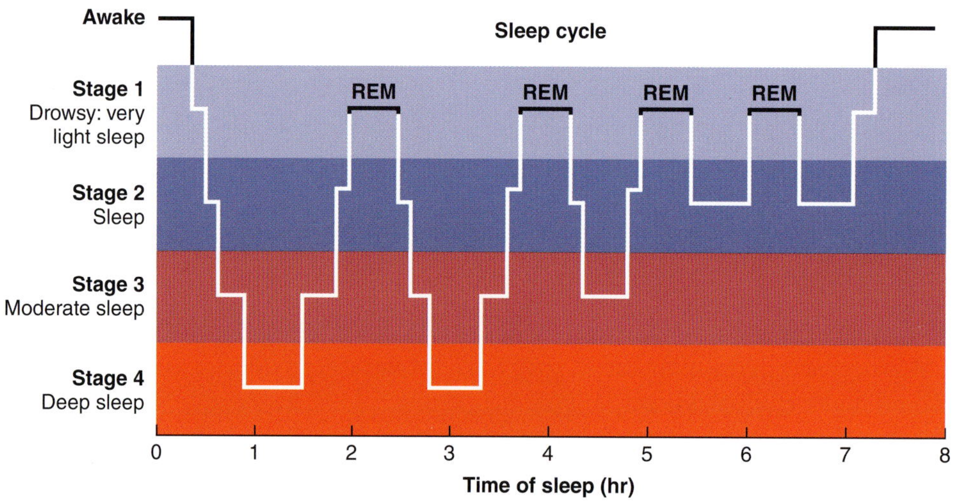


**Figure 4.4** The sleep cycle starts off with a two-hour cycle. As the sleep progresses, the cycles get shorter, with more time spent in the REM sleep stage.

Adapted by permission from Y.L. Meur, R. Duffield, and M. Skein, "Sleep," in *Recovery for Performance in Sport*, edited by The National Institute of Sport for Expertise and Performance, C. Hausswirth, and I. Mujika (Champaign, IL: Human Kinetics, 2013), 101.

4. *Deep sleep*. The brain only produces delta waves. People awakened during this stage will feel groggy and disoriented.
5. *REM sleep*. Breathing becomes more rapid and irregular. The eyes begin to jerk rapidly in various directions, and limp muscles become temporarily paralyzed. A complete sleep cycle lasts between 90 and 110 minutes. With each successive cycle, the REM stage increases in length.

Although there is some variation in how many hours each person requires to feel fully rested, research suggests that teens aged 13 to 18 should be getting around 8 to 10 hours of sleep per night and adults aged 18 to 60 should aim for at least 7 hours per night (Hirshkowitz et al., 2015). Unfortunately, many people report not getting enough sleep (Otte, Lalevich, Hollingsworth, Chernyak, & Manchanda, 2017), with about one-third of U.S. adults not getting the recommended amount of sleep each night (National Center for Chronic Disease Prevention and Health Promotion, 2020). Lack of adequate sleep can lead to an increase in stress and anxiety, along with other health ailments (Shuttleworth & Foster, 2020). During the wake cycle, cortisol levels rise; this rise is called the **cortisol awakening response** (CAR) and is affected by the amount of sleep you get each night. The less sleep you get, the more erratic your CAR numbers become (Vargas & Lopez-Duran, 2014). Erratic CAR levels have been associated with negative health outcomes such as the following:

- Type 2 diabetes
- Obesity
- Depression
- Increased levels of stress
- Impaired driving
- Poor school and work performance
- Increased risk of accidents

Stress can impact the quantity and quality of your sleep (Hu, Visser, & Kaiser, 2019), with stress during the day shown to accurately predict sleep quality at night (Akerstedt, Orsini, Petersen, Axelsson, & Lekander, 2012). This relationship is bidirectional: Lack of sleep is also associated with increased levels of stress (Chang et al., 2020). If you are tired, you will have lower mental stamina and ability to manage stress during the day, making it more difficult to fall and stay asleep at night, leading to poor sleep outcomes and a continued cycle of stress (Benham, 2010). This combination of high stress levels and sleep disturbances has been shown to have negative health outcomes, such as decreased cognitive performance, increased risk of infectious disease, and decreased mental health. One study conducted on female college students found that high levels of stress coupled with poor sleep were significant predictors of depressive symptoms (Lee, Wuertz, Rogers, & Chen, 2013).

Often, people simply don't prioritize sleep. To support adequate sleep each night, it is important to practice good **sleep hygiene**, or healthy practices that promote sleep. This includes acknowledging the importance of sleep, creating a schedule that allows adequate time for sleep, and establishing and maintaining a nightly sleep routine to make it easier to fall asleep and wake up at the appropriate times. The room where sleep occurs should be relaxing and conducive to sleep. It should be slightly chilly, quiet (or white noise only), and free of distractions. Other considerations include staying away from stimulants such as caffeine and nicotine before going to bed, which can work against the body's efforts in falling asleep. Using a smartphone or tablet or watching television in bed should also be avoided—these activities tend to stimulate the mind and may make it more difficult to fall asleep (Perrault et al., 2019).

**Prioritizing sleep requires a change in mindset to place sleep in a position of importance when managing your day.**

## Stress and Rest

How do you think about rest? Do you consider it a necessity to break away from the daily hassle and just allow yourself to be still? Or do you view it as a waste of time that can better be used doing something more meaningful? Many people have a difficult time justifying periods of rest during the day. However, rest is needed to perform your best: Without it, you will burn out and lose the ability to perform at optimal levels (figure 4.5).

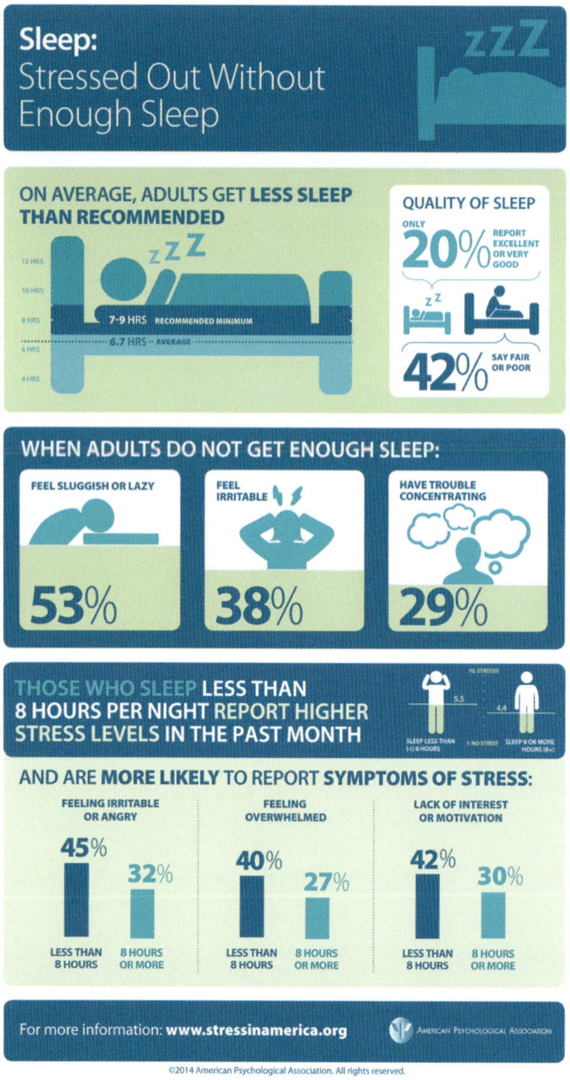


**Figure 4.5** Impact of not getting enough sleep.

From American Psychological Association. Available: www.apa.org/Images/2013-sia-Sleep-Infographic-1024_tcm7-166594.jpg.

**Rest** is defined as the cessation of activity necessary to maintain health and recover from illness and stress (Asp, 2015). Rest promotes a pathway to mental health, calm, and stillness (Helvig, Wade, & Hunter-Eades, 2016). Rest can also be active or passive: Active rest includes activities requiring focus, such as mindfulness, whereas passive rest is inactive and provides a short-term break or relief from an activity, such as napping.

What exactly is rest, however, can be difficult to measure. What may be considered restful for one person may not be for another person. For example, if you enjoy reading, then taking a 30-minute break to read a novel may be restful, but someone who does not enjoy reading would not find this restful. What exactly needs to be in place to be considered rest? One researcher conducted an exploratory study about rest and determined four attributes that must be in place for an activity to be considered rest (Allison, 1970):

1. The activity must provide freedom from mental stress.
2. The activity must be enjoyable to the person.
3. The person should derive pleasure from performing the activity.
4. The person should experience a sense of restoration from engaging in the activity.

Optimal performance is often the goal, whether the task is physical (e.g., a race) or mental (e.g., a big project at work). Regardless of the task, being able to perform at high levels can be achieved through a simple formula: Stress + rest = peak performance (figure 4.6). This formula posits that

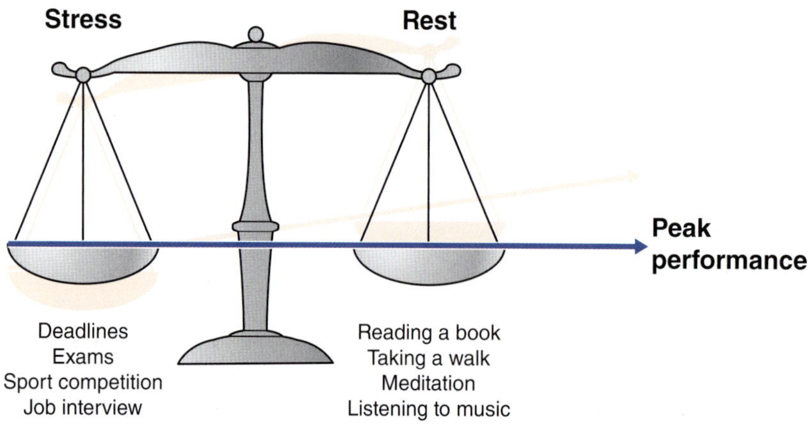


**Figure 4.6** The equation to promote peak performance includes finding a balance between stress and rest.

at low doses, stress can improve performance (as described in chapter 2). However, this period of induced stress must be followed up by rest—an element just as important as work (Magness & Stulberg, 2017). Too much work for too long without rest will lead to burnout and fatigue.

In today's fast-paced society, the notion of rest is often considered synonymous with *lazy*. This negative connotation is a common barrier for many to scheduling the rest they need for best performance, health, and growth. In actuality, however, people who are high performers tend to follow a three-step path that includes this necessary component: immersion, incubation, and insight (Magness & Stulberg, 2017). **Immersion** is a period of full engagement in the activity, wherein it is the sole focus of one's energy, time, and effort. This is followed by **incubation**, or time away from the activity used for rest and stillness. Lastly, the **insight** period is a time for reflection on the activity, allowing for emergence of new ideas and growth (Magness & Stulberg, 2017).

## Stress and the Relaxation Response

Another way to counteract stress is through the **relaxation response**, a state first described by Dr. Herbert Benson, a Harvard Medical School cardiologist studying the impact of meditation on the body. By allowing the mind to focus through a repetitive mental activity, the body is able to improve its functioning by decreasing heart rate, blood pressure, breathing, and metabolic rate, promoting natural healing and providing an opportunity for the body to rejuvenate (Benson & Klipper, 2009).

The relaxation response is achieved through a mindset that allows one's thoughts to be quiet. There are four elements that can help activate the relaxation response (Benson & Klipper, 2009):

1. *A quiet environment*. Choose a quiet environment without any distractions.
2. *A mental device*. Use a stimulus to help break away from thought. This stimulus can be repeating a single word or phrase, listening to a repetitive sound, or gazing at an object. Pay attention to the rhythm of your breathing.
3. *A passive attitude*. The most important part of the equation is developing a passive attitude. Ignore or disregard distracting thoughts by focusing on the mental device from step 2.
4. *A comfortable position*. Choose a comfortable position, such as sitting in a chair or the cross-legged lotus pose. It is not recommended to lie down because there is a tendency to fall asleep (which, while important, does not contribute to the relaxation response).

The benefits of the relaxation response have been documented in many areas. One of the main

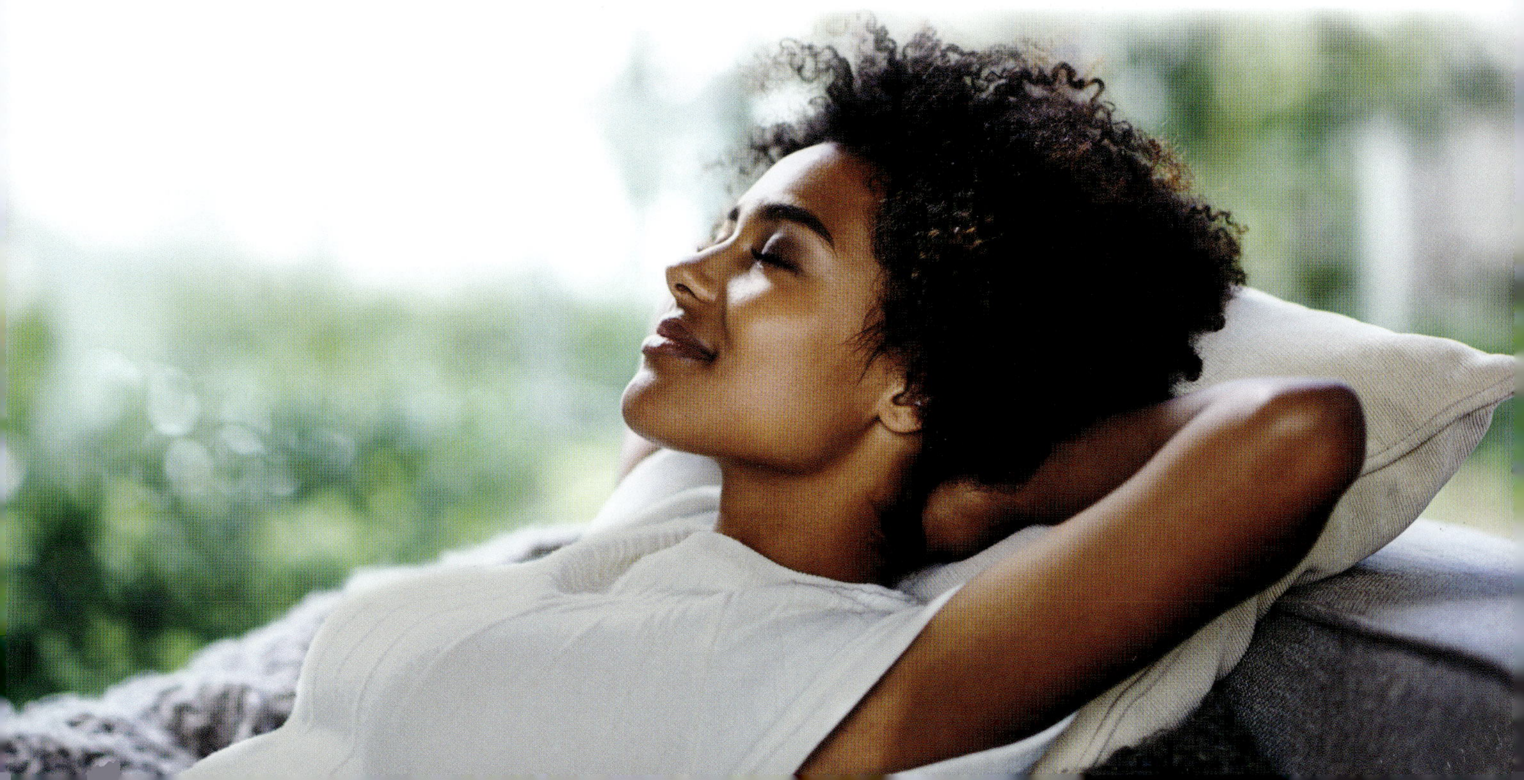

benefits has been to reduce stress on the body, but the relaxation response has also shown other health benefits. Results from one study found that patients who practiced the relaxation response twice daily for seven days prior to cardiac surgery experienced less tension and anxiety, felt reduced pain, and had fewer postsurgical complications (Irkham, 2022; Leserman, Stuart, Mamish, & Benson, 1989). The relaxation response may also help reduce anxiety and depression, both mental disorders that have been connected with stress. In a study on elderly patients, researchers found the relaxation technique helped reduce anxiety, depression, and sleep disturbances (Elsayed, Radwan, Elashri, & El-Gilany, 2019).

If the benefits from the relaxation response are so great, why don't more people do it? The number one reason given is not enough time. However, this practice doesn't require a huge time commitment; it requires only 10 to 20 minutes once or twice per day (Benson & Klipper, 2009). Like everything else in life, it becomes easier with practice.

**Being able to make time for relaxation is as important as making time to complete your homework. Make it part of your daily routine so it becomes a habit, much like brushing your teeth.**

## Stress Reduction Techniques: Massage, Acupuncture, and Acupressure

For many, the thought of getting a massage is indulgent. However, massages are beneficial to your health and have been shown to reduce levels of stress. During and after a massage, the body lowers its levels of cortisol and increases the activity of the parasympathetic nervous system (Fazeli et al., 2020). Both of those mechanisms help calm the body and reduce feelings of stress. Massage is also beneficial in reducing general muscle tension and lower back pain, both of which are linked to stress (Ben-Ami & Korn, 2020; Chou et al., 2017; Simao, Horing, Lima, Silva, & Alfieri, 2021). There are different types of massage, but studies suggest those that utilize moderate pressure have more positive benefits compared to light-pressure massage (Field, 2014).

Comparable to massage is acupressure, a treatment method used in Chinese medicine. Acupressure is based on the meridian theory, which says that energy (Qi) flows through invisible circuits in the body, and when there are disturbances in these circuits, mental and physical health are impacted (Honda, Tsuda, & Horiuchi, 2012). Acupressure uses pressure administered at certain points on the body to correct these imbalances, which can be performed by a professional or self-administered. Self-administered acupressure does provide a reduction in stress when performed consistently (Honda et al., 2012).

A cousin to acupressure is acupuncture. Acupuncture is based on the same principles as acupressure, but rather than using pressure points, tiny needles are inserted just under the skin to improve the flow of Qi (Sun et al., 2019). Acupressure works by inhibiting the sympathetic nervous system (Middlekauff et al., 2002). It is believed these needles stimulate the brain to release endorphins, which make a person feel euphoric. After the needles have been placed, a person is asked to rest for about 30 minutes to allow the treatment to take effect. This period of rest can provide a time of calm and promote relaxation.

One study divided participants into two groups: One group received a fake acupuncture treatment, and the other group received the real acupuncture treatment. After receiving treatments once a week for 12 weeks, both groups reported lower stress levels; however, the group that received the real treatment reported significantly lower stress levels, and the effects lasted longer compared to the other group (Schroeder et al., 2017).

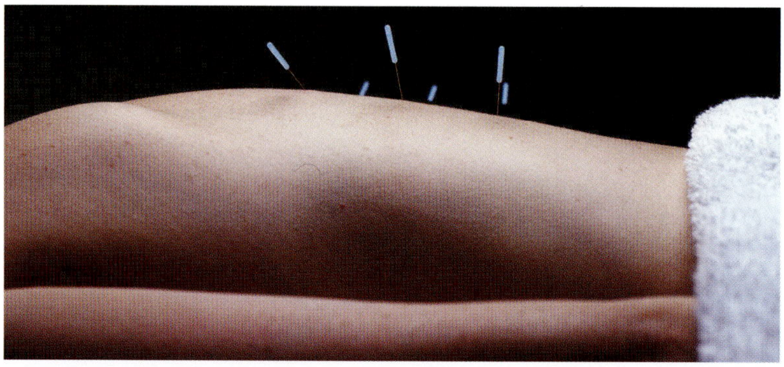

## Summary

This chapter analyzed the relationship between stress and physical health. People who engage in physical activity tend to have lower levels of stress and better overall health. Physical activity can help modulate stress levels and help people better cope with the stresses of daily life. The relationship between stress and food is a complex one. Although stress eating or eating hyperpalatable foods can reduce the short-term physical effects of stress, the long-term impacts of unhealthy eating on stress will be negative. Lastly, this chapter differentiated between rest, relaxation, and sleep, and identified the necessity of each in reducing stress and performing at optimal levels.

### ONLINE RESOURCES

Visit HK*Propel* to access audio supplements, worksheets, and vocabulary flash cards for this chapter.

### DISCUSSION QUESTIONS

1. Predict what would happen if all college students were required to participate in a physical activity class each semester. In your answer, include the benefits and challenges this would present.
2. What causes a runner's high? Describe the feelings associated with it and identify other activities that can encourage the same result.
3. What contributes to stress eating? What are ways to reduce the urge to stress eat?
4. What is the difference between rest and relaxation? Why are each important in relation to stress reduction? Why are both necessary to include in a daily schedule?
5. Discuss what is meant by the term *sleep hygiene*. Describe your own sleep hygiene. Design an ideal sleep hygiene environment and schedule.

5

# Emotional Wellness

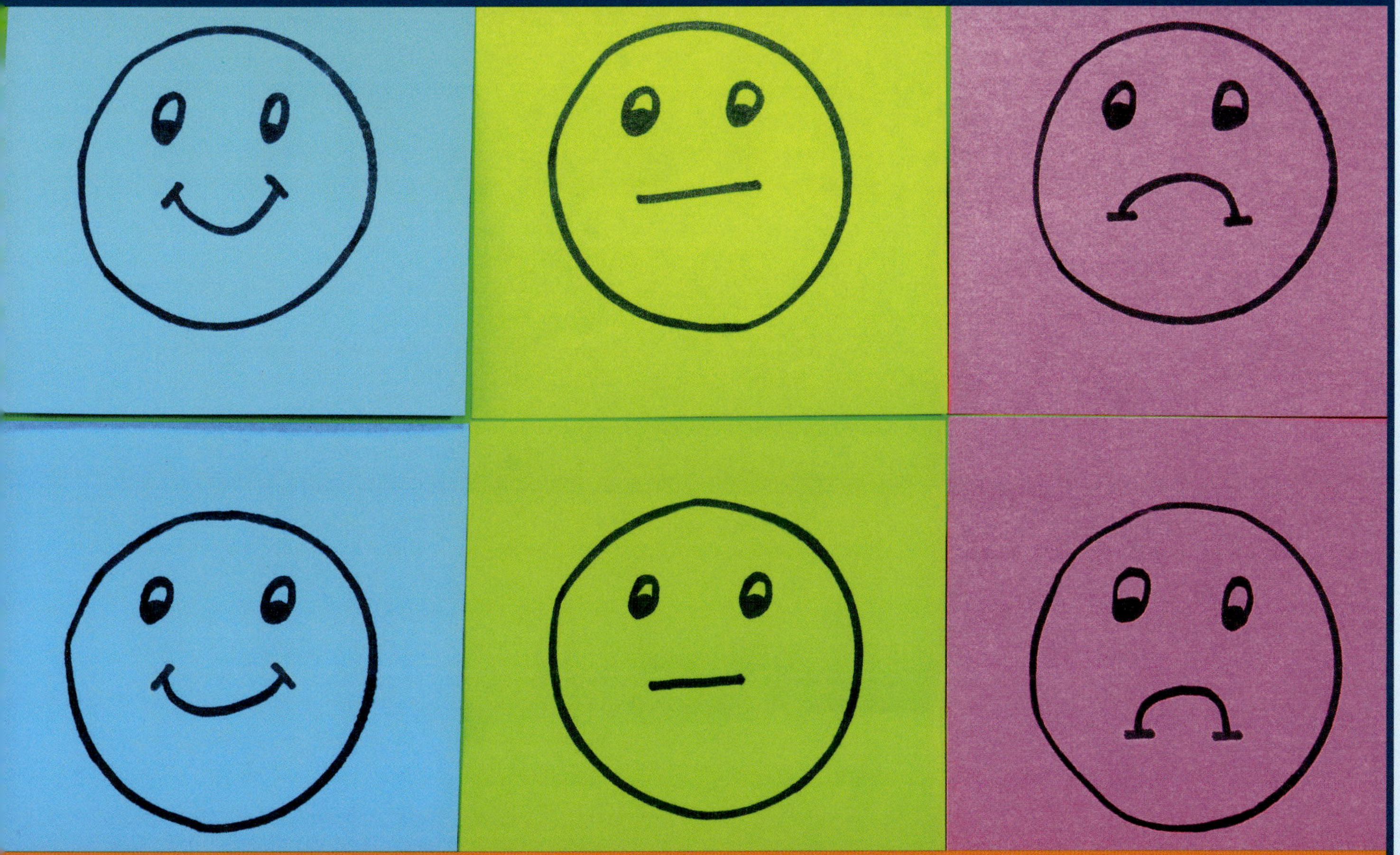

## LEARNING OBJECTIVES

After reading this chapter, you will be able to do the following:

- Describe the function of emotions
- Summarize the relationship between stress and emotional wellness
- Identify the basic emotions and their connection to stress
- Develop a plan for managing your emotions

# KEY TERMS

anxiety
emotional competency
emotions
external self-awareness
generalized anxiety disorder
internal self-awareness
interpersonal
intrapersonal
locus of control
optimism
positive self-talk
resilience
rumination
self-awareness
self-esteem
social referencing

Emotional wellness is the understanding and management of one's emotions. Many people think that being emotionally healthy means never experiencing sadness, but that is not the case—rather, emotional health is the ability to experience and manage all the different emotions (including sadness) so they do not control you or your behavior. To support emotional wellness, you should take time to reflect on your emotions. To begin, let's first learn where emotions come from and how they have adapted to help you survive. For the purpose of this textbook, *feelings* and *emotions* will be used interchangeably.

**Emotions** are a neurological response to stimuli based on your environment, relationship, circumstance, or mood. As discussed in chapter 3, emotions develop and form in the limbic system, which includes the hippocampus, amygdala, and hypothalamus. When you experience a sensory stimulation, the information is sent to the amygdala for processing. This information can be sent quickly or slowly depending on the situation. The quick route, or low road, carries information from the sensory organ to the thalamus to the amygdala, bypassing the cortex (i.e., "thinking area" of the brain) to allow for a quicker response. The slower route, or high road, goes from the sensory organ to the thalamus to the cortex and finally the amygdala (Ghai, Ghai, & Effenberg, 2018). This longer route provides more information for the brain to be able to better respond. For example, imagine you are walking home from campus on a dark night and you hear a noise behind you. Because the situation may be dangerous, your brain would transfer the information using the low road to allow you to respond quicker. If you were walking home using the same route during the day and heard a noise, your brain would most likely take the high road and provide your brain with more information about the situation. It is also important to remember that your prior experiences have shaped how you respond to external stimuli. For example, if you had once been robbed during the day, you may experience a low road response to both situations.

When emotions are sent through the low road, the response to those emotions tends to be reactive and immediate. They also tend to be fear based (discussed later in this chapter). However, there are ways you can train your brain to take the high road and allow more conscious thought into the emotion process, helping you to become less reactive. Imagine you are out on a date and someone bumps into you, causing you to spill your drink. If your brain were to take the low road, you would automatically sense danger and perhaps react by pushing the person back. On the other hand, if you were to train your brain to take more time to process information before reacting in situations that are not immediately threatening, you may find the person who knocked into you did so by accident and is ready to apologize and purchase you another drink. Learning how to slow down reactive emotions is the first step in learning how to manage emotions effectively.

The second step is learning how to identify the multitude of emotions being experienced. Have you ever witnessed a toddler having a tantrum? It is quite a scene. Toddlers have tantrums because they are unable to clearly identify their emotions. They do not have the vocabulary yet to say "I am frustrated," and the only way they can share what

**Understanding and identifying your emotions is a key step in learning to manage them.**

they are feeling is through an outburst of emotion. Being able to properly identify and communicate your emotions can help you manage them.

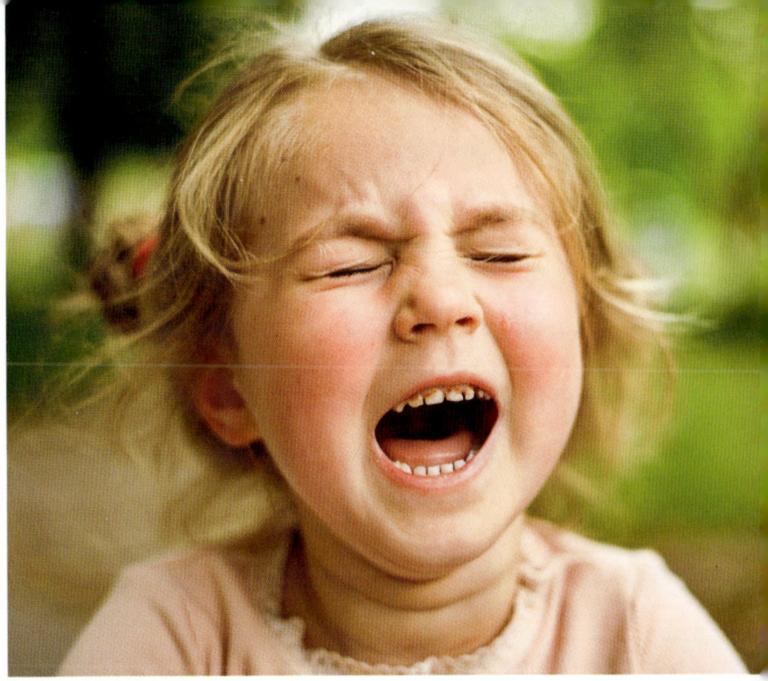

## Function of Emotions

Being happy tends to be the goal for many; however, being happy 100 percent of the time is not realistic or possible. You feel a range of different emotions to help you categorize your life's experiences (Bastiaansen et al., 2019). They help provide you with internal narratives and thoughts to identify experiences as pleasant or unpleasant. Although no one would choose to be sad, sadness exists to help identify the existence of happiness. Now consider the bigger question: Why do we have emotions at all?

> There are moments when I wish I could roll back the clock and take all the sadness away, but I have the feeling that if I did, the joy would be gone as well.
>
> **Nicholas Sparks**

In the beginning of life, emotions are the primary mode of communication between the parent and infant. Infants are intrinsically motivated to promote their attachment with a parent or caregiver and to use emotions to secure that attachment (Kerahrodi & Michal, 2020). Crying in an infant signifies an essential need that must be met. Initially, these needs are hunger, sleep, and soothing from pain or discomfort. Thus, emotions help you better understand yourself, they help you better understand others, and allow for others to better understand you.

Emotions serve **intrapersonal** functions to help guide your actions and allow you to act with minimal thinking required (Hwang & Matsumoto, 2022). For example, the fight-or-flight response can be triggered by fear and requires little to no thinking to activate. The emotion of disgust is similarly adapted—if you have ever cracked open a rotten egg, you know the smell would compel you to not eat that egg. Emotions also help guide our behavior. For example, receiving praise feels good, and because you like to feel good, you are more likely to continue the behavior to receive more praise. The same is true about negative emotions: If you didn't prepare well for an exam and performed poorly, you may feel bad about your performance. The next time there is an exam, you will remember how you felt bad about not performing well, which will motivate you to better prepare this time around. Finally, emotions also influence thoughts and memories. Consider a vivid memory: More likely than not, there is a strong emotion attached to it, whether positive or negative. Robust memories derive their strength from being attached to emotion (Hwang & Matsumoto, 2022).

Emotions also serve **interpersonal** functions and support our efforts to connect with others. Many nonverbal cues—your movements, facial expressions, and body language—express your emotions and convey meaning to others, such as your intentions (Hwang & Matsumoto, 2022). This emotional information can help keep you safe. For example, researchers found that children were able to identify happy faces significantly more quickly than fearful and angry faces (Zsido et al., 2021). This emotional adaptation may have evolved to help children quickly identify safe people when in need of help. Emotions also help regulate social behavior. For example, if a child is reaching for a hot plate, a tone of panic and fear while shouting "no" provides additional meaning and context for the child, which warrants direct notice more easily than a calm "no."

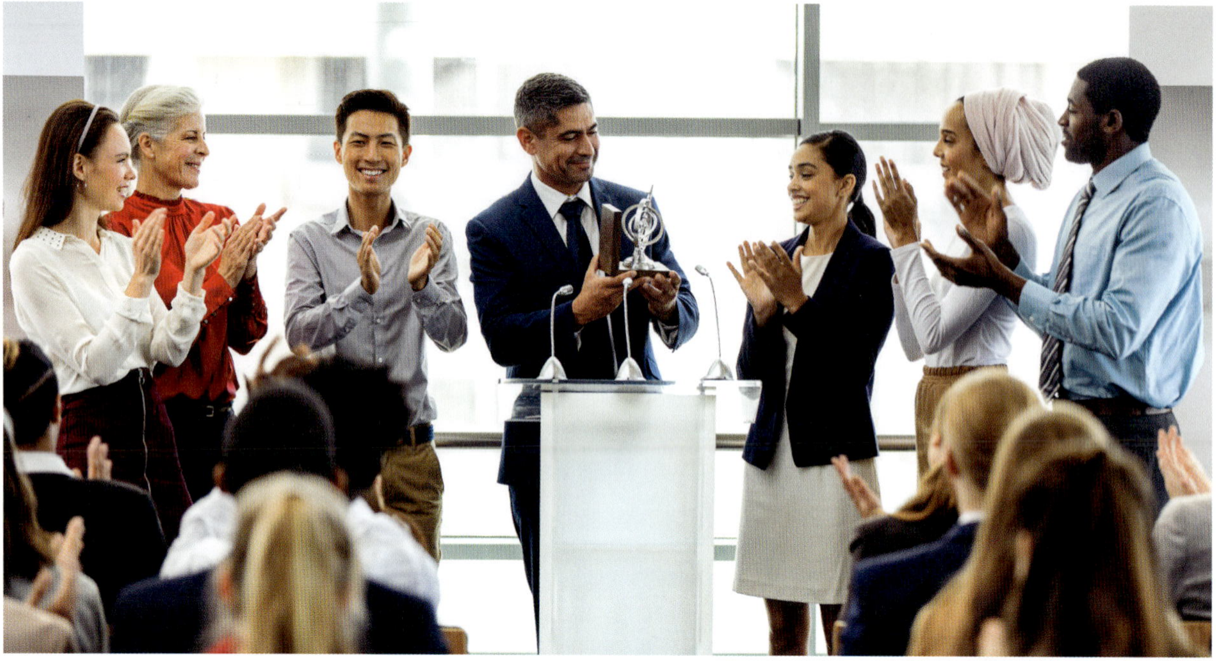

**Social referencing** is the process that helps you read the emotional cues of others in order to regulate your own behavior (Ehli, Wolf, Newen, Schneider, & Voigt, 2020). This process begins right at birth, with infants adjusting their own behavior using emotional cues from adults (Klinnert & Sorce, 1983; Tolksdorf, Crawshaw, & Rohlfing, 2021). Adjusting your own behaviors, thoughts, and emotions based on those of others helps you learn how to manage emotions and can also help keep you safe. Imagine you are walking down the block and you see people with fear on their faces running in the opposite direction. More likely than not, you would read the situation as dangerous and avoid that area too.

## Emotions and Stress

When experiencing stress, certain emotions like anger, shame, and anxiety are a common response (Du, Huang, An, & Xu, 2018). For example, high levels of stress have been associated with an increased risk for depression (Burrage, Marshall, Santanam, & Chantler, 2018). Similarly, those who are under a lot of stress may also be at an increased risk for anxiety (Vo, Chiu, Chuang, & Huang, 2022). During the COVID-19 pandemic, one study found that depression, stress, and anxiety were experienced by about one-third of the population (Salari et al., 2020).

Academic stress has also shown a positive correlation with anger, with some college students turning to substance use and abuse as a method to reduce these emotions (Du et al., 2018; Masood, Kamran, Qaisar, & Ashraf, 2018). A study conducted on college students also found a correlation between anger and alcohol use among those who had experienced sexual harassment (Wolff, Rospenda, & Colaneri, 2017). Overall, college students may be using greater amounts of alcohol to help deal with negative emotions (Sorid, Wedell, Herchenroeder, & Bravo, 2021).

As previously mentioned, most stress we experience today is invisible and derives from some type of internal pressure. You cannot see academic stress; it is not an animal charging at you. Rather, it may arise from the pressure of personal expectations, parental pressures, life stresses, or financial strain, as well as your own emotions. Negative emotional states can increase academic stress, whereas having high levels of emotional regulation can lead to decreased feelings of academic stress (Piryaei, Mohebbi, Khademi Ashkzari, & Khademi Ashkzari, 2017).

**College students often use alcohol to help them deal with difficult emotions.**

## Stressed Out at School

Junie has been stressed at school. When she comes home, she is awful to be around. She snaps at her parents and siblings and is generally in a foul mood. Junie decides to visit the university's wellness center for some help with stress management. At her first session, the counselor suggests she keep a journal of her emotions throughout the day. After one week, Junie goes back to the counselor, and they go over her journal. It is very evident that Junie is feeling angry during one of her lab classes. Junie's lab partner is often late and comes to class unprepared. Junie is angry and frustrated about doing her lab partner's work and her partner getting credit for it. Recognizing the situation that brought on the stress allows Junie to take a step back and figure out ways to handle it. Once she learns to manage that emotion and the situation causing it, Junie's whole outlook begins to change for the better. She is no longer burdened by her lab partner, and the anger she feels toward them dissolves. She is happier at school and at home.

Learning about your emotions can better help you manage them, therefore better supporting your emotional wellness. This leads to having higher levels of **emotional competency**, which refers to the ability to recognize, interpret, and respond to your emotions. It is the beginning of being more proactive and less reactive, which in return reduces stress. The following sections will present an overview of the different emotions and provide strategies to help manage those emotions.

## Basic Emotions

There are many different theories regarding emotions and the basic emotional response in humans. For this textbook, we will consider Paul Ekman's model of six basic emotions of fear, disgust, anger, sadness, enjoyment, and surprise (Ekman & Cordaro, 2011; Ekman, 1999). These emotions serve as the building blocks that can be combined to form other emotions (figure 5.1); they are common among all people and do not differ based on geography, ethnicity, or gender.

1. *Fear*. Fear is the emotion that occurs when you encounter something dangerous and your safety is in jeopardy.
2. *Disgust*. Some believe the origin of disgust came from disease or pathogen avoidance (Rozin & Haidt, 2013). Think of the face someone makes when eating something bad: This look tells you not to eat the same thing, thus signaling you to avoid potential danger.
3. *Anger*. This particularly strong emotion may be a reaction to danger and the desire to protect yourself.
4. *Sadness*. Sadness describes a range of emotions from disappointment to a deep despair. When someone around you is sad, it can evoke your empathy and cause you to share in the feeling of sadness, allowing connection with others (Shirai, Soshi, & Suzuki, 2021).

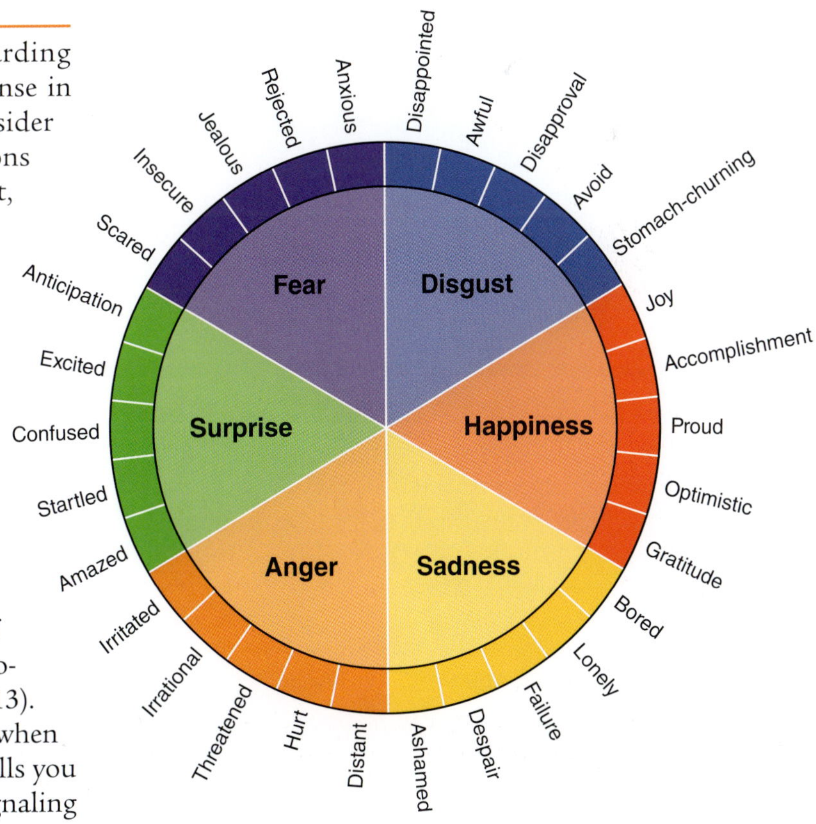


**Figure 5.1** The emotion wheel.

5. *Enjoyment.* Associated with a pleasurable state of being, enjoyment describes a continuum of emotion from contentment to intense joy.
6. *Surprise.* A brief emotion in response to something startling or unexpected.

## Negative Emotions

Although they might feel bad, negative emotions can serve an important purpose. They can signal that something is wrong and needs our attention; for example, feeling apprehensive when walking to your car late at night is your brain telling you to be aware of your surroundings. Negative emotions can also serve as motivation: Being frustrated over a poor test score tells you to change your behavior to improve your performance for the next exam. Negative emotions are not something to be avoided or ignored, which will likely only cause you more stress. Strategies to help you manage your emotions will be discussed later in this chapter.

**When negative emotions are high, it is best to take some time to calm down before making any decisions.**

### *Fear*

Fear is one of the most basic emotions. It occurs in response to a perceived threat, signaling you to be proactive to avoid potential danger or to act on a current dangerous situation. Dangerous situations can include those that place you in physical danger (think dark alley) or emotional danger (giving a speech in front of an audience). When encountering something that promotes fear, your body responds by increasing heart rate and muscle tension and reducing nonessential body functions. Sound familiar? This is the body's fight-or-flight response at work—in other words, fear sets off the stress response cycle.

There may be times in your life when you experience uncontrolled fear or fear that seems out of place. When fear becomes more centralized and chronic, it can lead to anxiety and other mental disorders. Before that happens, there are some questions you can ask yourself:

- How am I experiencing this fear in my body?
- What exactly am I finding frightening?
- Is this concern sensible?
- What is the worst possible outcome, and how could I prevent it?

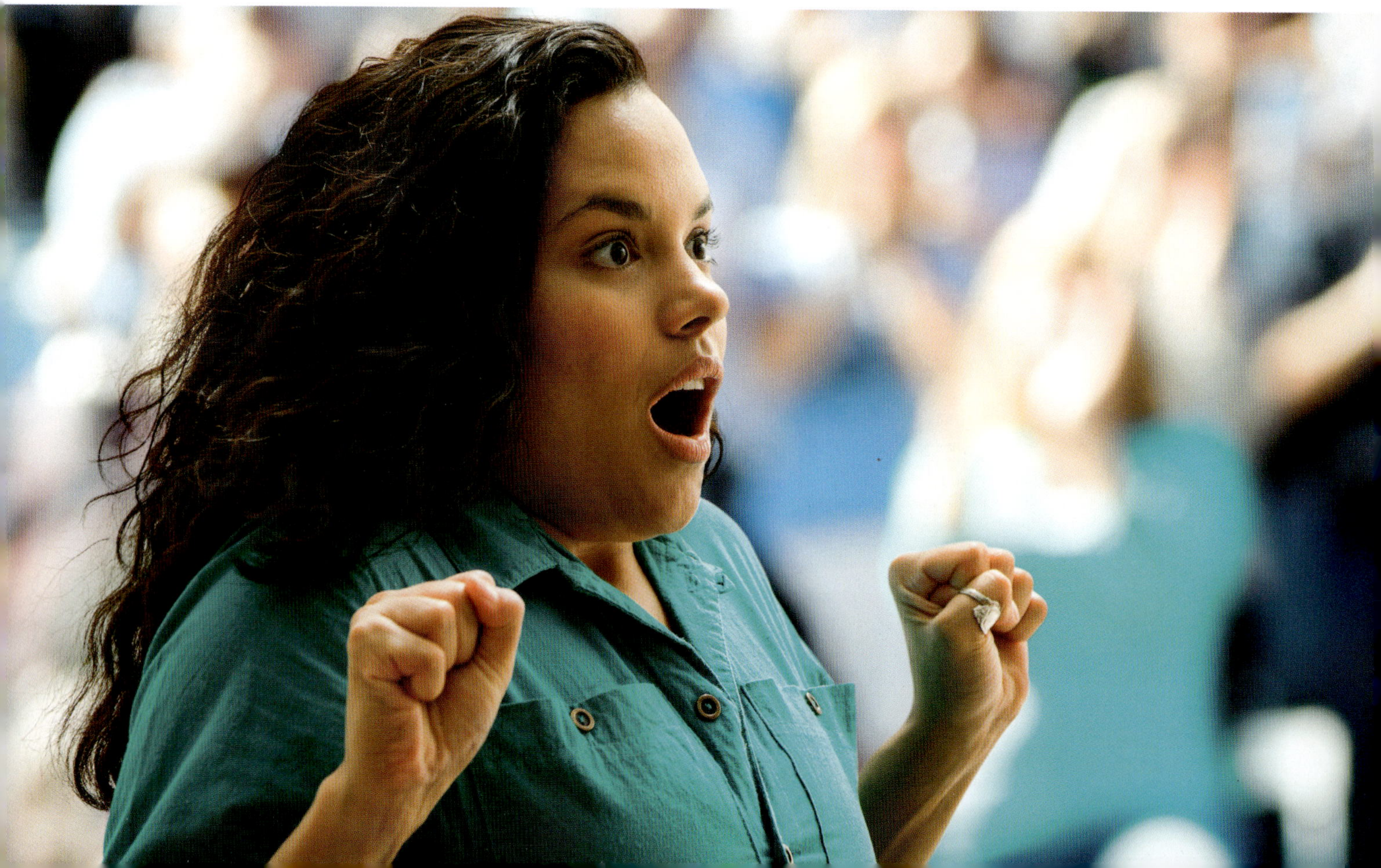

These questions will allow you to think about your fear and obtain a better sense of its root before anxiety takes over.

### Anger

How do you behave when you are angry? Do you yell at people and clench your fists? Or do you push it down and try to ignore it? Anger is a normal emotion that is experienced by all; whether it is seen as positive or negative is dependent on how well you handle anger. People who have a difficult time managing their anger tend to have problems within social settings, interpersonal relationships, and their own wellness (Shepherd & Cant, 2020).

Not surprisingly, anger is associated with stress. Think about the last time you were angry: Did your heartbeat increase? Did you blood pressure go up? Did your face get red? These are all physical signs of the stress response. The same health problems associated with high levels of unmanaged stress are also associated with unmanaged anger.

The instinctual way to handle anger is through physical outbursts. When people act out of anger, it tends to be through behaviors such as yelling, screaming, curling the hands into fists, and throwing things. Many people say they feel out of control during an angry outburst. This physical response may have served as an adaptation to be able to quickly respond to threats. Outbursts also provide an escape for the pent-up physical energy that builds during anger. After an outburst, the body can begin to return to normal and a person feels back in control.

However, unmanaged anger can lead some to suppress or repress their emotion. Suppressed anger is a conscious effort to control anger impulses by choosing to not express them: Although you are feeling angry, your facial expressions and body language do not convey anger. Repression, on the other hand, is an unconscious effort to ignore your anger impulses. When you repress anger, your brain is putting it away to deal with later. Anger, however, doesn't go away. Repressing it today means it is still present and will have to be managed.

Both unexpressed and repressed anger can lead to additional problems, especially with other people. Unmanaged anger takes energy and effort, preventing you from being fully present in the moment, which is associated with poorer relationship outcomes, decreased performance, and less satisfaction in life. Research suggests that people in relationships report higher levels of satisfaction when both partners practice emotional regulation (Bloch, Haase, & Levenson, 2014). In relationships among people with poor emotional regulation, studies suggest they were less satisfied with the relationship. Furthermore, when one partner displays anger toward the other, the receiving partner's anger levels increase, but their anger displays decrease; these higher levels of anger suppression are associated with lower levels of relationship satisfaction (Dworkin, Waldinger, Zimmerman, & Schulz, 2019). A study on nurses also found that those who had higher levels of suppressed anger had lower levels of job satisfaction (La & Yun, 2019). Research has found that those who repress anger have a lower ability to focus on the task at hand, with higher levels of anger associated with poor academic performance and achievement

## Boiling Over

Bree just moved to a new area and has been feeling a little down. She is still working on making new friends and just wants to fit in at work. She starts her day with a quick trip to grab a cup of coffee on her way to work. In line, a woman cuts in front of her, saying she is in a big hurry and running late. Bree is annoyed but acquiesces. On her way to work, a car cuts in front of Bree, causing her to spill a bit of her coffee on her pants. The nerve of some people! When Bree finally gets to work, a group of people walking to the building in front of her are talking loudly, and she feels ignored and invisible. They hold the door for one another and walk away. As she gets there, the door practically closes in her face. Bree can feel herself getting angry but continues to her desk. As Bree finally gets settled in, a coworker tells her she has a stain on her pants. Bree is about to share what happened when another coworker makes a joke about Bree's stained pants. Bree loses it and snaps at her coworker, and tears start streaming down her face. She can feel herself wind down and now just feels embarrassed about her outburst. Bree kept pushing down her anger until it erupted.

(Pekrun, Lichtenfeld, Marsh, Murayama, & Goetz, 2017).

Suppressed anger may also inhibit your ability to show empathy for others. Those who are suppressing anger have a more difficult time recognizing facial expressions and emotions, which makes it difficult to connect with others (Cristiano, 2019). Social connections help us share feelings, manage emotions, and value the connections between people, which can help reduce stress. A reduced ability to make and form these connections places you at higher risk for isolation and loneliness.

Learning to control your anger can be beneficial. Remember from chapter 3 that the stress response decreases your cognitive functioning—in a heightened state, your decision-making capabilities are not functioning optimally, and you don't always filter out things you normally wouldn't say. That is why relationship experts will often say not to try to solve problems while arguing. In the heat of the moment, it is sometimes best to walk away from the situation to calm down and think about the argument (not the anger). After calming down, you can come back and discuss the initial cause of the anger.

**Learning to manage your anger can help you maintain positive relationships.**

It is important to learn how to manage your anger so that it doesn't control you. When you are in control of your emotions, you acknowledge and deal with them directly. There are several ways to help manage your anger.

- *Relaxation techniques.* Take a few minutes to relax. Examples include meditation, yoga, repeating a mantra, and visualization.
- *Cognitive restructuring.* This technique focuses on changing the way you think (Tarmizi, Sugiharto, & Sutoyo, 2020). Stay away from all-or-nothing thinking. This includes phrases such as "you always" or "you never." This can lead you to become even more angry and is rarely the case. Instead, say how you are feeling and the specific behavior that caused you to feel that way.
- *Communication skills.* Anger can arise when there is a misunderstanding or someone doesn't agree with your viewpoint. Practice listening to what others are saying. Don't say the first thing that pops into your head; take time to think of your response before saying it. Reflect and use words that contain emotions.
- *Problem solving.* Sometimes anger arises from situations that feel out of your control. When this occurs, step back from the situation and think about what you can control. Problem solving uses critical thinking, questioning, and reflexive thinking to help make appropriate decisions.

Stress and the physical response to stress often accompany anger, working against your movement toward emotional wellness. Learning to manage your anger can reduce your overall stress. More techniques for managing emotions will be discussed later in this chapter.

## Case Study

### Anger Is Not Heart Healthy

One 20-year longitudinal study researching the impact of emotions on physical health measured the levels of anger expressed between married couples who engaged in 15-minute conversations on assigned topics ranging from enjoyable activities to areas of conflict. The researchers then invited the couples back every five years for health assessments. What they found was amazing: People who had the highest anger levels were shown to have more cardiovascular symptoms, which started showing up after the first five years of the study. Moreover, the cardiovascular symptoms among the group with anger continued to increase more rapidly compared to the other groups (Haase, Holley, Bloch, Verstaen, & Levenson, 2016).

#### Discussion Questions

1. Would you support emotional check-ups at yearly physical exams? Why or why not?
2. If you feel you have high levels of anger, where can you go to get help managing your emotions?

### *Sadness*

Sadness is another basic emotion and is associated with physical markers such as slumped posture, downcast eyes, and crying. These markers help alert others of your feelings, which can result in receiving emotional support to help you cope. It is important to note that sadness is different from depression. Depression is a chronic illness that limits emotional functioning. Sadness, on the other hand, is acute and within the normal spectrum of emotions.

Motivation levels can help predict to what extent a person will remain sad. For example, people with lower levels of self-esteem generally have reduced motivation to manage their sadness. They would prefer to listen to sad music and are less likely to engage in activities that are uplifting (Arens & Stangier, 2020). Sadness cannot be avoided, but how long you stay in this emotional state is within your control.

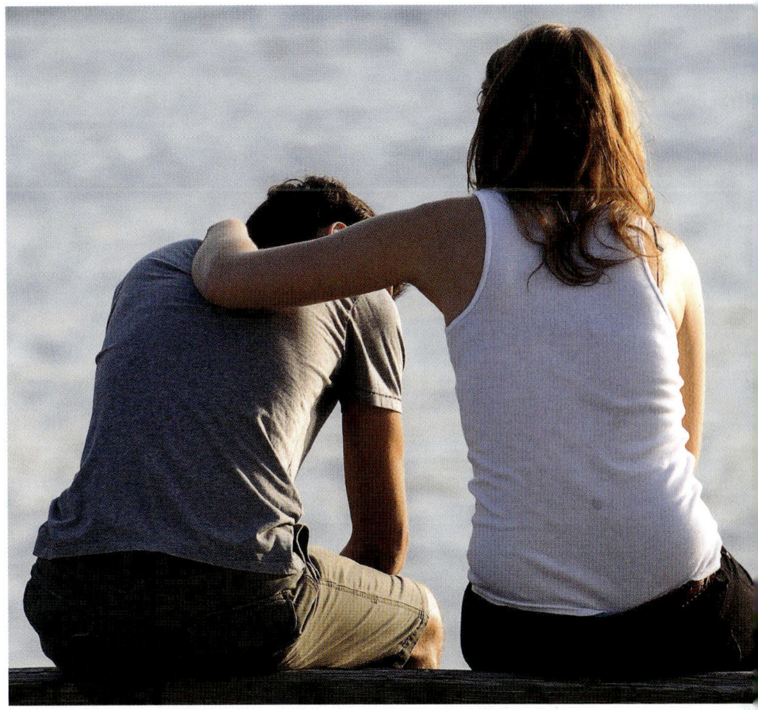

## Thinking Patterns and Emotions

How you choose to think about events can impact your emotional response to them. This section will highlight examples of thought patterns and their impact on emotions.

### *Rumination*

**Rumination** is a thinking pattern that revolves around thoughts and feelings about a negative event (Du et al., 2018). Rumination is different from reflection, which involves considering the cause of the situation and coming up with a plan to avoid the same consequence if encountered again. Rather, rumination involves repeatedly thinking about a negative event, increasing or supporting negative emotions and causing distress with no solution or learned experience. For example, let's say you received a text message while driving. You took your eyes off the road for a split second and—*bang*!—you hit the car in front of you. Thankfully, no one was hurt other than the cars. If you were ruminating about the accident, you would relive the accident in your head, feeling worse and worse about it. You are not coming up with a way to avoid a similar accident in the future; instead, you just wish it would have never happened. Generally, rumination magnifies negative emotions and distracts you from problem solving (Watkins & Roberts, 2020). If you were reflecting on the accident, however, you would acknowledge that your cell phone distracted you, and you might silence notifications while you are driving so you will not be distracted by your phone again. Rumination leaves you feeling down, whereas reflecting leaves you feeling hopeful.

**Rumination increases stress and can leave you feeling down, sad, or angry.**

### *Anxiety*

**Anxiety** is a state of nervousness in anticipation of a future threat. In this sense, it is both a thinking pattern and an emotion. As a thinking pattern, anxiety is the fear associated with some future threat (either real or imagined). As an emotion, anxiety is the tense foreboding feeling associated with some future threat. One study found that anxiety heightened a person's ability to recognize faces with angry or fearful expressions (Zein, Wyart, & Grezes, 2015). This enhanced recognition skill can possibly help clarify levels of threat and allow you to determine an appropriate course of action.

When you experience anxiety, your body responds by igniting the fight-or-flight stress response. If anxiety is uncontrolled and starts to

Case Study

## What Did the Doctor Say?

A few months ago, Kellan's doctor asked him to come in to discuss some test results. Kellan was nervous about the results, and as the appointment drew nearer, Kellan's anxiety worsened. At the appointment, the doctor discussed the diagnosis and treatment options and then told Kellan to go home and think about them. When Kellan got home, his partner asked him to summarize the doctor's visit. Kellan had a difficult time remembering what the doctor said and felt like he was missing much information that was shared during the appointment.

Kellan made another appointment with the doctor to go over the information again but this time invited his partner to join him. Kellan was better able to focus, but he also felt relieved to have someone else there with him to help process the information. When he returned home, he and his partner were able to talk about the different options, and Kellan's partner was able to fill in the gaps and provide additional clarity on the information presented.

Studies have shown that anxiety is related to a decrease in working memory performance (Huang, 2022). When people go to the doctor, they often experience anxiety, and the ability to be present and understand information provided may therefore be diminished. If you experience anxiety, bringing a friend, partner, or family member to your appointment to help you remember and process information can prove to be helpful.

### Discussion Questions

1. This case study presents an example of how anxiety can impede memory. How do you think test anxiety can impact test performance?
2. If you experience anxiety related to a specific event, what can you do to help reduce anxiety?
3. When was the last time you experienced anxiety? If you had to do it again, what would you do differently to reduce your anxiety level?

interfere with your daily life, it is then considered a problem. When anxiety becomes persistent—defined as experiencing it often over a period of six months—it is called **generalized anxiety disorder** (Mayo Clinic, 2018). There are other types of specific anxiety (e.g., social phobia, separation anxiety), which can interfere with daily activities. Although the causes of anxiety are different, the symptomology is the same: The body feels anxious and reacts by initiating the stress response.

## Positive Emotions

Positive emotions can help you cope with life's hurdles. Positive thinking evokes positive emotions and vice versa. Generally, people who think positively tend to also believe they control their future and are more willing to share their feelings and emotions with others (Stangor & Walinga, 2017). People who engage in positive thinking are more likely to report higher levels of life satisfaction. Life satisfaction supports optimal levels of wellness; those who report higher levels generally make more positive decisions regarding their health and wellness (Green, Noor, & Ahmed, 2020).

Many people confuse the terms *happiness* and *joy*. What does it mean to be happy? Many people, when asked what they want for themselves, will say happiness. How does one go about achieving happiness? One group of researchers proposed that happiness is influenced by three elements: intentional activity, set point, and life's circumstances (Lyubomirsky, Sheldon, & Schkade, 2005). They felt that 40 percent of happiness comes from engaging in intentional activities that contribute to your happiness. Of the two other categories, which are unmodifiable, 50 percent is from your set point (influenced by your genetics) and 10 percent is from your life's circumstances. More recent studies have similar interpretations that happiness in the form of life satisfaction and subjective well-being was most influenced by genetics (Nes & Roysamb, 2017). Additionally, happiness tends to be future oriented, meaning the future must align with your expectations for you to be happy. It is seen as a temporary state that will dissipate and may even leave you feeling dissatisfied or down. For example, lottery winners initially report higher levels of happiness and general well-being, but as with all feelings of happiness, they diminish after a period of time (Sherman, Shavit, & Barokas, 2020). Although winning the lottery may make life easier, it does not change a person's emotional wellness.

So, if you can't work on being happy all the time, what should you focus on? The answer lies in contentment, gratitude, and joy. Contentment can be imagined as a state of being. It can also be examined through the lens of having your physical and psychological needs met and feeling thankful for your life's circumstances (Cordaro, Brackett, Glass, & Anderson, 2016). Those who feel content are happy with what they have and do not feel a need to gather more possessions. Unlike happiness, which is temporary, contentment is sustainable. You can achieve contentment by practicing gratitude, setting small goals and achieving them, and examining your past achievements and accomplishments.

**Gratitude promotes positive emotions.**

Gratitude is another positive emotion that has been shown to support wellness. Gratitude is the ability to see and acknowledge the positive aspects in life. You can practice and develop gratitude in your life by giving thanks for everything you have. The more you practice being grateful, the more you will develop your own gratitude. Gratitude influences optimal wellness; those who are grateful are more likely to engage in decision making and behaviors that support wellness (Green et al., 2020).

Finally, joy is an emotion that is connected to an inner peace. Joy is not conditional on someone else's behavior or any external events. It is not based on money, material things, or relationships (unless you count the relationship you have with yourself). Joy is a deep sense of being good enough and wanting the best for those around you. When you have joy, you are in control of yourself and your thoughts and emotions. When you feel anger, sadness, or anxiety, you acknowledge those emotions and understand they will be short lived. As such, when you encounter stress, you are confident in your ability to manage it.

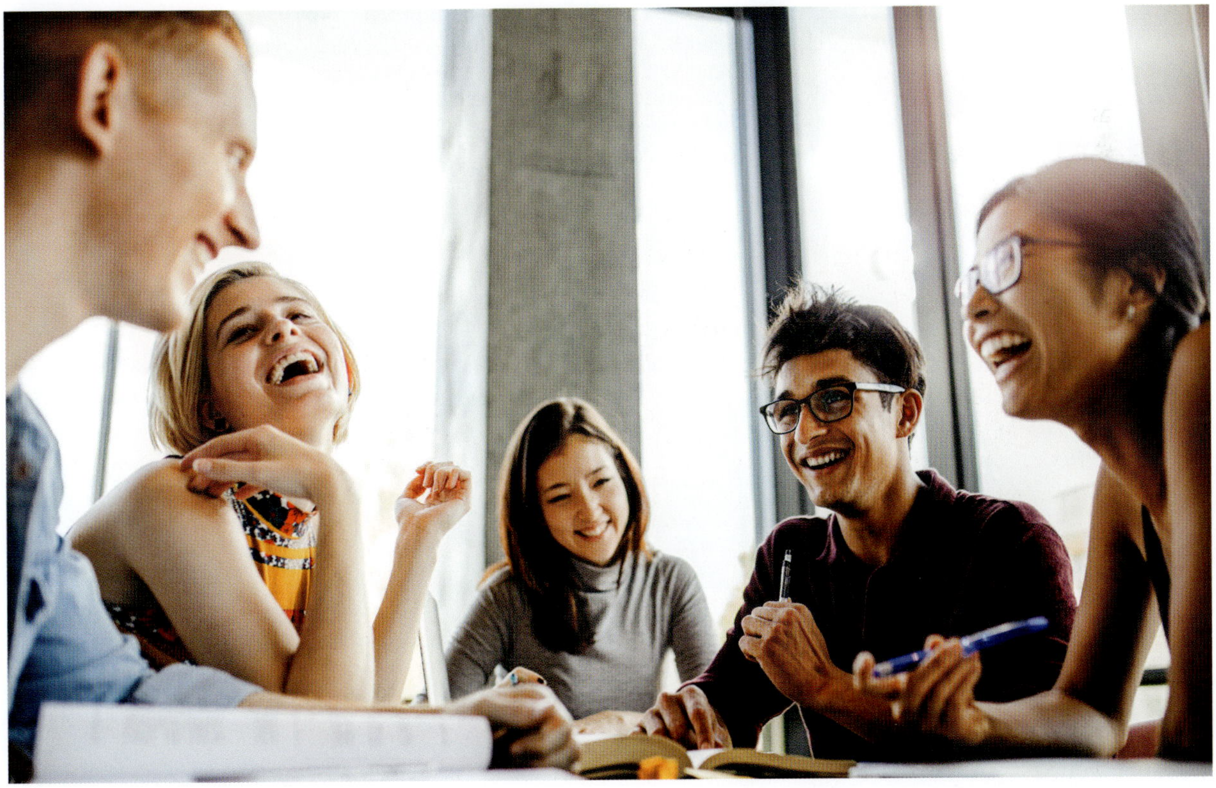

Research Spotlight

## Moving from Stress to Joy

Dr. Rozina Lakhani (2021) provides a framework for how to move from stress to joy using the initials CPR:

- Calm
- Process
- Respond

The first component in dealing with stress is calming the mind and body. You are not able to focus while body is in fight-or-flight mode, which is why it is necessary to calm down before proceeding. This can be achieved through meditation, yoga, or any activity that stimulates the parasympathetic nervous system. These techniques will be addressed in more detail in chapter 10.

The next step is to process what is going on by actively thinking about the situation that caused you stress. One such method, developed by Stephen Covey (2004), utilizes the circle of concern and the circle of influence. To use this technique, imagine a large circle in your mind: This is the circle of concern, containing everything that you really care about (figure 5.2). It is quite large, as you can imagine. Within the larger circle is a smaller circle; this is the circle of influence. This circle contains everything that you do have some control over (your situations and attitudes). Within that circle are the items you can proactively work to control (your words, thoughts, and actions). The space between the circle of influence and the circle of concern contains the things you care about but have no power over—everything from the actions of others to the weather. When you encounter stress, ask yourself the following questions (Lakhani, 2021):

- Is this thought inside my circle of influence? (If yes, act on it; this will reduce stress and lead to joy.)
- If not, is there something about this stressor I can do something about? (If yes, act on it.)
- If not, is my reaction to the stress hurting or helping me? (If it is hurting you, shift your focus to issues inside your circle of influence.)

Lastly, you will need to respond to the stressor. This is the response to stress you have chosen that will lead to stress reduction and leave a positive impact. The goal is to work on identifying and managing the stress you have control over, which leads you to joy (Lakhani, 2021).

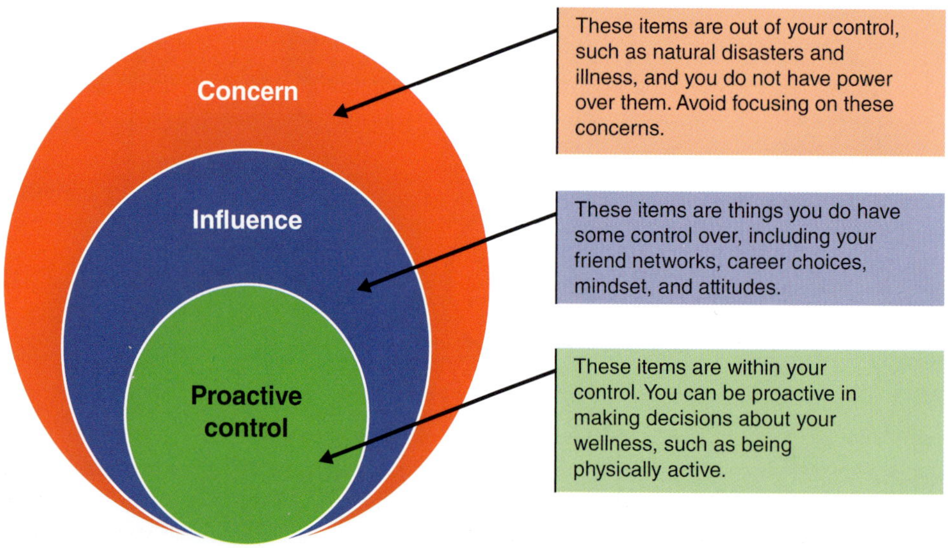


**Figure 5.2** Circles of concern and influence.

## Managing Emotions

Studies have shown a high correlation between stress and negative emotions (Du, Huang, An, & Xu, 2018). When you are under stress, your body is expending energy to initiate the stress response system, leaving you with less energy to manage your emotions. As a result, when we encounter emotions that we don't like, we tend to ignore, deny, suppress, or just poorly handle them.

Denial occurs when you refuse to acknowledge your emotions and try to go on as normal. However, when you deny your emotions, they do not disappear; they are only being pushed down temporarily. As you continue to push those feelings down, they begin to build up. As with anything that builds up under pressure, there will eventually be an explosion—in this case, an emotional explosion. Much like a real explosion, an emotional explosion will result in people running away to get out of the range of the blast.

Another common but harmful way to manage emotions is withdrawal. Sometimes engaging in life feels too tiring, and it seems easier to be alone. Other times, people withdraw when they are overwhelmed or ashamed of something. Withdrawal can lead to extreme loneliness, anger, and distorted thinking; it may also be an early sign of depression.

Some people handle difficult emotions by bullying others. Bullying is the repeated behavior pattern of using verbal or physical threats to show power over another person. People tend to turn to bullying when they don't feel good about themselves. Conversely, some people turn their negative emotions inward to engage in self-harm, which may include cutting, starving, or participating in dangerous behavior. Although it may seem counterintuitive, self-harming behavior allows someone to be in control over their emotional pain.

These harmful strategies all have one thing in common: They only serve to temporarily manage or disguise difficult emotions. Luckily, there are methods you can use to help you positively manage your emotions and keep them from bubbling back up to the surface.

### Pause, Acknowledge, Think, Help (PATH)

The Pause, Acknowledge, Think, Help (PATH) approach uses pauses to help you identify your emotions.

- *Pause.* When you start feeling something strongly, stop what you are doing. You may need to go for a walk or just sit quietly. This allows you to take a break from the strong emotion.
- *Acknowledge.* Take time to identify what you are feeling. Go through a list of emotions in your head and put a name to it, if necessary. It is important to be able to describe how you are feeling.
- *Think.* It is time to identify the causes or contributing events that resulted in your emotions. What happened that resulted in this reaction?
- *Help.* This is the actionable part of the approach. Now you can do something to manage the event that led to your strong emotion. If you are angry at a friend for not including you when they went out, talk to your friend about your feelings. If you are mad at yourself for not performing well on a test, you can make a plan to better prepare yourself for the next test. In this stage, you are taking active steps to deal with the event that led to your emotion.

### Managing Emotions for Better Relationships

Anytime you deal with other people—including coworkers, classmates, and friends—your emotions play a role. Unmanaged or poorly managed emotions can create stress in those relationships. This can also lead to unhealthy behaviors to temporarily reduce feelings of stress (alcohol consumption, overeating) that will not solve the problem.

For example, Robyn has been dating Zoe for a couple of months. She really likes her but feels a bit insecure in their relationship. When they go out one evening, Robyn feels jealous and angry that Zoe is talking to another woman, and she drinks too much alcohol to suppress her feelings. Unfortunately, she ends up arguing with Zoe and ruining their date. Alcohol does not do a good job of helping manage emotions.

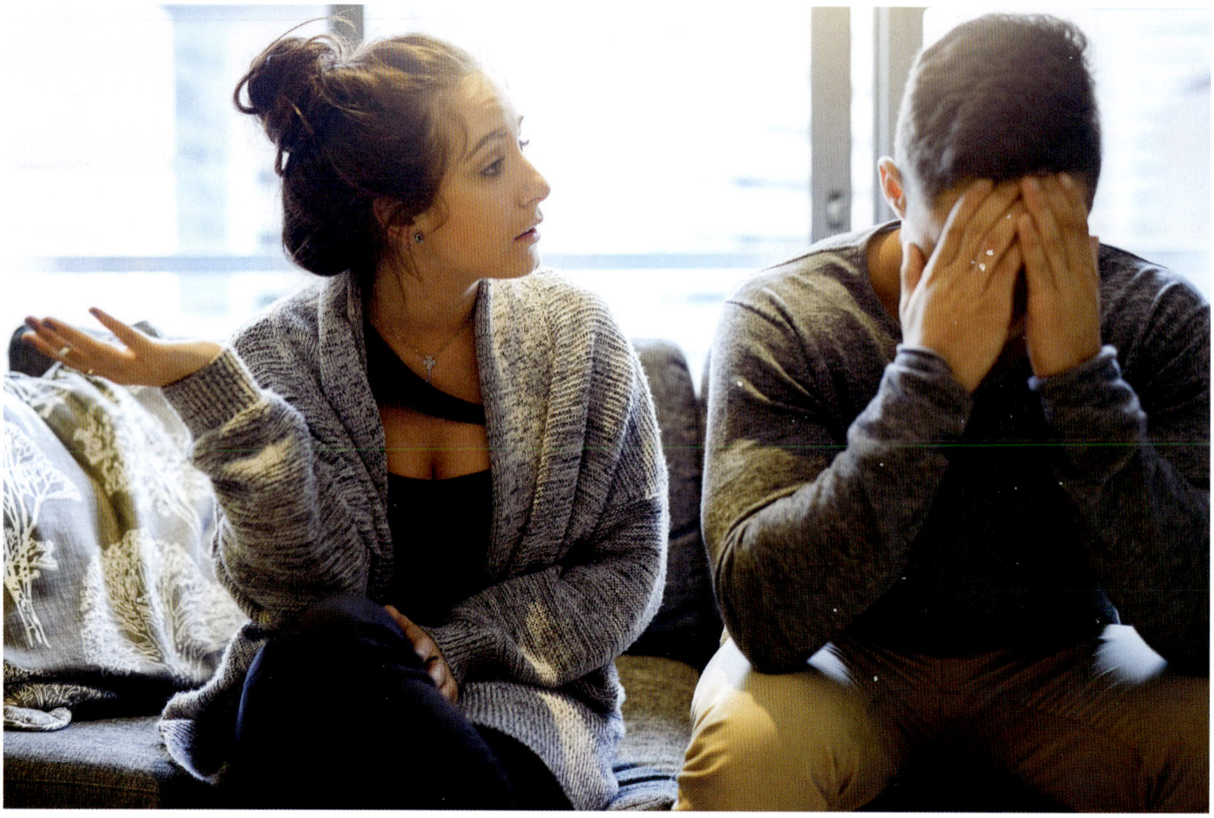

## Give Yourself a Time-Out

Anger and fear are two emotions that can be difficult to manage. Any type of strong emotion can elicit a stress response, putting you into a heightened state. Coupled with your brain's inability to engage your frontal cortex, which is responsible for logical thought, you become locked in an endless battle with that emotion. Imagine trying to engage a drowning person in a meaningful conversation. No matter how important your conversation may be—even if it were about how to use a life jacket—there is no way the person would be able to engage with you. They would be too focused on survival.

Strong emotions make your brain feel as if it needs to survive. Although you may not be in physical danger, your brain reacts as though there is danger present. One way of managing those strong emotions is to give yourself a time-out by removing yourself from the triggering situation. Giving yourself time to cool off allows your parasympathetic nervous system time to bring down your stress hormones, heart rate, and blood pressure. Time-outs are very useful to help you resume your thinking brain so you can make logical steps to manage the situation.

When you experience a strong emotion with another person, the conversation or argument tends to deteriorate as the emotions continue to build. Time-outs pause the argument to provide you time to stop and think about the situation. When you return, you are better able to have a constructive dialogue. Adults can benefit from time-outs too!

## Practice Accepting Your Emotions

There may be times in your life when it is difficult to accept your emotions. One way to practice accepting your emotions is to consider them from the outside. Pretend that you are asking a friend questions to better understand their feelings. What kind of questions would you ask (e.g., "How are you feeling?" "When did that feeling start?")? Asking yourself questions allows you to better identify your emotions and what contributed to them.

For emotions that are difficult to identify, a more detailed feeling wheel, shown in figure 5.3, can be a useful tool (Willcox, 1982). Being able to choose terms to label your feelings will help you share, address, and acknowledge your emotions. (You may notice the terms for primary emotions used here are different from the ones used previously in this chapter and in figure 5.1—recall that researchers have not agreed on common terms used to describe these emotions.)

**Ask yourself questions about your emotions to better understand them.**

## Seek Professional Support

There may be times in your life when you feel overwhelmed by your emotions and cannot self-regulate. A therapist can be helpful in this case by serving as a neutral party who can help you learn how to better manage your emotions (Soma et al., 2020). They can help address severe mood swings and work with you to discover the mechanism causing those swings. There are times when we are so close to our feelings and emotions that we fail to see the big picture. Think of it like viewing a painting through a magnifying glass: You will only be able to identify colors and brush strokes, but not what the painting is representing. A therapist can help you step back and see the bigger picture.

# Self-Awareness

**Self-awareness** is developed through inner reflection and attention to your conscious thoughts. It allows you to focus on yourself, paying attention to how well your thoughts, feelings, and emotions match your internal goals and standards. This can help you see yourself as others see you and better align your behavior to match who you want to portray. Those with high levels of self-awareness can objectively evaluate their own actions, feelings, and thoughts and can talk about their strengths and challenges to promote personal growth (Duval & Wicklund, 1972; London, Sessa, & Shelley, 2023).

There are two types of self-awareness: internal and external. **Internal self-awareness** includes being able to understand what impacts your thoughts, feelings, and emotions (Yilmaz, 2022), as well as how your thoughts, feelings, and emotions impact those around you. Having a strong sense of internal self-awareness has been associated with lower levels of anxiety and stress (Contreras, Edwards-Maddox, Hall, & Lee, 2020). In a study conducted on college freshmen, researchers investigating the impact of skills training found that self-awareness has the largest impact on social and academic adjustment, which includes lower levels of anxiety and stress (Manee, Khoiee, & Eghbal, 2015). This ability to think about what influences your emotions—and sometimes just the act of acknowledging your emotions—can help you better manage those emotions.

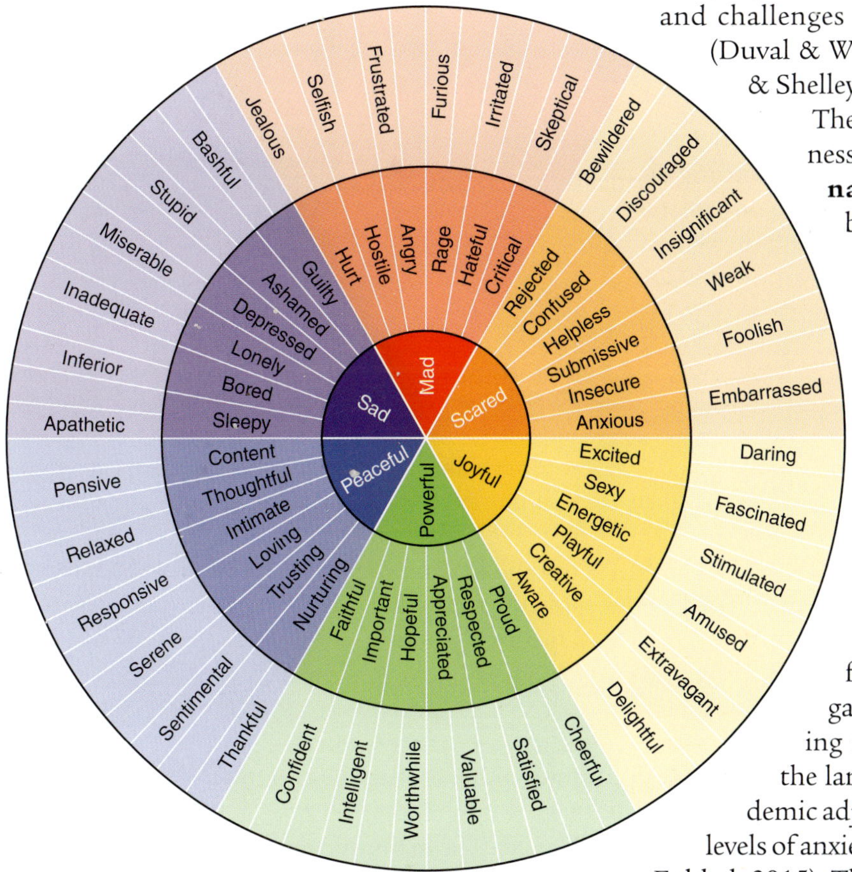


**Figure 5.3** The feeling wheel.

Adapted by permission from G. Wilcox, "The Feeling Wheel," Transactional Analysis Journal 12, no. 4 (1982): 274-276, reprinted by permission of the publisher (Taylor & Francis Ltd, http://www.tandfonline.com).

### Why Are You Mad?

Noah wakes up feeling anxious about his upcoming oral presentation. As he runs into his roommate, he snaps at him for not doing the dishes or taking out the garbage. As his roommate tries to apologize and explain, Noah just walks away and goes back to his room. Thinking about his current behavior, Noah realizes that perhaps he is in a bad mood because he is nervous about the upcoming presentation. Once he realizes this, he apologizes to his roommate for being rude and explains why he was upset. Though still nervous, he feels a bit better and goes about getting ready for the day. He talks to a few other students in class who also admit to being nervous. Noah feels a camaraderie with them and is comforted by the idea that others are nervous too. He goes on to present and feels he performed quite well.

If Noah hadn't thought about his behavior but had instead gone through the morning snapping at everyone he met, his bad mood would have likely continued as the day progressed. If so, how do you think Noah's presentation would have gone? Why?

The second part of self-awareness is **external self-awareness**, or the ability to understand how others view you (Yilmaz, 2022). Those who show high levels of external self-awareness also demonstrate higher levels of empathy, have better relationship skills, and generally relate better with others as a result (Blakely et al., 2022; Eurich, 2018).

Self-awareness is a skill that can be learned and developed. Here are some ways to improve your own self-awareness:

- *Ask "what" questions.* Instead of focusing on the *why*, ask questions that focus on the *what*. For example, if you did not do well on a paper and you were to ask your professor "Why did you give me a poor grade?" you may be given a few reasons why the grade was low. If instead you ask, "What steps do I need to take to get a better grade next time?" the answers would be solution based and allow to you focus your energy on performing better.
- *Believe in yourself.* Using positive self-talk and imagining yourself being successful can improve your confidence.
- *Learn from mistakes and failures.* Failure and mistakes are not the end game, but placeholders to help guide you in the right direction. For example, if you get the second step of a mathematical equation wrong, making the entire solution wrong, identifying your error and how to fix it is a learning opportunity. If you quit, you lose the opportunity to learn how to use that mathematical process and would most likely not be able to solve similar equations.
- *Practice mindfulness.* Take note of how you are feeling. Ask yourself, "what is causing me to feel this way?" This will help you better identify your feelings and emotions, which will help you better manage them (Yogeswaran & El Morr, 2021).

When you are in an emotionally aroused state, managing other things can seem impossible. Improving your self-awareness improves your ability to manage emotions, which can help you manage your stress. Ultimately, emotions are under our control.

## Resilience

**Resilience**, or the ability to adapt to difficult situations, is one of the foundations of emotional wellness. Being resilient doesn't mean that you will not experience emotional pain, but that you are able to acknowledge your pain and take steps to rebuild after the challenging event has passed. Resilience is a skill that can be learned, practiced, and strengthened.

Having resilience places you in a position of control. Although you do not have control over all circumstances, you do have control over how you respond in those circumstances. The **locus of control** describes whether you feel personally in control of your life. When

**Resilience is supported and strengthened by having an internal locus of control.**

you have an external locus of control, you see life as something that happens to you as a result of external events. On the other hand, if you have an internal locus of control, you feel in control of your circumstances.

When resilience is low, stress can harm your emotional wellness (Chow & Choi, 2019). It might result in such symptoms as the following:

- Depression
- Anxiety
- Becoming easily agitated and angered
- Feeling overwhelmed
- Not feeling in control

## Self-Esteem

**Self-esteem** describes your sense of self-worth and confidence. Self-esteem begins to develop at birth and is influenced by how you were raised. Although it can be developed and nurtured, self-esteem is generally stable.

Someone with high self-esteem generally feels confident in life and has a strong sense of identity. They have a sense of security in their environment and feel a sense of belonging within their community (Kowalczyk, Aydin, Gulcz, Mela, & Roszak, 2022). Conversely, people with low self-esteem have lower levels of motivation and performance and are more likely to give up on something that requires work and has a learning curve. This is especially true after experiencing failure: In their eyes, failure is a result that cannot be changed. Additionally, failure further hurts their self-esteem (Rector & Roger, 1997; Zarrin, Gracia, & Paixao, 2020). Moreover, those with low self-esteem are more likely to show greater emotional responses to negative feedback and are less adept at managing their emotions (Rector & Roger, 1997). They generally feel that stress is out of their control and that they have no power to alter the events causing stress. The additional burden of these negative feelings then further contributes to stress.

Stress can negatively impact your self-esteem. When not managed well, it places undue burden on you and takes away feelings of confidence and worthiness. However, having a high level of self-esteem is related to better stress management techniques and ultimately, lower levels of stress (Kaplanova, 2018). For example, when ice hockey players were taught strategies to improve their self-esteem, their levels of stress went down. These lower levels of stress were maintained during competition, which resulted in improved performance (Kaplanova, 2018).

Improving your own self-esteem may help you feel more confident in managing your stress—it may even improve your confidence in your ability to practice stress management techniques. The following are some ways you can strengthen your self-esteem (Mayo Clinic, 2020):

- *Become aware of negative thoughts.* Actively challenge those thoughts. Treat yourself as you would a friend. Say kind things to yourself. Be supportive and encouraging.
- *Focus on the positive.* Use positive self-talk and acknowledge your positive traits. What are you good at? What challenges have you already overcome?
- *Enjoy life.* Find things you enjoy and do them. Spend time with people and activities that make you happy.
- *Learn to say no.* Say no when you are asked to do things you do not want to do. Do not overburden yourself fulfilling the requests of others. Practice being assertive.
- *Improve your physical health.* It is easier to feel good about yourself when you are actively moving toward physical wellness (see chapter 4). Making the decision to improve your health can also improve your feelings of self-esteem.

## Choosing Optimism

People respond to stress differently. Some will feel discouraged and give up. Others will see it as a challenge and thrive. What can help us move from being discouraged and giving up to feeling challenged and motivated to move on? Choosing positive outlooks and emotions can help you deal with the daily stressors.

Having the right frame of mind can lead to emotional wellness. Do you consider yourself a pessimist or an optimist? **Optimism** is an inclination to have positive expectations for the future.

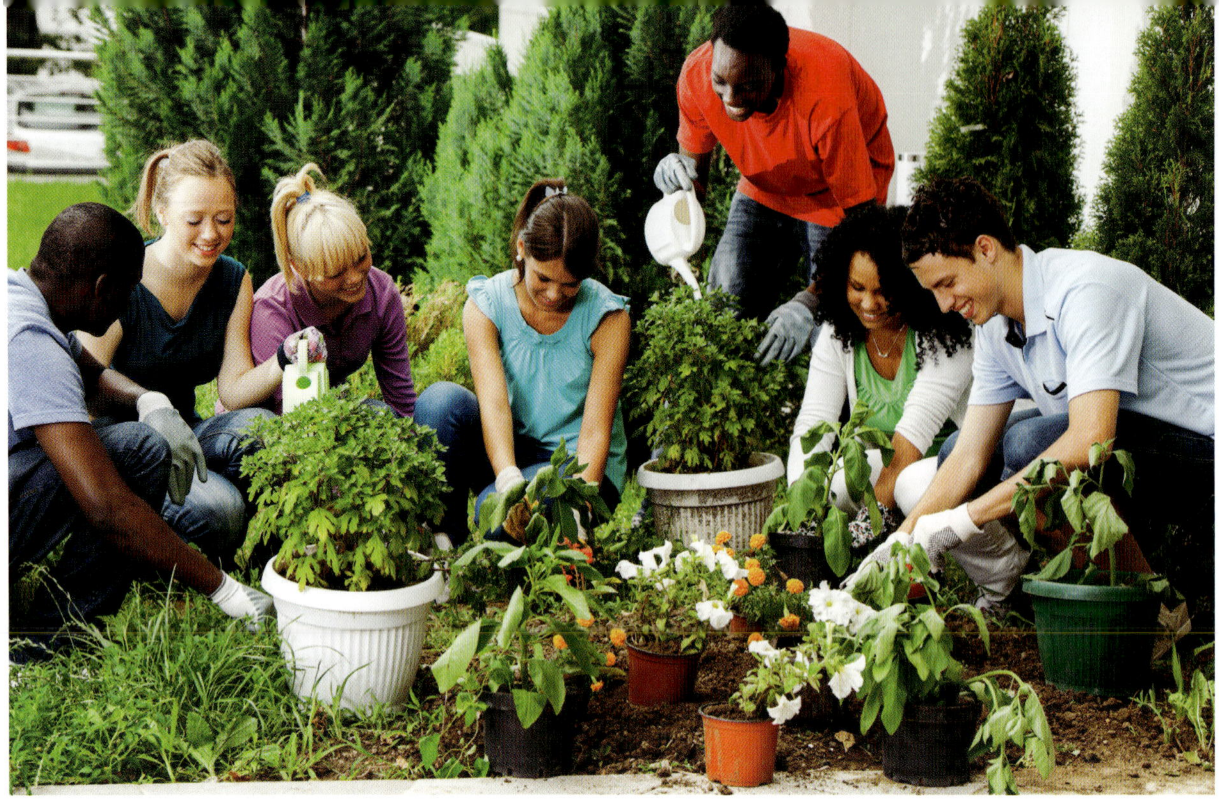

An optimist tends to have a positive outlook on life and expect positive outcomes, as opposed to a pessimist, who views life from a negative perspective and tends to expect the worst. Although at times pessimism can be beneficial (e.g., planning ahead for obstacles), an optimist is generally more open to new ideas and experiences. Being optimistic is related to lower levels of stress, higher levels of motivation, slower disease progression, and higher engagement in healthy behaviors, as well as overall better physical and psychological well-being (Baumgartner, Schneider, & Capiola, 2018; Puig-Perez, Hackett, Salvador, & Steptoe, 2017). Optimistic people have been found to have lower cortisol responses and lower blood pressure levels under stress compared to pessimistic people (Levy, Heruti, & Avitsur, 2019; Terrill, Ruiz, & Garofalo, 2010). Optimism also helps promote a parasympathetic nervous system response that encourages the body to return to normal prestress levels.

There are several factors linked with optimism that work to help reduce stress and its impact. First, those who are optimistic generally tend to practice healthier behaviors, such as following a healthy diet, scheduling regular doctors' visits, and engaging in regular physical activity (Puig-Perez et al., 2017). As discussed in previous chapters, these behaviors work to reduce stress. Optimism also supports motivation. If you feel optimistic about a task or assignment, you are more likely to be motivated to complete it and see the positive outcome. Additionally, optimism increases your level of engagement when completing work or tasks (Puig-Perez et al., 2017).

**Being more engaged and optimistic about a task may help reduce the stress associated with that task.**

Generally, people who are optimistic feel they are in control of their life and outcomes. They view life's challenges as achievable and work to address and mitigate those challenges (Avvenuti, Baiardini, & Giardini, 2016). As a result, work doesn't get left undone or put aside for later, both of which contribute to stress.

Although to some degree optimism is a personality trait you are born with, it can also be cultivated with practice. Some ways to encourage a more optimistic outlook include the following:

- *Practice mindfulness.* Practicing mindfulness can improve many different areas of your life and will be seen throughout this textbook. Focusing on the moment can reduce regret over the past or worry about the future.
- *Practice gratitude.* Instead of focusing on what you don't have, gratitude encourages thinking about what do you have in life. A gratitude journal is an exercise that involves writing down the things you are grateful for each day.

- *Pay attention to positive emotions.* The simple act of writing down your positive emotions has been shown to increase optimism. This takes attention away from the negative emotions and places prominence and weight on the positive ones.

## Positive Self-Talk

During each encounter, task, and performance you engage in, you maintain inner dialogue about the task at hand. Your negative inner dialogue (such as "I can't do this" or "I will never understand this problem"), known as thought distortion, may work to protect you from possible failure by encouraging you to give up. However, if you continue, you will make it hard on yourself to try new and challenging things. **Positive self-talk** is using your inner dialogue in a manner that promotes self-esteem, uses optimism to support your efforts, and encourages you to try new things. Even if you fail, you can use positive self-talk such as "I see what I did wrong; next time, I won't make the same mistake" to reflect on your experience and learn from it.

When you are under stress, positive self-talk can be used to reduce feelings of anxiety and give you a better sense of control over the situation. It allows you to prepare for stress and gives you the confidence you need to effectively manage it. Those who use positive self-talk strategies have been shown to have lower levels of self-reported stress, feel more capable of managing stress, and believe their stress management skills will lead to better outcomes (Olyaiekhachic, Bozorgnejad, Haghani, Khayeri, & Seyedfatemi, 2020). One way to think of positive self-talk is to think of yourself encouraging a friend. We tend to be very hard on ourselves, but when we see a friend doing the same thing, we can show them compassion and kindness.

**Think of your inner voice as a friend and direct it to be kind and supportive.**

Being able to recognize your own thought distortion is a great way to start thinking about changing those patterns. The following are some strategies to help you increase your positive self-talk. Common thought distortions and more specific ways to overcome them are described in more detail in the next chapter.

- *Identify negative self-talk situations.* Are there certain situations that you know will bring about negative self-talk? Perhaps you get nervous taking tests and become self-critical or have anxiety about meeting new people and talk down to yourself at a party. Being able to identify these traps can help you prepare for these events and use language that is compassionate and supportive.
- *Identify specific reasons why your negative thoughts are false.* For example, if you think "I can never do it," consider a time when you thought something was too hard but you succeeded. After some practice (lots of practice), you will find yourself naturally finding evidence to counter negative thoughts.
- *Practice positive affirmations.* Practice saying (out loud or to yourself) positive affirmations or statements that promote self-empowerment. It may seem silly to talk to yourself at first, but with practice, it will become second nature. Examples of positive affirmations include:
    - "I can do this."
    - "I am doing my best."
    - "I am in charge of my own happiness."
    - "I love myself for who I am."
    - "I am worth it."
    - "I am grateful."
- *Create boundaries.* There may be people in your life who are a negative influence or bring out negative self-talk. Give yourself permission to separate yourself from these people. Surround yourself with people who are kind and encouraging, and remove or limit the time you spend with people who bring you or others down.

## Laughter

Have you heard the phrase "laughter is the best medicine"? It seems there is some truth to that saying: Laughter has been shown to improve both physiological and psychological health outcomes. It has been shown to decrease levels of cortisol, epinephrine, and growth hormones, as well as to help reduce depressive symptoms and improve overall mood (Yim, 2016). What exactly is laughter and how can a person increase laughter in their life?

The research describes two types of laughter. The first is spontaneous laughter, the type that is associated with a trigger (such as seeing something funny or hearing a joke). The second type is simulated laughter, which is voluntary (think of a person performing a fake laugh). As you can imagine, laughter therapy would be difficult to initiate if the focus is on creating spontaneous laughter, which requires subjective stimuli. Simulated laughter therapies therefore involve exercises like clapping, dancing, vocalizing laughter-like sounds, and breathing exercises; these have been shown to reduce depression and stress and improve overall emotional wellness (van der Wal & Kok, 2019).

In the past, many sitcoms had laugh tracks or live audiences that would laugh during the funny scenes in order to give viewers the feeling that they are part of the show. The thought was that hearing others laugh gives you permission and encouragement to laugh. However, laugh tracks have fallen off in popularity in more recent years, perhaps to our detriment: One study found that listening to other people laugh has been shown to have positive effects on stress (Fujiwara & Okamura, 2018). Maybe those laugh tracks will make a comeback.

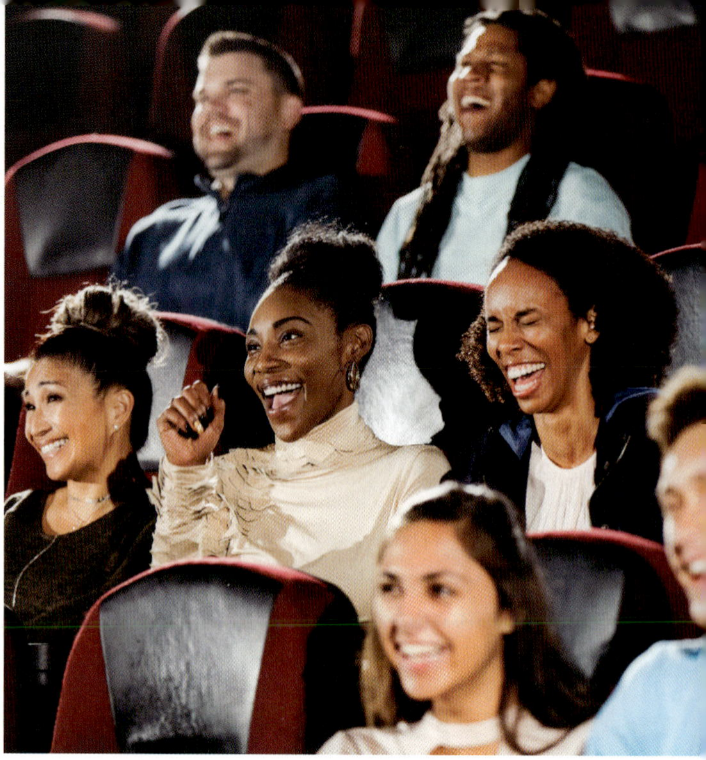

## Summary

Your emotional state can have a large impact on your levels of stress. Negative emotions such as anger, anxiety, and fear can serve as a barrier to managing stress, creating a cycle of increased stress and increased negative emotions. On the other hand, positive emotions can give you the confidence to better manage your stress. When stress is caused by something outside of your control, learning how to manage your emotional response can help you focus on things that are directly under your control, leading to better stress management.

## ONLINE RESOURCES

Visit HK*Propel* to access audio supplements, worksheets, and vocabulary flash cards for this chapter.

## DISCUSSION QUESTIONS

1. What is anger, and how does it contribute to stress? What are specific ways you can manage anger?
2. How does learning to be more aware of your emotions contribute to stress management?
3. Of the ways to improve emotional wellness presented in this chapter, which one resonates most with you? How will you incorporate that strategy into your daily routine?
4. Describe the impact self-talk has on your ability to manage stress and emotions.

6

# Intellectual Wellness

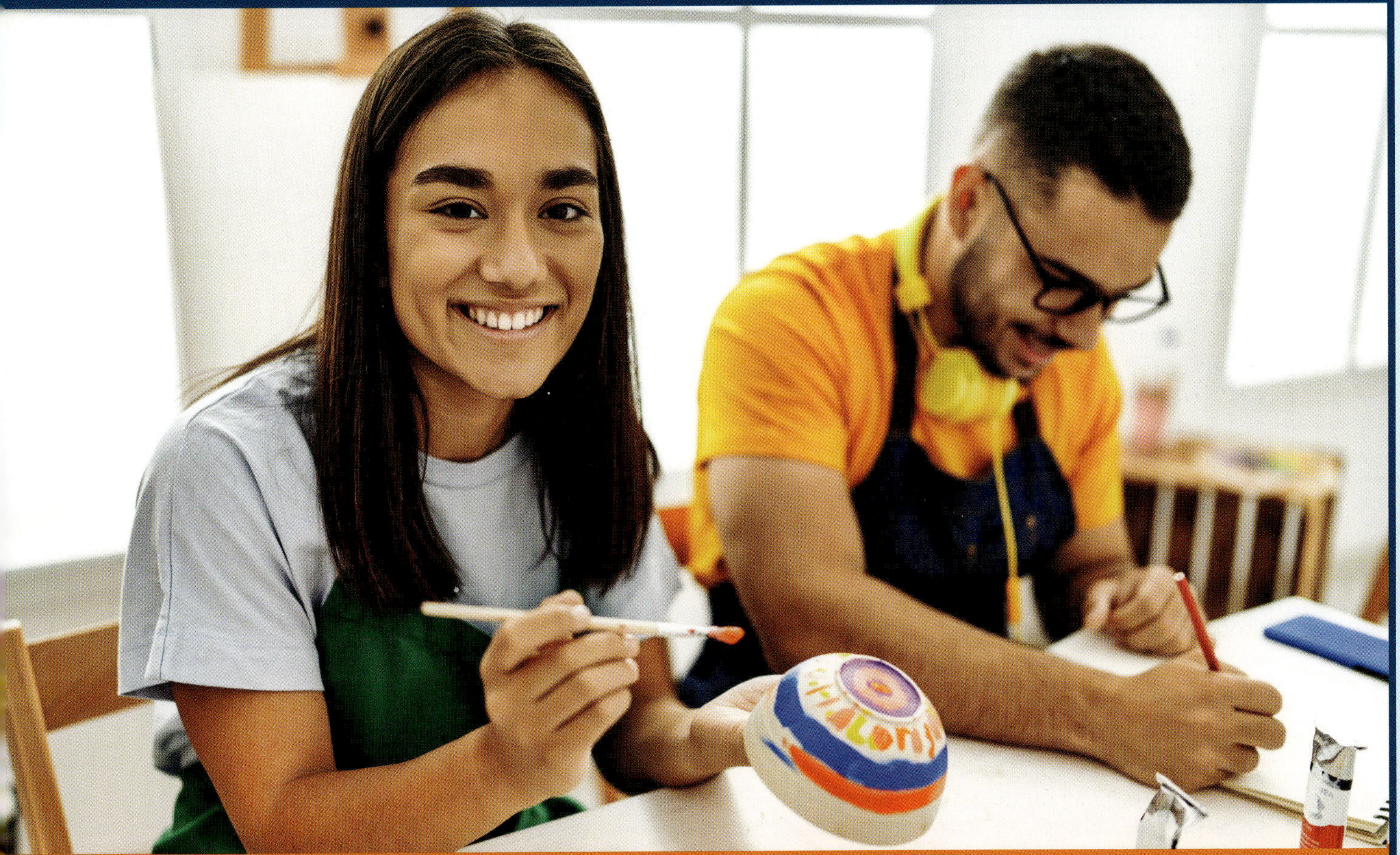

## LEARNING OBJECTIVES

After reading this chapter, you will be able to do the following:

- Define intellectual wellness and identify ways to improve it
- Explain the relationship between stress and intellectual wellness
- Construct a personal goal using the SMART goal principles
- Utilize the five-step problem-solving technique
- Utilize reframing, the ABCDE model, and affirmations to change distorted thinking
- Describe the difference between a growth and fixed mindset

# KEY TERMS

affirmations
creative thinking
distorted thinking
divergent thinking
goal disengagement
goal reengagement
goal-setting theory
growth mindset
mental imagery
neuroplasticity
reframing
visualization

Intellectual wellness is a person's ability and desire to continue learning throughout a lifetime. It includes being open to new ideas, being able to think critically, and being creative. Like other areas of wellness, intellectual wellness is a continuous action that shifts as you engage in different experiences. Intellectual wellness can also be referred to as lifelong learning. Imagine you are looking for a new doctor: You likely want a doctor who attends conferences and reads scientific journals to stay current in the field, rather than one who hasn't done much to stay up-to-date since medical school.

Like the body, the mind requires exercise to stay fit. Actively engaging your brain makes it work more efficiently and effectively and helps neurons form new connections, resulting in a decreased risk of age-related mental decline (Melnyk, 2018). Children are usually excited to ask questions and learn more about the world around them. As adults, we tend to be quieter about our interest, but you can learn to embrace your natural curiosity—every time you learn a new skill or challenge your way of thinking, you are improving your intellectual wellness. However, stress impedes your ability to learn, think, and be creative. This chapter will identify the ways stress can harm intellectual wellness, describe ways to enhance your intellectual wellness, and present intellectual strategies to manage stress.

## Benefits of Intellectual Wellness

The more you engage in activities that promote intellectual wellness, the easier those activities become. This is because working your brain makes it function better, just like exercising a muscle (Zechner, Pratt, Barrett, Dreker, & Santos, 2019). Intellectual wellness enhances memory power, recall, and concentration (Wickramarathne, Phuoc, & Albattat, 2020). Compare your first semester at college to a later semester. Did you find it getting easier? Part of this is likely a result of improved time management strategies, but another part is your improved ability to focus and learn.

**The more you use your mind, the easier learning becomes.**

As one ages, mental productivity and functioning declines, and the risk for Alzheimer's disease and dementia increases. Engaging the mind can help reduce the risk of developing those diseases (Zhang et al., 2021). In a longitudinal study, the Rush Memory and Aging Project, researchers found that cognitively active seniors were 2.6 times less likely to develop dementia than seniors with less cognitive activity (Bennett et al., 2013). The more you engage your mind, the less likely you are to lose functioning.

## Intellectual Wellness and Stress

Studies have shown three main effects of stress on creative thinking and intellectual wellness: inhibition, promotion, or an inverted U-shaped function (Wang et al., 2019). The inverted U-shaped function, also known as the Yerkes-Dodson law, was presented in chapter 2. This law posits that optimal levels of stress promote motivation and increase creativity levels in the brain. When stress is too low, motivation and arousal are decreased along with functioning; when stress is too high, creative thinking and cognitive functioning are impaired.

Let's highlight this example by looking at a study conducted on rats (Joesl, Pu, Wiegert, Oitzl, & Krugers, 2006). Researchers trained rats to find a raised platform while swimming in a water maze

Research Spotlight

## Time Pressure and Creativity

Most employers want to hire creative problem solvers who can get the job done, but researchers have found that creative thinking can be hindered or promoted by the perception of stress in the workplace. If the stressor is perceived as a positive challenge, creative thinking and idea generation are improved. On the other hand, if stress is perceived as a hindrance, creative thinking is diminished (Ren & Zhang, 2015). Similarly, a time crunch or deadline can serve to either promote or hinder work and creativity: When the stressor holds meaning to an employee, it creates a condition where creativity can flow (Yu & Wang, 2022). Teresa Amabile, a professor at Harvard Business School, explains four stress conditions at work and how they relate to creativity (Amabile, 1988; Ramos, Figueiredo, & Pereira-Guizzo, 2018):

1. *On a treadmill*. The work is high pressure but low in meaning. An example of this type of work is on a production line, where the task is highly repetitive and stressful but not very engaging intellectually or creatively.
2. *On autopilot*. The work is low pressure and low in meaning. These jobs have low amounts of stress but also low amounts of creativity.
3. *On an expedition*. The work is low pressure but high in meaning. Creativity also thrives in these positions.
4. *On a mission*. The work is high pressure but is also high in meaning. This is a fast-paced and stressful environment, but creativity also thrives here.

Even if your job feels like being on a treadmill or on autopilot, there are ways to find meaning in your work. Consider how your job fits into the big picture and how it helps others. You are in control of how you choose to perceive your work and your role. Set small achievable goals for yourself and be proud of your accomplishments. This will make the job more enjoyable and allow you to nurture your creative side while encouraging optimal levels of stress.

and measured the increase in the stress hormone corticosteroid to determine the amount of stress the rats experienced (which is positively related to the memory of the maze up to one week after training). The researchers then lowered the temperature of the water to induce additional stress. Again, the increased levels of corticosteroid hormones were positively associated with memory. However, this only works to a certain degree—when the corticosteroid levels became too high, memory decreased, and the rats were unable to find the raised platform in the maze. This highlights how memory and learning are positively associated with stress only up to a certain threshold. Individual thresholds can vary based on stress management techniques and genetics. This example may help explain why some people experience an increase in creativity after procrastination and attribute the motivation to stress.

For others, however, increased stress can negatively impact intellectual wellness. In a study to determine how stress impacts creative thinking, researchers found that stress reduces the brain's ability to initiate the early phases of creative cognition, which impedes the ability to write; this is commonly known as writer's block (Wang et al., 2019).

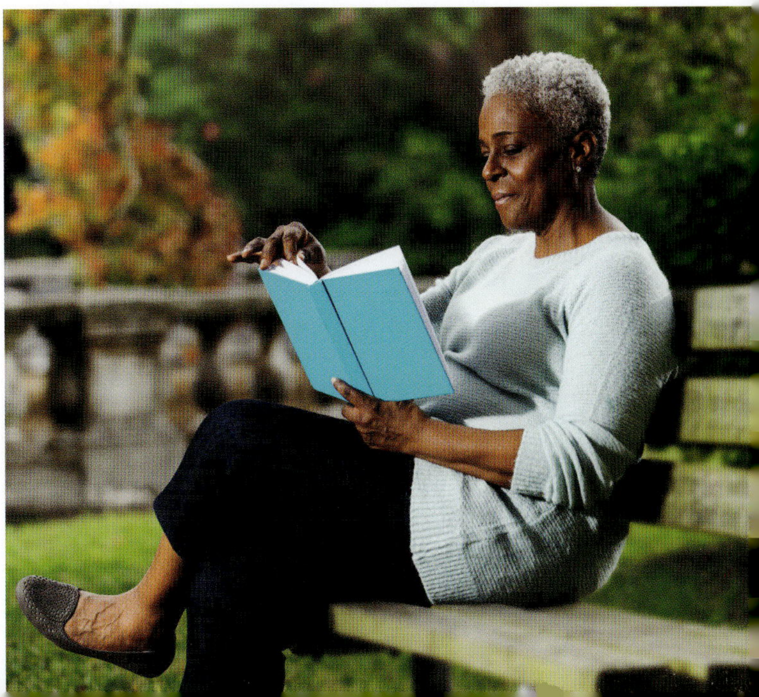

## Enhancing Intellectual Wellness

Regularly engaging your brain enhances your intellectual wellness—but what exactly does it mean to engage your brain? One college professor used to tell his class that calculus is like weight-lifting for the brain. Fortunately for most of us, there are many different ways to engage the mind to promote intellectual wellness.

**Creative thinking** is the ability to gain new insight on an issue and to generate original and useful ideas (Wang et al., 2019). It encourages an openness to others and helps facilitate communication. For these reasons, it is one of the most sought-after job skills among employers (Ritter, Gu, Crijns, & Biekens, 2020). Creative thinking is an important part of intellectual wellness because it enhances self-awareness (Bell, Limberg, Jacobson, & Super, 2014). Utilizing creative thinking can help you manage stress by allowing you to view problems through a variety of lenses.

One aspect of creative thinking is **divergent thinking**, or the ability to consider ideas from different perspectives. In his blog, Nick Wignall (2018) identifies ways to practice and improve your divergent thinking skills.

- *The "many uses" exercise.* This exercise involves taking an object and coming up with alternative uses for it—for example, Wignall's list of alternative uses for a paper clip includes power cord organizer, SIM card opener, Easter egg holder for dyeing eggs, shower head declogger, and bookmark (Wignall, 2018). What other uses can you come up with?
- *10 new ideas.* Every day for a week, come up with 10 ideas within a given category—for example, 10 ideas for vacation spots, science fiction books, bedroom layouts, and so forth.
- *Daily headlines.* At the end of the day, take a few minutes to go over the highlights of your day. Who were the major players? What were the points of drama or conflict? Come up with three headlines to summarize your day.
- *Articles on trial.* Read an article each day and come up with a question to ask the author that challenges their conclusion. Give yourself bonus points if you come up with an alternative conclusion.
- *Automatic to alternate thoughts.* This technique asks you to identify your automatic thoughts and try to generate alternatives to that thought. Automatic thoughts can be problematic because they become habitually negative and tend to assume the worst. For example, if you get cut off on the road, what is your automatic thought? Many people would swear at the other driver and get angry. What are some alternative thoughts? Perhaps that person is rushing to the hospital or a job interview. Or maybe they simply didn't see your car.

These exercises can also help you develop your ability to see things from multiple perspectives. Moreover, they can broaden your ability to communicate with others as you make efforts to see the world through their lens.

> **Allowing yourself to view an issue from a different perspective without judgment can provide you with a better understanding of the issue.**

Another way to enhance your intellectual wellness is to learn new things, which keeps your brain actively engaged. You might learn a new language, pick up a new instrument, or start a new hobby. You can also play puzzle or logic games. These can be enjoyable experiences that engage your brain at the same time. Lastly, practice self-reflection. Allow yourself to have some quiet time to reflect on your day, life, or just one problem.

## Goal Setting and Stress

Part of intellectual wellness is being able to set goals for yourself and create a plan to achieve those goals. Not knowing which direction to go in life can be very stressful. Goal setting transfers an idea from abstract to concrete, providing you with insight on which path to follow to get where you want to be. Let's say you are late to a friend's party, but you have lost their address. You know approximately where they live but not the specific location; although you have a general idea

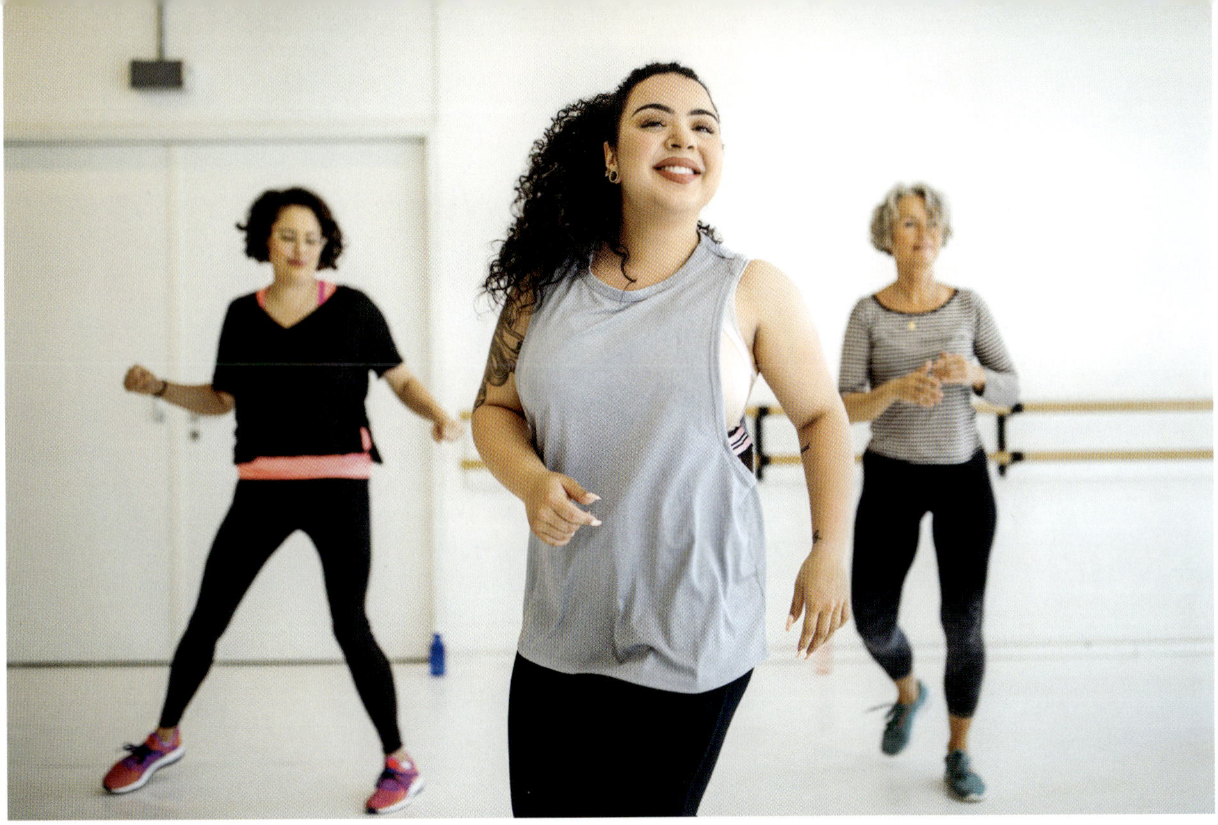

The more defined and specific your goal, the easier it is for you to map out your course.

of which direction to go, the only way to find it is to drive around feeling stressed. Goals operate the same way. The vaguer your goal, the harder it is to create a plan to achieve it. This causes additional stress as you make wrong turns in your attempt to reach your goal. However, if your goal is specific, you will know exactly where you are going.

Setting goals has been shown to improve academic performance, cognitive learning, and intrinsic motivation and can help make you more adaptable to change (Belenky & Nokes-Malach, 2012). However, goals can also be a source of stress. Recall that stress is a response to change, and the act of setting a goal is, in itself, creating change in your life. Even when the goal is positive and will enhance your life in the long run, it creates stress because it is a change to your everyday routine.

Not all goals are the same. There are large goals and smaller goals, important and less important goals, and long-term and short-term goals. Each of these will produce different amounts of stress. If your goal is to reach 10,000 steps in one day, it would probably not produce a lot of anxiety because it is short term and achievable. However, if the goal is set to reach 25,000 steps in a day, you may experience higher levels of stress. And if your goal is to run a marathon in two weeks—which may not be realistic or achievable—it can be a major source of stress. Making unrealistic goals sets you up for failure, which can cause you to feel bad about yourself and increase your stress.

Similarly, some goals are more important than others. If your goal is to finish college and today is your very first day, you may feel some anxiety because the end seems very far away. On the other hand, if your goal is to attend all of your classes this week, this probably doesn't feel as daunting. This section will identify ways to set realistic and manageable goals to help you reduce stress.

Many important goals we set for ourselves are long term. One way to help the brain cope with setting long-term goals is to set smaller goals that will help move you closer to accomplishing your long-term goal. For example, if your long-term goal is finishing college, setting smaller goals for each semester can help you focus on the now (figure 6.1). This provides you with a sense of control and an opportunity to celebrate your accomplishments every time you achieve a smaller goal.

Providing meaning to your goals may also work to reduce stress. Research shows that understanding why a goal is important to you provides the additional motivation to achieve it (Creed, Sawitri, Hood, & Hu, 2020). For example, many students have the goal of completing a college degree to

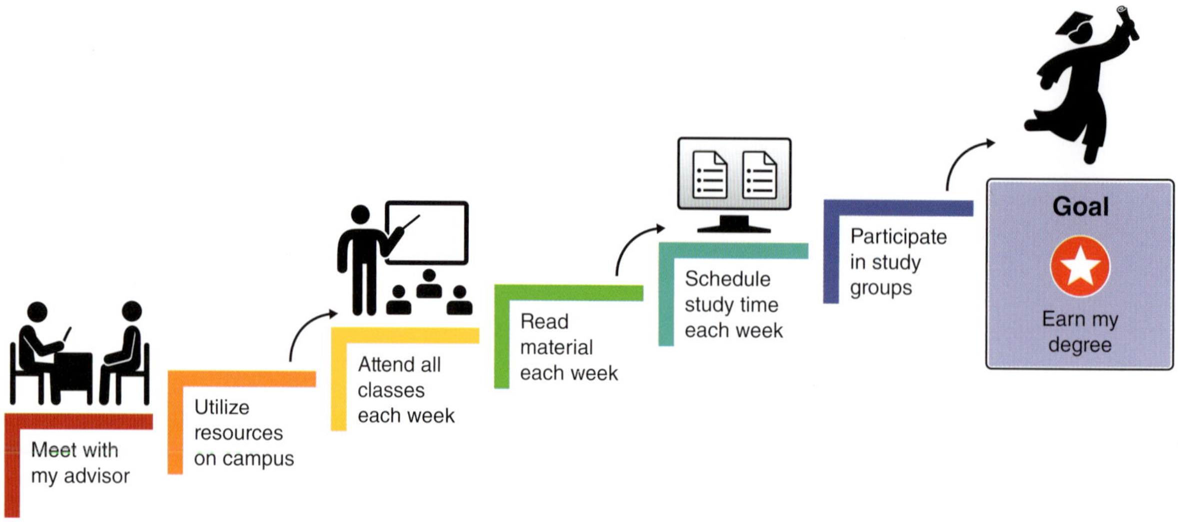


**Figure 6.1** Start with small goals and work your way toward larger ones.

help them get a job that can provide some financial stability and security. Career indecision, or having no clear goal of what to do after college, is related to higher levels of stress among students. Not surprisingly, career indecision among students in college was also associated with lower work efforts toward obtaining a college degree.

What you tell yourself about your goal can reduce or heighten the stress surrounding that goal. If you are constantly telling yourself that you will not achieve your goals and then give up on them, you will most likely feel heightened levels of stress. Additionally, if you choose not to set goals to avoid feeling disappointed, daily meaning and engagement may be lowered. The following are some guidelines that can help you maintain motivation and a sense of accomplishment in goal setting (Locke & Lathan, 2019).

**It is important to develop your ultimate "why" when setting goals for yourself. It will help improve your efforts toward achieving your goal and minimize stress along the way.**

- *Set the right goals.* Make sure you are following the SMART guidelines for setting goals (described in the next section).
- *Take small, measurable steps.* Create smaller short-term goals along the way to help you get closer to your long-term goal.
- *Reward yourself along the way.* Acknowledge your effort and success and celebrate your accomplishments.
- *Consider slip-ups to be part of the process.* Cut yourself some slack when you fall short. Talk to yourself as you would a friend.

When deciding on what type of goal to set, take a few minutes to think about your current state of mind. If you feel stressed or overwhelmed, it may be best to set goals that will take items off your plate and make your load lighter. If, on the other hand, you have normal amounts of stress, you may want to identify things you want to achieve and set goals to achieve them.

**Goal-setting theory** states that realistic and challenging goals contribute to better task performance (Aarts, 2019). If you set goals that are too easy or too difficult, you will not feel motivated to complete them—just like Goldilocks, they must be just right to help support motivation and your effort in achieving them. The following elements should be considered when setting goals (Buenaventura, Fajatin, Samaniego, Villagracia, & Reyes, 2022):

- *External factors.* The factors surrounding you can help or hinder you in achieving your goal. What supports do you have? What barriers will you face? How can you manage those barriers to help you achieve your goal?

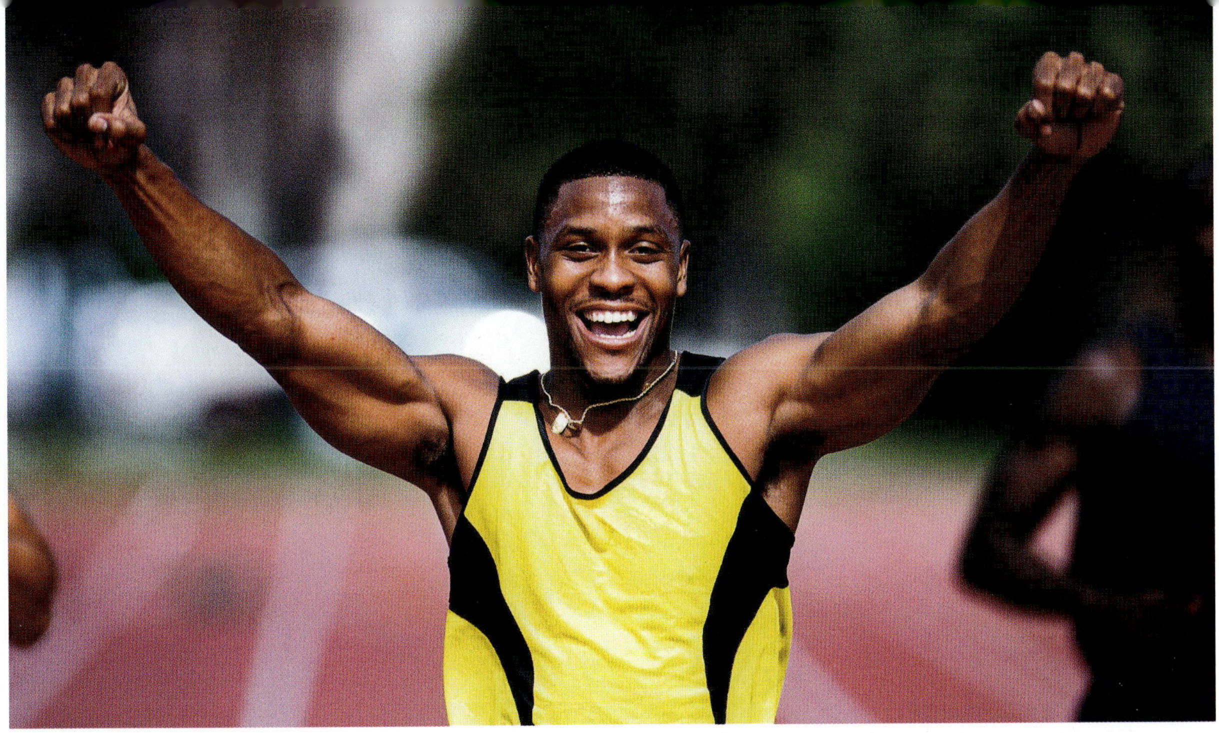

- *Clarity.* Is your goal clear and concise? Do you know exactly what it means and stands for?
- *Challenge.* Goals should be challenging, but not too challenging. Does your goal feel achievable or out of reach?
- *Self-efficacy.* Self-efficacy is your belief in your ability to achieve your goals. How confident do you feel that you can reach your goal? Do you feel you have the necessary skills to obtain your goal?
- *Commitment.* The more committed you feel, the greater the likelihood of achieving your goals. Some ways to help you remain committed include setting routines, seeking out inspiration, and keeping an eye on the big picture (Locke & Lathan, 2019).

As you work toward your goal, it is important to recognize and applaud your efforts. What have you done today, this week, or this month to bring you closer to your goal? Acknowledging the work you have put in and celebrating small successes will help you build momentum toward reaching your goals.

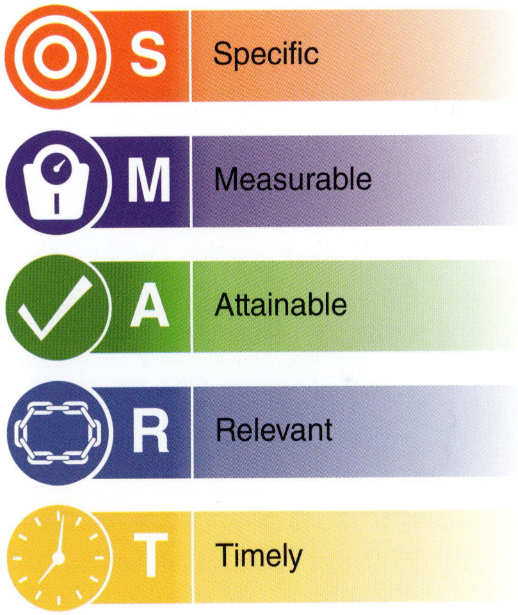


**Figure 6.2** Use the SMART acronym to help you devise clear and manageable goals.

## SMART Goals

SMART goals are a method to help you write effective and manageable goals that are specific, measurable, attainable, relevant, and timely (figure 6.2). This may seem like a lot of steps to write a goal, but it is worth it! SMART goals are effective because they help make goals concrete and attainable, moving you from a mentality of wishing for something to a mentality of doing something (Lathan, 2011).

### Specific

Your goals should be specific and should focus on the behaviors and actions you will take to reach your goal. For example, rather than "be more

## A SMART Meditation Goal

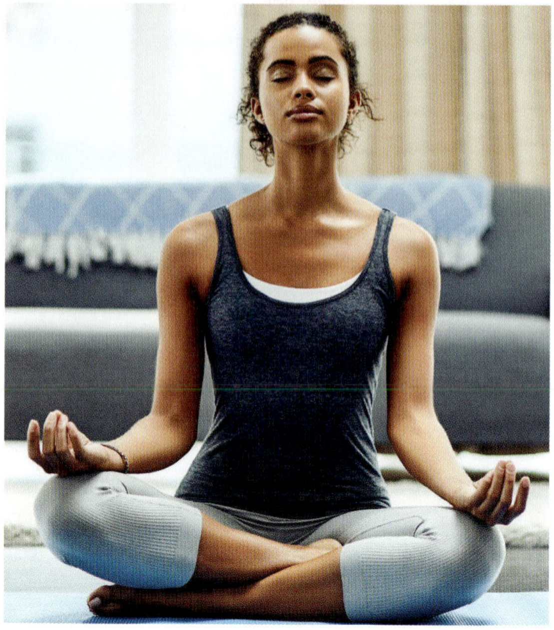

Let's say your goal is to reduce stress in your life. What would reduced stress look like? A more specific goal would be that you will practice meditation to reduce your stress.

How will you measure your progress? If you have never meditated and begin by attempting one hour each day, you will likely try it for a day or two, get frustrated, and give up. Remember, your goals should require effort but be within your reach. However, meditating for three minutes each day is achievable. Your goal could state you will practice meditation for three minutes in the morning at least five days a week.

The goal of meditating is relevant and important to you because you want to reduce stress in your life. This provides meaning to the goal, which will fuel your motivation to achieve it.

Finally, how will you know when you have achieved your goal? You have provided no end date to assess your accomplishment. You will practice meditation for three minutes in the morning five days a week for the next four weeks. At the end, you will reconsider your stress levels to evaluate whether your engagement in meditation has met your ultimate goal of reduced stress.

active," a specific goal might be "I will train to run a 5K." Questions to ask yourself to create a specific goal include:

- What do I want to achieve?
- What behaviors will I engage in to reach my goal?

### Measurable

Your goals need to be measurable—that is, they should contain some type of number or measurable quantity to help you track your progress and determine when you have completed the task. Let's return to your 5K goal. How long and how often will you train? These pieces are important to allow you to know when you have reached your goal. For example, perhaps you will run for 45 minutes three days a week. Questions to ask yourself to create a measurable goal include:

- How will I know if I am on the right path to achieving my goal?
- What numbers can I use to measure my goal?

### Achievable

Your goals need to be achievable. They should be difficult enough to keep you motivated, but not so difficult they are unrealistic. Running a 5K is likely doable with moderate training. Now let's say you want to run a marathon in one month and you have not run or engaged in any meaningful exercise in the past five years. This goal is not realistic and you are likely setting yourself up for failure. Think about your goal as an apple on a tree that is just within your reach, but you need to stand on your tiptoes and stretch. This is how your goal should feel. If the apple is too high in the tree, you will not be able to reach it no matter how you stretch. This is an unattainable goal. Questions to ask yourself to create an achievable goal include:

- Am I being realistic?
- Do I have the means or tools to reach my goal?

### Relevant

Your goals should be relevant to your life. Create goals that are important and meaningful to you. If the goal has no personal meaning to you, it will be difficult to stay motivated. Questions to ask yourself to create a relevant goal include:

- Does this goal fit into my life plan?
- Does it help me get closer to achieving something important to me?
- Am I excited about reaching this goal?

### Time Bound

Goals need to be time bound—that is, they need to have an end in place. For example, your goal could be to run for 45 minutes three days a week for eight weeks (following a program on a running app), at the end of which you will enter a 5K race. It is best to put these dates in your goal to allow you to see the end point. Questions to ask yourself to create a time-bound goal include:

- What is the time frame to accomplish my goal?
- Are there tasks I need to accomplish first?
- Can I break the goal into smaller chunks?

There may be times when you realize that your goal is simply not obtainable and you will have to quit. When you realize your efforts to achieve a goal will not be fruitful, it is best to reduce your effort and commitment, called **goal disengagement**. After you have disengaged from the goal, it is time to work on creating a new and attainable goal, called **goal reengagement**. In this process, you recommit to achieving a new goal with a new purpose. Being able to drop a goal that is no longer serving you and focus your energy elsewhere will help you better manage your stressors.

## Problem Solving

Think about the last time you encountered a problem. Did you feel stressed? How did you go about solving the problem? Did you approach it systematically or just wing it? Learning how to manage problems can help reduce stress and make life's challenges more manageable. Effective problem solving engages your intellectual wellness and critical thinking skills. The following steps will help you improve your problem-solving skills.

**You can practice techniques to help you become a better problem solver.**

### Step 1: Defining the Problem

First, you must clearly define the problem. This is the most important part of the process because you cannot begin to solve a problem without having a clear understanding of it. Consider the following example: Your English midterm grade is a D. It would be easy to say that getting the D is the problem, but that doesn't explain the issue and will not assist in finding a meaningful solution. Why you are getting a D? Is it because you are not attending classes? Is it because you have not handed in assignments? When considering the cause of the problem, you realize that your writing skills need improvement. Now you can come up with strategies to improve your writing skills, leading to an improved grade in class. When problems are ill-defined, they tend to be solved in a way that doesn't address the real problem so that you find yourself facing similar problems in the future. For example, you might have just asked the professor for extra credit, but you would have found yourself continuing to earn poor grades for

### SMART Goals, Workdays, and Stress

Think about your normal day. Do you start each day unsure of how it will go? Or do you begin with a goal and work to achieve that goal? Research shows that setting daily goals can create and support a positive work environment while reducing stress and fatigue.

The process of daily goal setting can help you create a plan to perform your daily tasks more efficiently. It helps provide focus and a sense of accomplishment each day, reducing the stress related to the daily demands of life (Weintraub, Cassell, & DePatie, 2021). Spend a few minutes at the beginning of each day thinking about what you would like to accomplish. Identify the barriers to obtaining that daily goal and ways to overcome those barriers.

your writing in other classes. Ask yourself the following questions to help you define the problem:

- What is the problem?
- What is contributing to the problem?
- What parts of the problem do I have control over?

> If I were given one hour to save the world, I would spend 59 minutes defining the problem and one minute solving it.
>
> **Albert Einstein**

## Step 2: Brainstorm Ideas

Now that you have your problem defined, you can start thinking of solutions. Try to come up with as many ideas as you can for solving the problem. For this step, there is no judgment—look at the problem from all angles, and do not limit the possibilities. In the previous example, you have defined the problem as a lack of writing skills. Some ways to solve the problem might include the following:

- Hire a tutor
- Utilize the college's writing center
- Talk with professor about ways to improve
- Create a study group with students from the class
- Ask the professor if you can revise past assignments
- Drop the class and take it again the following semester

## Step 3: Analyze the Solutions

Now is the time to pass judgment on the ideas. For each idea, and consider the following:

- Will it solve the problem?
- What are the advantages of this solution?
- What are the disadvantages of this solution?
- Will the solution cause any new problems? If so, what are they?
- How do you feel about this solution?

Using the solutions from step 2, an analysis could provide you with these points:

- Hire a tutor
  - Expensive—would need to work more hours or get a different job to afford one
  - Would help with writing skills
  - Would work around my schedule
- Utilize the college's writing center
  - Free
  - Would have to go during their open hours, may not be as convenient
  - May have to wait in a long line
  - May feel rushed
  - Unsure about the process
- Talk with professor about ways to improve
  - Nervous about talking with the professor
  - Would be personalized help
  - Would probably improve grade
  - Professor may offer other options I haven't considered
- Create a study group with students from the class
  - Don't know that many students in class
  - Nervous about telling people I am not doing well in class
  - Others in class might also benefit from a study group
  - Would be nice to get to know other students in class
- Ask the professor if I can revise past assignments
  - Nervous about talking with the professor
  - Need to read the syllabus carefully to review the course policies
  - Would improve my grade
  - Might learn from specific writing mistakes
- Drop the class and take it again the following semester
  - Would alleviate my stress about my grade

- Would feel like a failure this semester
- Already paid for class and would have to pay for it again
- Would have to admit to my parents that I was going to fail a class

### Step 4: Take Action

After analyzing your list, choose the best solution (or two) for your problem. In our example, you can choose two options. First, you decide to speak with the professor about ways to improve your grade. You will then utilize the college's writing center to help you improve your writing skills.

### Step 5: Reflect

After using a solution, reflect on its effectiveness. The following questions can help guide your reflection:

- Did it solve your problem?
- Were any parts of the problem still around after implementing the solution?
- What parts of the solution worked well? What parts didn't work well?
- If you had to do it again, what would you have done differently?

Utilizing a problem-solving process tends to lead to better solutions, ultimately reducing stress as the outcomes show positive effects in your life. A study on male students found that those who underwent problem-solving and stress management workshops were less likely to become dependent on alcohol or drugs compared to those who didn't undergo workshop training (Abdi & Sharyati, 2019). This can be attributed to possessing better coping skills, which reduces their likelihood of turning to alcohol and drugs to manage life's problems.

Consider again the example of getting a D on your English midterm. Let's say you didn't utilize the problem-solving process and eventually failed the course. One potential outcome may be that you feel depressed about failing, start using alcohol to manage your depression, and begin to skip other classes. As this continues, you are now facing additional problems, and your stress continues to rise. The problem-solving process allows you to take control and find solutions (Rastogi et al., 2018). You will find that using this process gets easier with more repetition. You may also find your problems weren't as big as you initially imagined.

## Changing Distorted Thinking

"I will never be good at math!" "I overslept and now the whole day is going to be awful!" Have you ever said these things to yourself or heard them from others? These are examples of what is commonly referred to as **distorted thinking**. Distorted thinking may have evolved as an ancient adaptive behavior to keep humans aware of dangerous environments or alter our experiences with previous trauma (Gilbert, 1998; McCarroll, 2017). However, in modern times, these distorted thought processes do not serve the same purpose and only result in increased levels of emotional stress by putting a negative spin on events and experiences (Jha et al., 2021).

### Identifying Thinking Distortions

When you are under stress, you are more likely to engage in distorted thinking because it is what you have always done (Skalski, Konaszewski, Bussing, & Surzykiewics, 2022). This section will help you recognize 10 common types of thinking distortions and ways to overcome them.

#### *Type 1: Polarized Thinking*

This type of thinking, also called *all-or-nothing thinking*, occurs when everything is viewed from the perspective of one of the two extremes—completely good or bad—with no middle ground or gray area. Those who engage in polarized thinking do not recognize that something can be both good and bad, and they generally allow one negative element to ruin their perception of an entire event. For example, let's say it is raining the morning of your wedding day, but it is expected to clear up in the afternoon. If you engaged in polarized thinking, you would surmise that your outdoor ceremony is ruined and cry the entire day. As you can imagine, this type of thinking would cause a lot of stress and give you little control over the outcome.

One way to combat polarized thinking is to think about the things you can control and acknowledge what is going right. For example, you

> **By shifting your focus to positive things, it allows you to change your thinking pattern and focus on the good.**

can tell yourself, thank goodness the rain will stop this afternoon, and then make plans to reduce the impact of the morning rain by having the wedding planner get there early to wipe down the chairs and lay a runner on the wet grass. In this example, you would experience less stress and have a more positive experience.

### Type 2: Overgeneralized Thinking

In this type of thinking, you take the conclusion of one event and apply it to all events. Take Madison, a softball player who has struck out in the first inning. Madison tells herself she is no good at softball and will strike out for the rest of the game. This type of thinking assumes a negative outcome and produces stress.

To counteract overgeneralized thinking, tell yourself that not meeting your expectation one time does not mean it will always be that way. For example, Madison could tell herself she will do better next time and visualize hitting the ball next time she is up to bat.

### Type 3: Mental Filtering

People who engage in mental filtering will only remember the negative aspects of the event, filtering out the positives. To revisit the wedding example, let's say the ceremony goes quite smoothly despite the morning rain. However, when thinking back on the day, you only remember how stressed you felt while it was raining before the ceremony. This continuous loop of negative thinking promotes stress.

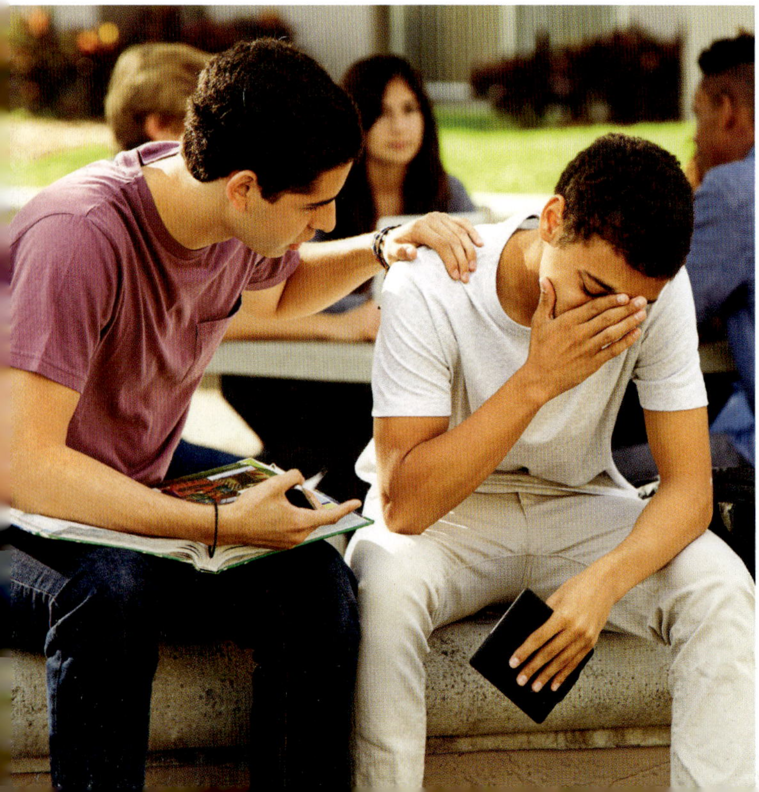

To help avoid this type of thinking, try focusing on the positives of the event. Even if something was truly terrible, look for the silver lining. Perhaps it allowed you to learn something about yourself or provided you with a different perspective. No matter how small, it is important to identify positives in your experiences.

### Type 4: Disqualifying the Positives

This is similar to mental filtering, but in this case, you discredit the positive events in your life and reframe them as negative. For example, let's say you get asked on a date by a person you have a crush on. As you get ready, you start telling yourself your crush must have asked you out because they feel sorry for you or had nothing better to do with their time. These types of thoughts turn what should be a positive situation into a stressful one.

Combating this type of thinking uses the same techniques as mental filtering. Focus on the positives and give yourself credit for them. In the previous example, you could reflect on the positive encounters you have already had with your crush to allow yourself to feel excited and nervous. Use those feelings to think positively about the upcoming date.

### Type 5: Jumping to Conclusions

This occurs when people jump to negative conclusions that are not based on any fact. For example, imagine you pass by a classmate while walking to class and you try to make eye contact and wave, but your classmate just walks by. You wonder what you may have done to upset your classmate and conclude that they do not really like you. This negative assumption can lead to stress based on little evidence.

You can fight those feelings by keeping your thoughts in check. Ask yourself, "Am I sure?" "What makes me think this is true?" Ask yourself if there could possibly be another reason your classmate didn't acknowledge you. Perhaps they were listening to music and not paying attention to their surroundings.

### Type 6: Catastrophizing

This type of thinking occurs when you blow one small piece of evidence out of proportion. Let's say your friend Xavier has a cough, and his doctor tells him it is probably a virus and that he should begin to feel better within a week. After a week, however, Xavier still has a cough. Xavier has now convinced himself it must be lung cancer and has started making funeral plans. This is catastrophic thinking and leads to extreme stress.

If you experience catastrophic thinking, tell yourself there is no reason to assume the worst. Remember times you assumed the worst was going to happen but it didn't—one small negative does not predict other larger negatives occurring.

### Type 7: Identifying With Emotions

In this thought distortion you are assuming that your emotions reflect the objective truth. Think back to the example of getting a D on your English midterm. You might feel discouraged and tell yourself you will never be any good at writing. One poor grade does not mean you are no good at something. It merely means you need to work on a particular skill to improve it. When you find yourself identifying with your emotions, take a step back, acknowledge how you are feeling, and remind yourself emotions are temporary. Create an argument against the emotion. For example, if you feel dumb, remind yourself of your successes and the good grades you have gotten in the past.

### Type 8: Using "Should" Statements

These are statements you tell yourself about the way things should be or what you should have done ("I should have studied today" or "I should be able to run a marathon by now"). Although you may want to do certain things, using "should" is negative self-talk that will only bring you down and increase your guilt and stress if you can't—or don't—accomplish them. Rather, reflect on the activities you have completed. If there is something you need to do, plan time to complete it, focusing on the elements that are under your control.

### Type 9: Labeling

Generally, labeling yourself or others is a negative distortion. For example, you might tell your partner they are a lazy slob because they left their clothes on the floor and not in the hamper. How do you think this makes your partner feel? Just because the clothes didn't make it to the hamper doesn't mean it is a character flaw. The same goes for yourself: If you are struggling with a college class, it doesn't mean you are dumb—rather, it serves as a reminder that this is hard stuff and you need time to fully understand it. Next time you find yourself labeling yourself or others, take a moment to make thoughtful and positive reflection statements.

### Type 10: Personalizing

This distorted thinking occurs when you attribute external experiences to your own influence. For example, if you are hosting a party at your house, you may feel obligated to make sure everyone

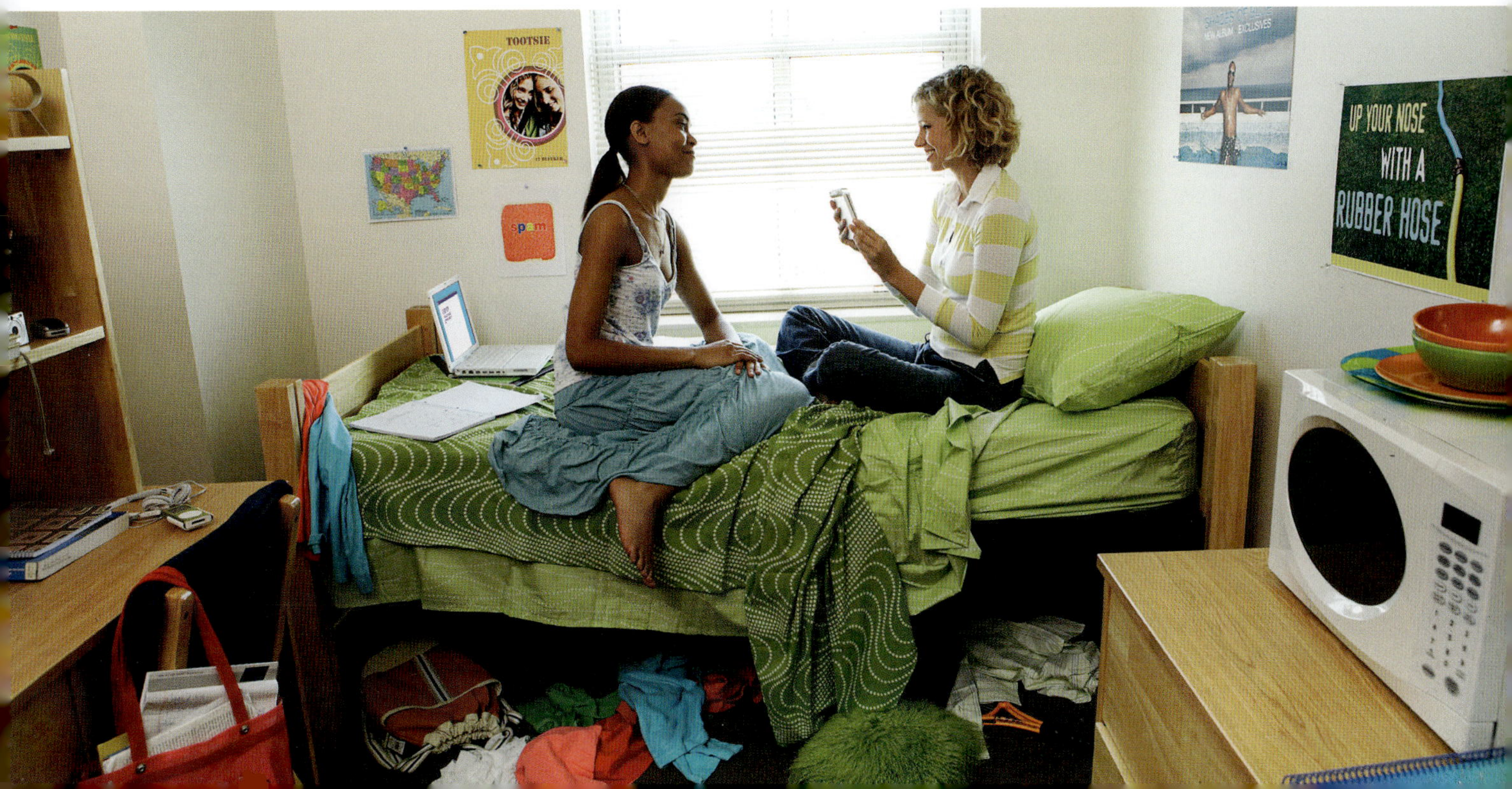

**It is important to continually practice strategies to overrule thought distortions so that your mind doesn't resort to distorted thinking when you are under stress.**

has a good time. This can cause you a lot of stress by making you feel responsible for the experiences of others, which are not under your control. You can set the stage for a nice party by decorating, introducing people, and offering delicious food, but ultimately, whether someone has a good time is not up to you. When you find yourself taking everything personally, start identifying all the things that are outside your control. This will help keep you grounded.

## Reframing

**Reframing** is a technique that can be used to reduce distorted thinking and is described in each of the 10 common distorted thinking categories. It is a technique that is often used in cognitive behavioral therapy and can be very helpful in breaking the cycles of negative thinking and stress (Surmai & Duff, 2022). Here are the steps to start practicing reframing (Harris, 2021).

1. *Start noticing your distorted thinking.* When you find yourself engaging in distorted thinking, take a few moments to identify the problem thought and try to categorize it. As you start noticing your distorted thinking behaviors and patterns, you will find it gets easier to notice them. Sometimes just acknowledging and defining the distorted thought is enough to change the thought
2. *Evaluate the evidence behind your thought.* Consider the distorted thought and provide evidence that disputes your negative thinking, no matter how small. Are you telling yourself you will never be any good at math? Think of previous experiences that show you are good at math. Perhaps you aced an earlier test, or you were able to correctly calculate the tip percentage on your last restaurant bill.
3. *Practice compassion.* We tend to be hard on ourselves, even though we would never use the same harsh language or have the same expectations for friends. When you are being hard on yourself, think about what you would say to a friend. For example, let's say you joined a club at college. At the first meeting, you felt nervous and spoke to a few people but really didn't engage with anyone. Afterward, you tell yourself no one talked to you because you were so boring. Now, if a friend told you the same story, would you tell your friend they are boring? Probably not! You would tell them they were probably just nervous and need to try to be more social next time. You would remind them what a good friend and person they are and how people like to be around them. Use the same kind language for yourself.

Practicing these strategies helps the mind turn to them under stress because they have become familiar. Reframing has been shown to reduce the impact of stress on the body—one study found that those who used reframing to help manage stress showed lower increases in heart rate and blood pressure in response to stress conditions compared to those who didn't use reframing (Liu, Reed, & Vickers, 2019). Other mental techniques to help you manage stress are presented in the next section.

## Using the ABCDE Model

The ABCDE model was created by Albert Ellis, the founder of rational-emotive behavior therapy. Like the reframing technique, it is designed to change distorted and negative thought patterns and help people take better control of their emotions. The ABCDE model consists of the following steps (Muller & Greif, 2022):

- *Activating event or situation.* What event or experience triggers the negative or harmful thoughts? Why does this event trigger negative thoughts? How and when did the negative thoughts begin with this situation?
- *Beliefs.* What are your negative thoughts attached to the event? What do you say to yourself? How do you feel when you encounter the situation? What is running through your mind at this time?
- *Consequences.* This is the starting point to understanding how the negative thoughts

Case Study

## Fear of Flying

Like reframing, the ABCDE approach helps you better your beliefs about certain events or experiences. Consider Beth, who experiences stress when flying. She has only flown a few times in her life, but every time she does, she feels tense and fearful. Beth begins the ABCDE process to help her identify and change her emotions as they relate to airplane travel.

- *Activating event.* The emotions are triggered by flying in an airplane.
- *Beliefs.* Beth is afraid; she feels as though the plane will crash and she will die.
- *Consequences.* As a result of her fear, Beth hates flying. She has missed out on several family reunions because of this fear. Her honeymoon is coming up and she wants to be able to relax on the airplane to their destination.
- *Disputation of beliefs.* Beth begins to research plane crashes and statistics. The chances of being in a plane crash are extremely low. Airplane travel is safer than riding in a car. As she continues her research, she has a better understanding of planes and their safety.
- *Effective new approach.* Beth begins to talk positively to herself about flying. She tells herself she is excited to go on their honeymoon. She imagines what it would feel like not to be afraid on the plane and what it would mean to be able to attend her family reunions more frequently.

Beth got on a short flight and found she was better able to manage her fear. She worked hard to remain positive and, as a result, had a better experience.

### Discussion Questions

1. How does the ABCDE approach help with irrational fear?
2. What is something you are frightened of? Describe your fear. How did it first develop? What is your response when you encounter your fear? How have you changed your behavior to avoid your fear?
3. Use the ABCDE approach to reframe your fear.

impact your life. What are the emotions you experience because of your negative thoughts? What do you feel are the consequences of your negative thoughts? How do they impact your behavior?

- *Disputation of beliefs.* This is the stage where start to challenge your beliefs. Identify the negative thoughts or self-talk you engage in. Actively think of past experiences that counter your negative thinking. How do the current beliefs serve you? How do they hinder you? What would it feel like to have different beliefs about the situation?
- *Effective new approach.* Think of new and positive ways to respond to the situation. How does this new approach make you feel? What would happen if this continued?

## Practicing Affirmations

**Affirmations** are self-affirming statements meant to promote self-confidence and self-efficacy. They include statements such as "I've got this!" "I can do it!" and "I look great!" They can reduce stress by shifting your mind from a lacking or negative perspective to a positive and self-promoting one. Envision a basketball coach talking to the team in the locker room at halftime. Which do you feel would be the better way to approach the team?

- *Option 1.* "All right, team, we made a few mistakes in the first half, but you all really came together. You can do this. We have been practicing these plays the entire year. I have faith in all of you."
- *Option 2.* "You all really bombed this. What happened to all the plays we practiced this

year? Have you forgotten them all? I just don't know what to say. I am disappointed in the way you have all played thus far."

The coach may be better off if they selected option 1. It focuses on the team's strengths and can bolster everyone's self-confidence, which can help them improve on the court. Studies suggest using affirmations can be effective in helping you succeed.

Affirmations can also be used to help you be more proactive in how you approach stressful situations. Imagine Aiden, a young professional, who gets very stressed during his morning commute. Aiden often engages in yelling, name calling, and gestures, and by the time he arrives at work, he feels completely frayed. The next time Aiden leaves for work he can say, "I will remain calm and unaffected while I drive this morning." This allows Aiden to think about how he wants to react and help ground him when he encounters traffic.

Affirmations have been shown to improve a person's well-being and sense of confidence, which can serve as protective factors against stress. People who utilize positive affirmations generally have higher levels of pleasure, enjoyment, and comfort (Sharouni et al., 2022). For example, in a study of high school students, the group who received daily positive affirmations showed significantly lower levels of perceived stress compared to the group who didn't receive them (Morris, 2020). Affirmations may give you more confidence in your ability to tackle your stress head on, which is a much more effective coping mechanism.

**You can use affirmations as part of your daily routine.**

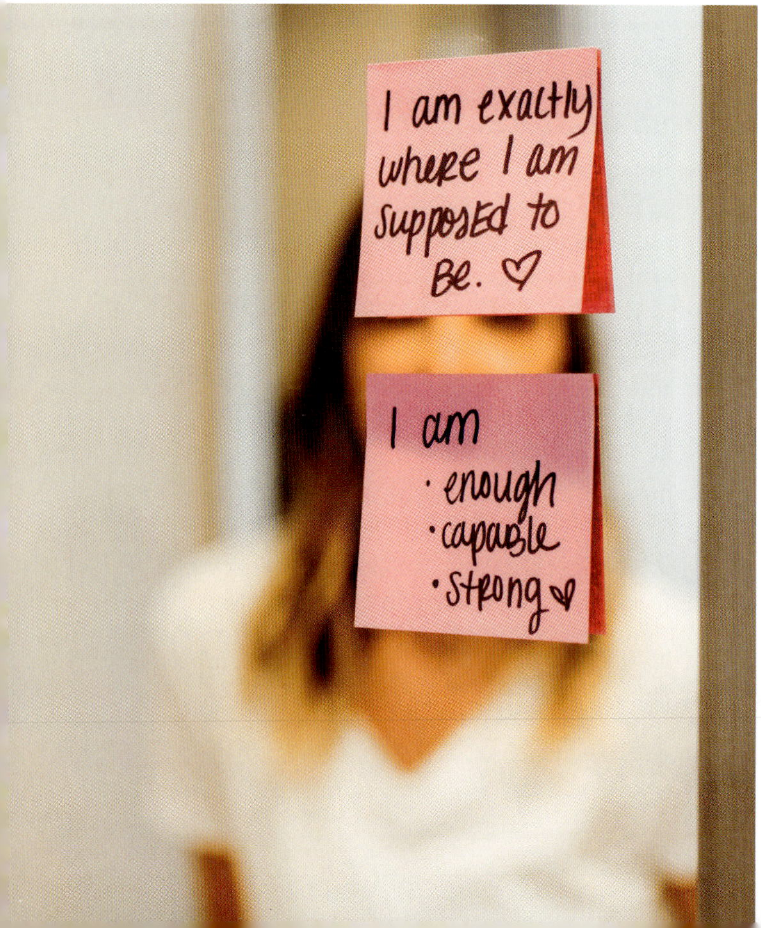
I am exactly where I am supposed to Be.
I am
· enough
· capable
· strong

Affirmations can help you gain better control of your life. You can start each day by telling yourself you are enough, and you are going to have a great day. (Remember, however, that affirmations are not a magic pill: You can tell yourself you will grow wings and fly, but it will not make it come true.) Use them as a tool for positive change. Do you want to raise your confidence before a class presentation, control your anger when driving, improve your self-esteem, improve your productivity, or overcome a bad habit? Once you have picked the category, write out a positive affirmation. Use a statement of fact, not a desire ("I am worthy," not "I want to be worthy"). Start using your affirmation and repeat it several times each day with feeling. Examples of positive affirmations include:

- I can do this!
- I enjoy working with my group.
- I am not afraid to stand up for myself.
- I am proud of myself.
- I will remain calm the next time I speak to my roommate.

## Resilience and a Growth Mindset

As discussed in chapter 5, resilience is the ability to cope with difficult situations and successfully adapt to the changing world. Your level of resilience comprises a few factors, including the ways you view and engage with the world, the availability and quality of social resources, and your coping strategies. People with high levels of resilience have been shown to better manage adversity (Garcia-Leon, Perez-Marmol, Gonzalez-Perez, Garcia-Rios, & Peralta-Ramirez, 2019). They are able to reflect on past events (even traumatic ones) to acknowledge the significance of the event and how the experience changed them (Crane,

Research Spotlight

## Mental Imagery and Visualization

**Mental imagery**, or the ability to produce a visual representation in the mind, is a technique that has many uses. It occurs most often when dreaming, but some people can bring up images in their mind and manipulate those images. **Visualization** is an active process that uses mental imagery as the primary tool to conjure up images and scenes in the mind. Visualization can be a powerful tool to manage stress and works in a couple of ways. First, it provides the brain with practice before a stressful event. Athletes often use mental imagery before an event to reduce stress and even improve their performance (Yadolahzadeh, 2020). Secondly, visualization can provide additional motivation to fully embrace and engage in an upcoming event (Renner, Murphy, Ji, Manly, & Holmes, 2019). For example, you may practice visualization to mentally prepare for a class presentation you are feeling nervous about. In your mind, you are wearing your chosen outfit. You confidently walk up to the podium and give your speech. When you finish, the entire class erupts with applause. After going through this scenario several times, you begin to feel more excited and less stressed.

Visualization works because the brain has a difficult time differentiating between reality and imagination, reacting to both in similar ways (Madu, 2019). When you have already walked through how you want to feel and perform during an activity, your brain essentially thinks it is doing the same activity again, and your actions will most likely follow that mindset.

Searle, Kangas, & Nwiran, 2019). Resilience has also been shown to serve as a protective factor against some mental health conditions such as anxiety and depression (Parvar, Ghamari, Pezeshkian, & Shahriarirad, 2022; Setiawati, Wahyuhadi, Joestandari, Maramis, & Atika, 2021).

**Resilience is being flexible and adaptable to changing situations.**

Resilience is partially inborn, but it can be developed and nurtured (Feldman, 2020). Studies have shown resilience can be fostered through education, particularly when problem-based learning methods are employed (Walsh, Owen, Mustafa, & Beech, 2020). Recall the problem-solving skills presented earlier in the chapter. These same skills can also enhance your resilience by giving you the space and tools to handle problematic situations, rather than passively experiencing them.

> It is not the strongest of species that survives, nor the most intelligent. It is the one that is most adaptable to change.
>
> **Charles Darwin**

Many techniques presented earlier in this chapter, such as using affirmations and learning how to combat distorted thinking, can be used to build resilience. The following behaviors are more helpful tools that can be used to strengthen your resilience.

- *Recognize the impermanence of difficulties.* Remind yourself that stress is temporary and that unpleasant experiences will not last forever.
- *Recognize setbacks as opportunities for growth.* Understand that failure is an opportunity to change what you are doing to obtain a different result.
- *Recognize you have tools to manage stress.* Have confidence in your ability to manage stress.
- *Recognize that many things are out of your control.* Stop dwelling on things that are out of your control.

One of the best tools to help develop your own resilience is to adopt a growth mindset. A **growth mindset** is the belief that intelligence is a changeable trait that can be improved with effort. People who adhere to a growth mindset see struggle as part of the path to developing intelligence and are more likely to take on challenging material as a result (Limeri et al., 2020). Many studies have

## Neuroscience and Neuroplasticity

A growth mindset is supported by the study of **neuroplasticity**, the brain's ability to rewire itself as a way of adapting to the environment. Every time you experience something new, your brain actively reorganizes itself in response, growing new neural networks and connections that speed the transmission of impulses (Puderbaugh & Emmady, 2022).

When you first learned addition in grade school, you required visualization to begin to understand the concept of adding numbers. You probably even counted out loud. As you practiced, you were able to add more quickly until it became close to automatic, especially for single-digit numbers. In this example of neuroplasticity, practice allowed your brain to form new neural connections related to addition.

Many of the techniques discussed in this chapter are based on the idea of neuroplasticity. For example, practicing the ABCDE technique can help the brain form new connections so that the initial response to an event is positive, not negative. Practicing these techniques helps the brain better adapt to the environment in a manner that supports health and well-being.

Some ways to encourage neuroplasticity include the following (Legg, 2020):

- *Playing video games.* Video games help develop hand–eye coordination, visual and spatial navigation, decision-making and problem-solving skills, and cooperative skills. Games that use virtual reality tend to have the strongest impact (Ekechukwu et al., 2021).
- *Learn a new language.* Learning a new language improves cognitive functioning. One study found that learning a new language increases the density of gray matter and white matter in the brain (Rossi, Cheng, Kroll, Diaz, & Newman, 2017). Gray brain matter is associated with areas in the brain related to language, attention, memory, emotions, and motor skills. White brain matter is associated with better problem-solving skills, creative thinking skills, reading comprehension, and multitasking ability.
- *Make some music.* Engaging in musical training has been shown to improve neuroplasticity (Olszewska, Gaca, Herman, Jednorog, & Marchewka, 2021). Music can also boost mood, learning, concentration, and focus.
- *Travel.* Experiencing new places can enhance your cognitive flexibility and creativity. Learning about new cultures helps you become a better communicator and improves your ability to see the world from different lenses and frameworks (Kartoshkina, 2022).
- *Exercise.* Research suggests exercise can help improve fine motor coordination and brain connectivity (Lin, Tasai, & Kuo, 2018). Exercise also improves blood and oxygen flow to the brain.
- *Create art.* Making art can help you develop your creativity, work through emotions, and obtain deeper insight. Artistic abilities can be developed and improved through practice (Vaisvaser, 2021).

---

shown that students who believe in the growth mindset outperform those who feel intelligence is an innate ability that cannot be changed (Smiley, Buttitta, Chung, Dubon, & Chang, 2016). Additionally, those who believe in a growth mindset see mistakes as a learning opportunity and think of them as part of the learning process (Murphy & Gash, 2020).

People with a fixed mindset, on the other hand, tend to see mistakes as an indicator of failure, avoid challenges, and give up when they encounter struggle (Limeri et al., 2020). Research shows students with a growth mindset are better able to manage stress and have higher levels of academic success compared to those with a fixed mindset (Mosanta, 2019). Refer to table 6.1 on the differences between a growth and fixed mindset.

Having a growth mindset allows you to learn from your successes and mistakes (figure 6.3). When encountering stress, those with a growth mindset are not intimidated and actively work on finding ways to cope. A person with a growth mindset is focused on the process, whereas a person with a fixed mindset is just focused on the result. A growth mindset places value in the process, which is completely under your control, and not the outcome, which may only partially be under your control (Ronkainen, Kuusisto, & Tirri, 2019).

**Table 6.1** Growth Mindset Versus Fixed Mindset

| Growth mindset | Fixed mindset |
|---|---|
| Embraces challenges | Avoids challenges |
| Perseveres in spite of failure | Gives in to failure |
| Believes people can increase their intelligence or skills | Believes intelligence and skills are something you are born with |
| Wants to learn | Believes they already know everything |
| Accepts and embraces criticism | Dismisses criticism |
| Is inspired and motivated by the success of others | Is threatened by the success of others |

Adapted from Campbell, Craig, and Collier-Reed (2020).

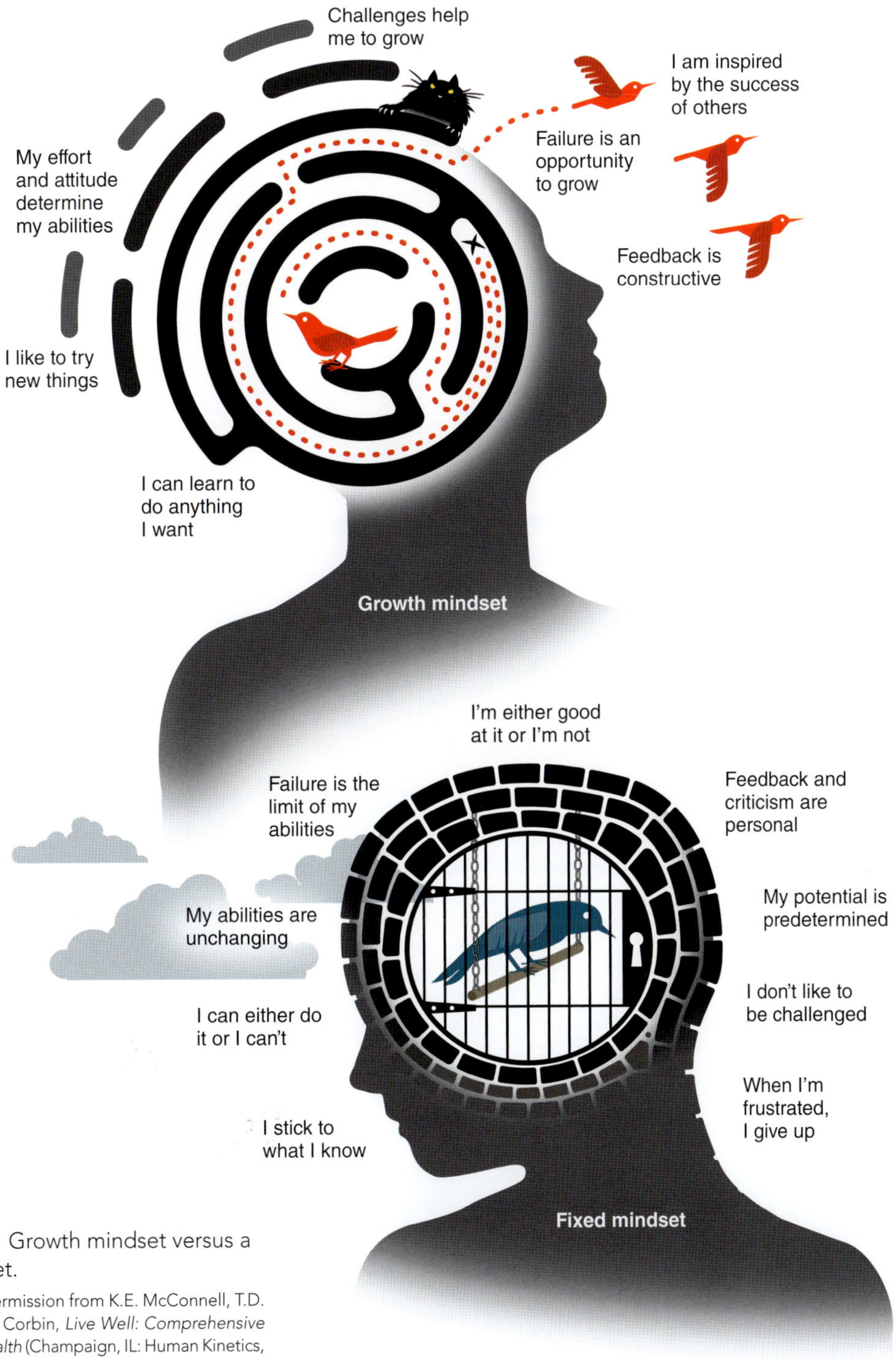


**Figure 6.3** Growth mindset versus a fixed mindset.

Reprinted by permission from K.E. McConnell, T.D. Farrar, and C.B. Corbin, *Live Well: Comprehensive High School Health* (Champaign, IL: Human Kinetics, 2024), 313.

Carole Dweck, a professor of psychology who developed the theory of growth mindset, recommends the following to help you move toward a growth mindset (Dweck, 2006).

- Where are you currently on the continuum between a growth and fixed mindset? Think about how you understand intelligence and learning. This is your starting point.
- Explore why you want to develop a growth mindset. What is motivating you to want to change your mindset? What is your purpose?
- Find examples of others who have developed their growth mindset. Talk with friends, teachers, and family members to see if anyone has worked on developing their own growth mindset. Ask about the strategies they used.
- Understand your own limitations. Having a growth mindset doesn't mean you can do anything. It is understanding your limitations and setting realistic goals for yourself.
- Start changing how you talk about things that are hard or difficult. Instead of saying things like "I can't" or "that's too hard," say "I am not great at this yet, but I am getting better." When something is hard or difficult, it means you are learning.
- See your challenges as opportunities. Life will always provide you with challenges—instead of cowering away from them, meet them head on.
- Reflect on your failures and how you can learn from them.
- Stop seeking approval from others. Be comfortable with yourself and the progress you are making.

## Summary

Intellectual wellness describes the ability and desire to continue learning throughout a lifetime. It includes the ability to think critically and express yourself creatively. Stress can negatively impact intellectual wellness by inhibiting creativity and production. However, when managed well, stress can serve as the motivation to improve intellectual wellness. Certain behaviors and thoughts can harm your intellectual wellness, including setting uncertain goals, engaging in distorted thinking, and having a fixed mindset. You can combat these behaviors and improve the functioning of your mind with techniques such as goal setting, problem solving, adopting a growth mindset, and reframing negative thoughts. Practicing techniques to improve your intellectual wellness supports neuroplasticity by helping the brain make new and stronger neural connections to better adapt to the environment.

## ONLINE RESOURCES

Visit HK*Propel* to access audio supplements, worksheets, and vocabulary flash cards for this chapter.

## DISCUSSION QUESTIONS

1. Explain the difference between intellectual wellness and intelligence.
2. Describe how reactions to stress can reduce our levels of intellectual wellness.
3. Everyone engages in distorted thinking at some point. What is an experience you have had with distorted thinking? Walk through the ABCDE technique with your distorted thought.
4. Describe the relationship between stress and creativity.
5. Would you consider yourself to have a growth or fixed mindset? How did you come up with your answer? What are ways to encourage a growth mindset?

7

# Social Wellness

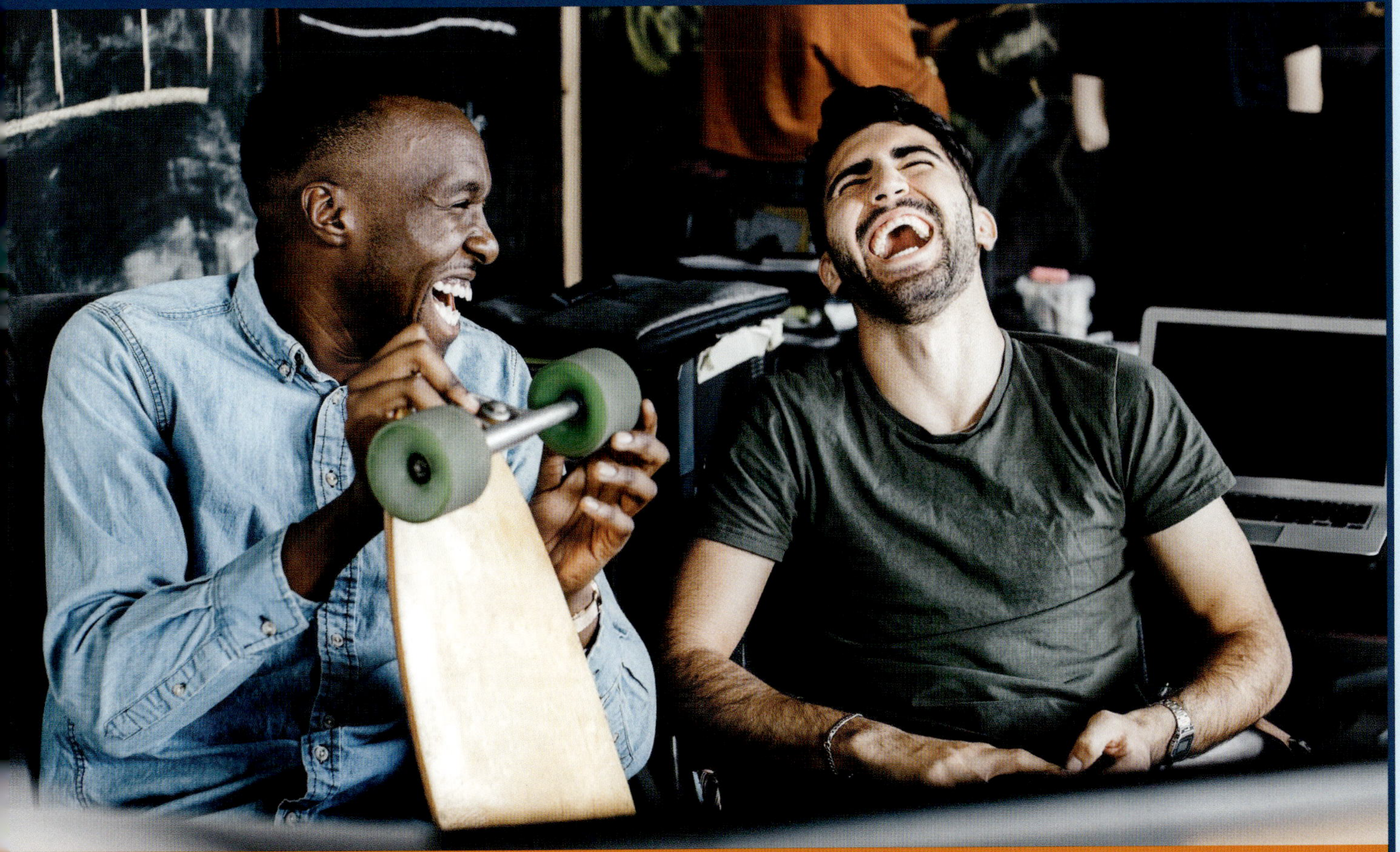

## LEARNING OBJECTIVES

After reading this chapter, you will be able to do the following:

- Identify ways to improve social wellness
- Evaluate the impact a social support network can have on stress and overall wellness
- Explain the benefits and detriments of social media on social wellness
- Recognize the characteristics of healthy and unhealthy relationships

# KEY TERMS

- avoidance
- connotative meaning
- denotative meaning
- emotion-focused coping
- euphemism
- interpersonal communication
- loneliness
- nonverbal communication
- perceived social support
- problem-focused coping
- received social support
- reflective listening
- social network
- social support
- stress buffering hypothesis
- verbal communication

Aristotle once wrote, "Man is by nature a social animal." It is believed that social relationships have helped humans evolve. About 2.6 to 1.8 million years ago, people began to share resources with other members in their group, resulting in stronger social bonds and a greater chance of survival (The Smithsonian Institution, 2020). These relationships are just as important today as people across the globe rely on one another to share their resources.

The relationships you have with people around you are known as your **social network**. Do you feel your dealings with other people are generally positive or negative? To what extent is there reciprocity in your relationships—that is, do you give as much as you take? How well do you know and interact with those in your social network? Do you share power with those in your social network? Do you provide social support to one another?

Social wellness is the ability to form and maintain healthy relationships with others. The power of social connections cannot be underestimated. They help us feel connected to others, our community, and our world. Being around others provides you with **social support**, which is the extent that others in your life help you and provide a buffer against adverse life experiences. Social support comes in a variety of different forms, including the following (House, 1981):

- *Emotional support.* People who offer emotional support enhance your sense of self-worth. They provide positive affirmations and listen to you. They are the ones who offer hugs, pats on the back, and a shoulder to cry on when needed.
- *Informational support.* This type of support promotes intellectual growth and a growth mindset by helping you make informed decisions. This can come from a variety of avenues, including news reports, social media, friends, and the Internet.
- *Tangible support.* This type of support involves sharing resources. This may include a parent giving you money when finances are tight or a friend helping you move into your new apartment.
- *Belonging support.* This type of social support helps you feel as though you belong. This can include being part of a sports team, study group, or a sorority or fraternity. It is important to feel a sense of belonging to help ward off feelings of isolation.

It is important to have social support that is both high quantity and high quality (Spohr, Suzuki, Marshall, Tasman, & Walters, 2016). High-quantity social support is readily available when needed, whereas high-quality social support is prosocial and supportive of improving health outcomes. Both have been shown to be associated with a reduction in risk behavior.

## Benefits of Social Wellness

Maintaining your social wellness can help improve your overall health. People who are chronically ill have better health outcomes and a decreased risk of mortality when they participate in social groups and maintain positive and strong social connections with others (Umberson & Montez,

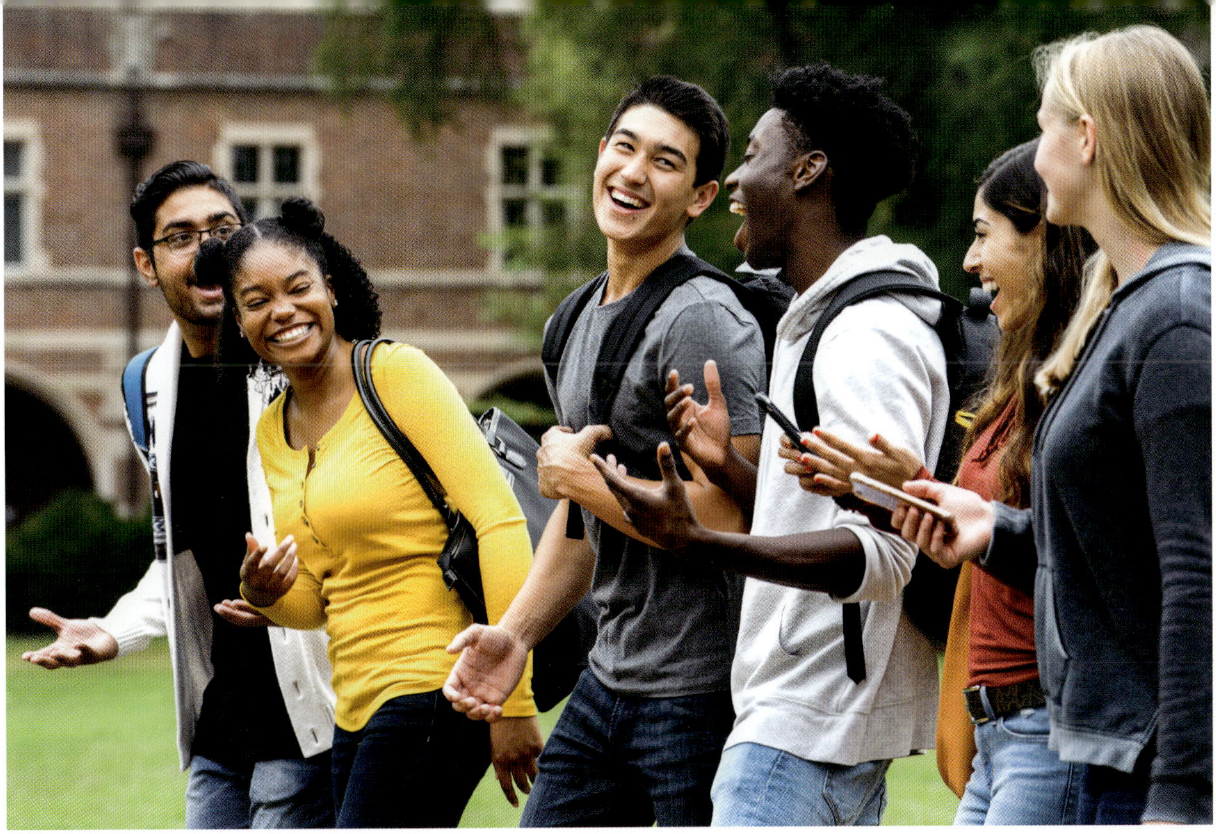

2010). On a study conducted on people with breast cancer, those who had stronger social support experienced less anxiety and reported better recovery outcomes (Bibi & Khalid, 2020). There are groups for many topics ranging from Alcoholics Anonymous (AA) to grief support. You can search for these groups on the Internet or ask your college advisor. They will be able to point you in the right direction.

Having a strong social support system can also help with stress management. People who feel they can talk about their worries and problems with friends and family report lower levels of perceived stress compared to those who do not have a social support system (Wu et al., 2021). College is a time that it is common to experience loneliness; some studies show that up to 60 percent of college students experience loneliness (Counts & John-Henderson, 2020). Most colleges offer services such as student counseling, peer tutoring, academic clubs, and social gatherings to help students feel supported and ultimately perform better. In a study on college freshmen, social support was determined to help lower perceived stress (McLean, Gaul, & Penco, 2022). Likewise, high levels of social support have associated with higher levels of academic success (Maymon, Hall, & Harley, 2019).

## Social Support and Stress

The **stress buffering hypothesis** posits that having a strong social support system can help reduce or eliminate the negative impact of stress (Gellert et al., 2018). Social support can be measured as either perceived or received support. **Perceived social support** asks a person to estimate their level of social support. **Received social support**, on the other hand, focuses on how often different forms of social support are received. In other words, perceived social support is based on how much social support a person feels is available when they need it, whereas received support is what they actually get (Riu & Guo, 2022). Many studies have found that of the two, perceived social support provides more protection against stress and better supports wellness compared to received social support (Szkody & McKinney, 2019).

**Just knowing you have support available when you need it is enough to give you that extra boost of confidence to manage life's challenges.**

Perhaps counterintuitively, high levels of received social support may result in an overreliance on others to solve one's problems (Pilcher & Bryant, 2016). Consider a college student who does not know how to do their own laundry because a parent has always done it for them. Received social support can be considered similar to an indulgent parent: When you know someone will always be there to help you, you may not learn to do things for yourself. Similarly, high levels of received social support have been associated with higher rates of depression and lower self-worth (Pilcher & Bryant, 2016).

People with adequate levels of social support may already possess effective stress coping mechanisms. For example, those who have more perceived social support feel more in control of stressful events and tend to manage stress more effectively compared to those with lower perceived levels of social support (Pilcher & Bryant, 2016). Likewise, people with higher levels of resilience report reduced levels of perceived stress (Garcia-Leon, Perez-Marmol, Gonzalez-Perez, Garcia-Rios, & Peralta-Ramirez, 2019).

Resilience is generally formed during the early years of life. Babies who have secure attachment bonds with their parents show higher levels of resilience, which may contribute to the ability to form positive relationships with others later in life, leading to increased levels of perceived social support. On the other hand, babies who do not form secure attachments show lower levels of resilience and have a difficult time trusting others (Ortiz, Horner, Sato, Nelson, & Lamas, 2023). Thus, the type of relationships you form early in life influence the type of relationships you have later in life.

The ability to form social networks and build trusting relationships with others is a key developmental task during the college years (Chickering & Reisser, 1993). One study found that female college students who have interpersonal relationships have higher levels of academic success (Chang, Chou, Hsieh, & Huange, 2020). Furthermore, students who have social support have better grade point averages, have higher retention rates, and are happier at college (McNaughton-Cassill et al., 2021).

**Students who feel more connected at their institutions are more likely to be academically successful and to graduate from those institutions.**

Consider your own experience at college. Do you make an effort to connect with classmates? Do you attend events on campus? The simple act of talking with other students about your concerns or worries can help reduce or alleviate your stress.

## Emotion-Focused Coping and Problem-Focused Coping

In 1984, Lazarus and Folkman created a model describing two types of stress coping mechanisms: emotion-focused coping and problem-focused coping. **Emotion-focused coping** is dedicated to analyzing how a person manages and regulates their emotions when under stress (Stanislawski, 2019). This method doesn't focus on managing the stressor; rather, it focuses on managing the feelings that occur because of the stressor. **Problem-focused coping**, on the other hand, focuses on the problem that is causing the stress.

Emotion-focused coping can be positive or negative. Positive emotion-focused coping utilizes positive self-talk, self-kindness, and self-compassion. These characteristics have been associated with decreased levels of perceived stress (Brenner, Heath, Vogel, & Crede, 2017; Doron et al., 2014). On the other hand, negative emotion-focused coping mechanisms, such as self-criticism or self-blame, can lead to increased levels of stress and anxiety (Stanislawski, 2019).

Problem-focused coping can also be separated into two categories: problem solving and problem avoidance. In problem solving, one would actively engage in creating and implementing a plan to solve the problem that is causing stress. Those who engage in problem solving tend to have high confidence in their problem-solving skills and a sense of personal control over their problems (Pretorius & Padmanabhanunni, 2023). This is associated with reduced levels of distress and overall improvements in mental health. Alternatively, people who engage in **avoidance** avoid, deny, or minimize the problem or give up on trying to solve it, which has been linked to greater amounts of distress (Madigan, Rumbold, Gerber, & Nicholls, 2020). For instance, people who tend to procrastinate are practicing avoidance. When you avoid the problem through procrastination, the associated stress may increase as the deadline nears (Sirois, 2023).

## Problem-Focused Coping and Social Drinking

Shane is feeling ashamed because he performed badly on a test, and he decides to go out with friends to a bar to help cope with those feelings. This is an example of problem avoidance because Shane is using alcohol to ignore the problem (his poor test performance) rather than doing anything to solve it. Although it is too late for Shane to change his grade, there are still options for Shane to address his problem. He can ask the professor to see his graded exam so he can learn from his mistakes. He can create a better plan for studying for his next test. These problem-focused coping skills would reduce Shane's stress and prevent the problem from occurring again.

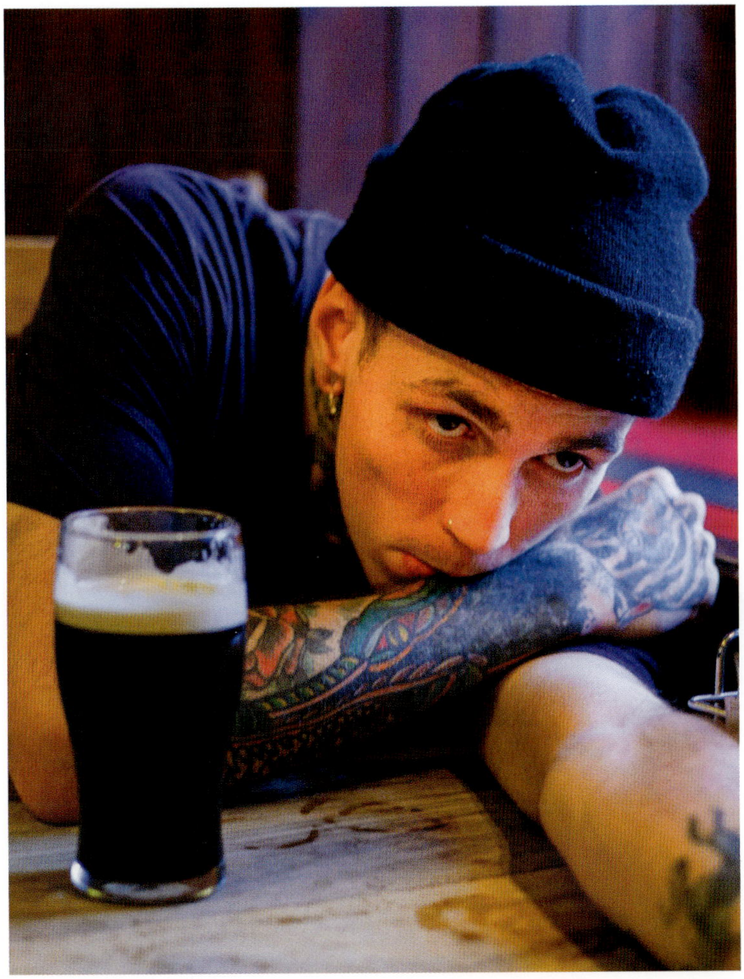

People with higher levels of social support tend to use problem-focused coping skills to manage their stress (Agbaria & Mokh, 2022). Similarly, having strong social support may serve as a tool to help people manage stress from a problem-focused perspective. Having strong perceived social support has been associated with increased levels of self-esteem, which may lead to an increase in self-confidence to solve problems and manage stress (Wang, Cai, Wian, & Peng, 2014).

## Problem-Focused Coping and Social Support

Ava has positive social support from a few close friends and her parents. She is having some problems with her job and feels she is not appreciated or valued at work. When she expresses her feelings to her social support network, they suggest talking with her manager and work with Ava to come up with a script.

This example highlights how a social network can help support the problem-focused coping method. If Ava didn't have social support to lean on, she might have just quit her job to manage the negative feelings associated with her work. But when she engaged her social support network, they were able to help her identify the problem and come up with ways to manage it.

## Decision Making

Positive social support has also been shown to help reduce risky behavior and have positive influences on your decision making. For example, one study found that adolescents with a social support network showed reduced behaviors associated with substance use (Heerde & Hemphill, 2018). Other studies have found similar outcomes of reduced risky behavior (Pilcher & Bryant, 2016).

Having a strong sense of self-control is related to lower rates of risky behavior. When you feel in control, you are less likely to be impulsive and make poor decisions. On the other hand, having lower perceptions of self-control can lead to an increase in risky behaviors. When under stress, your ability to make sound decisions is reduced. The problem-solving process you learned in chapter 6 cannot function as it should and is often ignored or rushed. As a result, you are more prone to making quick and impulsive decisions—which may not be the best decisions.

The relationship between stress, decision making, and risky behavior can be partially explained by looking at the brain circuitry involved in decision making. When under stress, the area of the brain that is responsible for decision making is affected (Friedman et al., 2017). In this situation, the brain is unable to measure out the costs and the benefits of a specific action and tends to go for the high-benefit (and often high-cost) decision. High levels of social anxiety also increase the likelihood of engaging in risky behavior when under stress. On the other hand, people with low levels of social anxiety will reduce their level of risk-taking behavior when under stress.

Engaging in risky behaviors is associated with increased levels of physical and mental harm. Examples of risky behaviors include unsafe sexual practices, driving under the influence of alcohol, staying up all night partying when you have an exam the next day, or cheating on a partner. These practices can result in harms such as getting a sexually transmitted infection, failing an exam or class, or losing a meaningful relationship. Early engagement with risky behavior has been associated with poorer health and emotional outcomes later in life (Reynolds et al., 2013).

**Learning how to effectively manage stress can reduce your likelihood of engaging in risky behavior and help you make better decisions for yourself.**

## Isolation

When social support is lacking, **loneliness** can occur. Loneliness is a feeling, not a condition of the environment. As such, people can feel lonely in a crowded room. Loneliness is based on the quality and quantity of social relationships—or lack thereof (Hu, Zheng, & Huang, 2020). Loneliness has a detrimental impact on social functioning. People who feel lonely tend to be shyer, more anxious, and more socially awkward. These behaviors tend to reduce the chance of positive social interaction. People who experience loneliness may further withdraw from social interactions and connections, which further exaggerates feelings of loneliness.

The act of being separated from others and prevented from making connections is detrimental to physical, mental, and emotional health. In prison, for example, the most severe punishment for inmates is isolation. Some argue that solitary confinement is necessary to keep other prisoners and guards safe, reduce dangerous behavior, and help maintain control of a prison facility (Chadick, Batastini, Levulis, & Morgan, 2018). However, because the effects have been shown to be more harmful than helpful, others argue that solitary confinement should be abolished from the prison system (Kapoor, 2020). Studies have found that people released from prison who spent any time in isolation were 24 percent more likely to die in the first year after being released compared to those who did not spend any time in isolation (Brinkley-Rubinstein et al., 2019). Some people develop psychiatric symptoms after being in solitary confinement for a period. These problems can persist even after being released from prison (Reiter et al., 2020).

Although this is an extreme example of isolation, it is meant to highlight the negative impact of loneliness on health outcomes. Research has shown a relationship between isolation and increased mortality (Herring, 2020). People who report higher levels of loneliness also report poorer levels of health, limited physical abilities, and increased negative health diagnoses (Jessen, Pallesen, Kriegbaum, & Kristiansen, 2018).

Research Spotlight

## Social Isolation and Stress

The COVID-19 pandemic was a great source of stress for many. Fear of the virus led to an increase in mental disorders, including stress-related disorders. Studies have found that social isolation increases levels of distress, which was more common among younger people. One study examined distressed rates of younger adults (18 to24 years old) and compared them with older adults (over 65 years old). They found almost half of the younger adults compared to less than 10 percent of the older adults scored very high on experiencing psychological distress (Every-Palmer et al., 2020). During the initial stages of the pandemic, poor health outcomes were associated with higher levels of stress, anxiety, and depression (Ozamiz-Etxebarria, Mondragon, Santamaria, & Gorrotxategi, 2020). The increased symptoms of stress and anxiety also began to rise significantly about two weeks after lockdowns, suggesting that shorter periods of isolation have fewer impacts on psychological health. Those with preexisting chronic diseases or mental illnesses were more susceptible to these negative psychological impacts (Ozamiz-Etxebarria et al., 2020). Lockdowns have also contributed to an increase in alcohol consumption, suicidal thoughts and behaviors, and family violence.

These restrictive measures decrease social connectivity, resulting in increased levels of distrust among others (Pietrabissa & Simpson, 2020). The pandemic has caused us to consider others as potential threats to our health, resulting in purposeful effort to maintain social distance. As such, even when the threat of COVID-19 is eliminated or reduced, many people still avoid social interactions. This may result in an inability to form new social relationships and a deterioration of existing relationships, which may ultimately lead to higher generalized levels of social isolation. This can have serious health impacts: People who report high levels of loneliness and social isolation are at an increased risk for all-cause mortality (Ward, May, Normand, Kenny, & Nolan, 2021).

Furthermore, feeling lonely may also impact how you perceive and react to stress. People with higher levels of loneliness tend to have heightened responses to smaller stresses and rate them as more disruptive compared to people who do not feel lonely. This may be explained by increased feelings of vulnerability: People who are lonely lack a social support system, making stress seem more threatening (Freedman & Nicolle, 2020).

This overactive stress response places a lot of strain on the body and can lead to other health conditions. Those suffering from loneliness generally have fewer stress management skills and may lack the motivation to utilize those skills they do have (Gifford, Fouche, & Beadle, 2021). As such, people who experience loneliness have higher rates of chronic stress compared to those who are not lonely. Furthermore, loneliness can be seen as a predictor of chronic stress later in life (Gifford et al., 2021).

**People who are lonely rate threats as more dangerous than they are.**

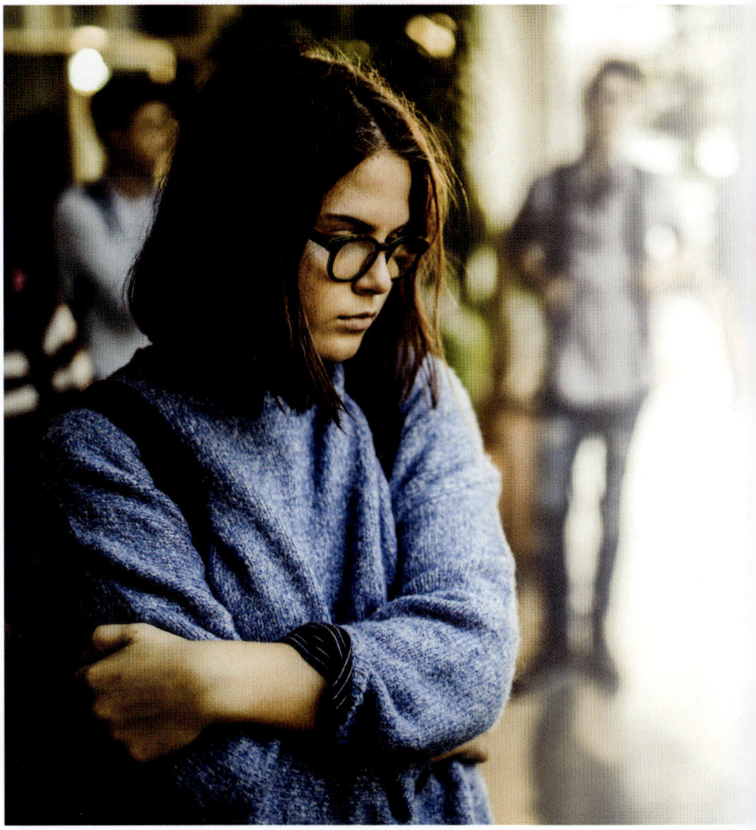

## Increase Your Social Support Network

As you age, your social circles will change based on your life circumstances. For some, childhood friendships remain strong throughout a lifetime. For others, these relationships change as they mature. Both are completely normal and can highlight the different needs of different people. There may be times in your life when you feel that your goals and priorities have shifted away from those of your friends. Sometimes major life events, such as marriage or parenthood, create a wedge with friends who are in a different place in life. Thinking about your social support network and identifying ways to update and maintain it can serve as a stress reliever that is worth its weight in gold.

One way to improve your social support network is to meet new people. For some, this is easy, whereas for others, it seems like a daunting task. Here are some ways to meet new people:

- *Attend or get involved in your religion.* Attend services or volunteer at your place of worship. Join a social committee or study group. You will meet people who have similar ideologies, which can serve as a foundation for a friendship.
- *Join a gym or attend fitness classes.* Whether you are just beginning or an old pro, working out with others can help you meet people and encourage you to attend those fitness classes.
- *Volunteer.* This is a great way to serve your community and meet new people. There are many organizations that welcome volunteers and make it fun.

Finally, let go of negative influences. There may be times in your life when one of your friendships turns negative. Perhaps the person makes you feel bad about yourself or is engaging in activities that no longer interest you. It is okay to let go of those relationships and build new ones.

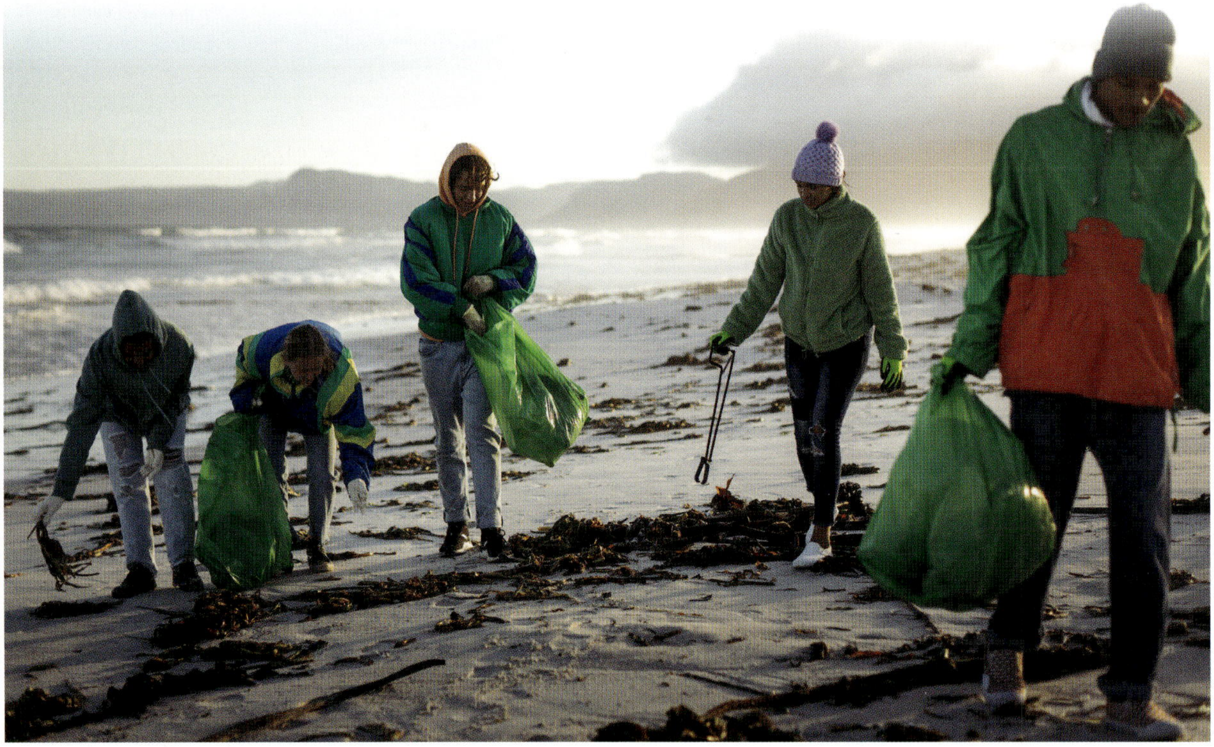

## Social Media

Technology has made it possible to meet and engage with others across the globe, both asynchronously and in real time. With the ever-increasing use of social media, people are spending more and more time online, spending an average of 2.5 hours on social media each day (Buchholz, 2022). Consider your own social media usage. Are you spending more or less time online than the average person? How does it impact your day? Generally, do you feel good about yourself after engaging in social media?

Social media can be seen as a virtual social support arena. For example, if you are going through a rough time in college, you can find a variety of resources offering emotional support for college students. You can also search for ways to increase your success at college, which would be geared toward informational social support. Finding a group to provide extra help with homework would satisfy tangible social support. Finally social media can help you find groups to join on campus, which would work on your belonging social support.

Studies show that receiving virtual social support from others is just as effective as real-life support to reduce stress (Kothgassner et al., 2019). For this reason, there is a growing trend to utilize social media to help create social support networks. For example, although it is generally accepted that breastfeeding is best for both the mother and infant, less than 25 percent of infants are exclusively breastfed at six months (Skelton, Evans, & LaChenaye, 2020). One of the factors related to breastfeeding is stress, which is caused by factors such as lack of sleep, having unclear expectations about breastfeeding, and needing additional support for breastfeeding (Skelton et al., 2018; Skelton et al., 2020). New mothers often feel isolated as the primary caregiver as well, which leaves little time to cultivate and maintain friendships. Social networking sites dedicated to breastfeeding can help new mothers share knowledge, tips, and support and provide a sense of belonging (Skelton et al., 2018). Studies have found that belonging to these social media support groups can increase breastfeeding initiation and maintenance, reduce feelings of stress, increase maternal confidence and self-esteem, and improve health outcomes for both mother and child (Skelton et al., 2020).

Transgender youth are another group at higher risk for stress and other negative outcomes because of a perceived lack of social support (Selkie, Adkins, Masters, Bajpai, & Shumer, 2020). Compared to cisgender youth, transgender youth are at a higher risk for suicide, anxiety, and depression. Social media platforms and online communities can help provide different types of social support to transgender adolescents they may not have access to in their own community. Other examples of online social support include finding resources and support for a chronic health condition or information about scholarships and financial aid. There are social networking sites for every need and interest.

Social media does have its drawbacks. People who spend many hours on social media each day generally have a more sedentary lifestyle, which increases risks such as depression, cardiovascular disease, and generally poorer health outcomes (Suciu, 2021). Additionally, high amounts of social media use can impact sleep quality and quantity, which can have an effect on health.

Problematic social media use is associated with an increase in stress, anxiety, and depression (Lin, Namdar, Griffiths, & Pakpour, 2021). Currently, there is no common definition, but problematic social media use is the preoccupation with and the addictive desire to use social media, coupled with a loss of control over behavior (Griffiths, Kuss, & Demetrovics, 2014). Men and women show different patterns of social media use. Men tend to engage in online gaming and gaming forums with the goal to gain knowledge, whereas women tend to engage in social comparison and seek personal feedback (Twenge & Martin, 2020).

Learning how to manage and reduce your own social media use can keep it from becoming a problem. Consider the following tips.

- *Be positive.* When you comment on other people's posts, be positive. Ask yourself whether your comment is kind or helpful. Being positive will make others feel good as well as yourself.
- *Be in the moment.* Many people worry about documenting the present moment and forget to enjoy it. Instead of taking pictures of your dinner at a trendy restaurant while it gets cold, enjoy your food. If you really want to take a picture, do so quickly and then put your phone away. Research shows that using media (such as

**Regardless of how you choose to use social media, excessive use can lead to poorer health outcomes.**

Case Study

## Social Media Is Not Real Life

People tend to compare themselves and their lives to the images portrayed on social media. When you scroll through social media, others' lives seem to be full of fun and interesting activities, romantic partners appear to be completely devoted to each other, and many people have no blemishes, body fat, or wrinkles. In reality, the images portrayed on social media are usually altered to portray the best version of oneself. In fact, these images are sometimes so retouched that you wouldn't recognize the real person. Comparing yourself to these images may make you feel dissatisfied with your body, attractiveness, and life status (Tiggemann & Anderberg, 2019).

Research shows that social media users are impacted negatively when they compare themselves to these images (Vandenbosch, Fardouly, & Tiggemann, 2022). Many people get stressed because they are not able to look like the images posted on social media, even though these images are not real. They start to become obsessive about their looks, which places them at a higher risk for disordered eating and exercise (Wilksch, O'Shea, Ho, Byrne, & Wade, 2020).

A recent campaign called Instagram Versus Reality is a social activism effort that compares side-by-side images of a "perfect" picture and the unedited version or a similar unedited picture of the person (Tiggemann & Anderberg, 2019). This helps people better understand that the ideal images are not real—they appear that way because of perfect lighting, poses, camera angles, and photoshopping. When these side-by-side images are shown, it results in lower levels of body dissatisfaction.

### Discussion Questions

1. Many young people use social media to determine what is beautiful. How would you educate these people to broaden their ideas of beauty?
2. Do you think restricting young people's use of social media is an effective strategy to combat negative self-image? Explain your answer.
3. Should photoshopped or retouched images be labeled as such? If so, how would it impact your own ideas of beauty? Would you support this action? Why or why not?

taking pictures) can diminish your memory of the event later on (Tamir, Templeton, Ward, & Zaki, 2018). Enjoying the moment in the here and now will help you remember the event later.

- *Don't compare yourself to others.* When you look at images and press the "like" button, take a moment and think about what you like about the image. Does it put the person in a nice light? Is it a beautiful landscape? Don't compare yourself or your own experiences to it. Acknowledge the image and move on.
- *Choose positivity.* Follow people, places, and things that bring you joy. Stay away from negative influences. Even if a person's negativity is not directed at you, consider unfollowing that person to help maintain positive influences in your life.
- *Stay off social media at night and in the morning.* Avoid ending the day on social media, which can impact the quality of your sleep. Also try not to wake up and engage with social media before getting out of bed; seeing something negative first thing in the morning can contribute to negative thought patterns throughout the day. Try starting the day with meditation, prayer, stretching, or affirmations to support a positive mindset.
- *Focus on your purpose.* Instead of mindlessly scrolling through feeds, set an intention. What are you trying to do? What are you trying to accomplish? Being more mindful of your activity can help you be aware of your own thoughts and feelings as you engage with social media.

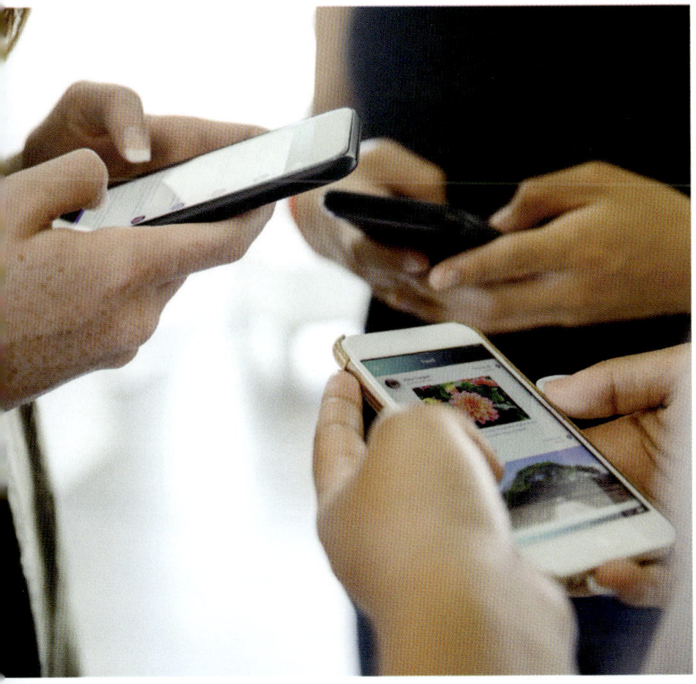

- *Hang out with your friends in person.* Sometimes it is too easy to put our friends on the back burner to focus on social media or engage with them only online. Make time to spend with your friends face to face.

Social media, like anything else, can be both beneficial and harmful depending on how you use it. Being intentional and mindful of your social media use can help you maintain healthy habits to support your well-being.

## Relationships

Your relationships with the people who surround you, including family, friends, and peers, are an important component in your life and your journey to wellness. Unfortunately, there are times in our lives when our relationships with others are unhealthy. Learning how to recognize healthy and unhealthy relationships can help you better cope with life's stressors.

### Healthy Versus Unhealthy Relationships

Humans are social creatures; we rely on relationships to help us cope with stressors and be more productive. Additionally, people who are in healthy relationships have better health outcomes and a decreased risk of mortality (Mertika, Mitskidou, & Stalikas, 2020). The key to these benefits is a *healthy* relationship: Although all relationships have some healthy and unhealthy components, a healthy is one that you feel safe in physically, mentally, and emotionally. This section will highlight the characteristics of healthy and unhealthy relationships, present signs of an unhealthy relationship, and provide some tips for ending an unhealthy relationship.

Healthy relationships with others can help you feel supported. Just being in the presence of your romantic partner can help mitigate the stressors in your life—among women, getting a hug from their partner during a stressful event was shown to reduce cortisol output and lower perceptions of stress (Berretz et al., 2022). Another study showed that women rated a laser stimuli as less painful when they had a romantic partner with them than when they were alone (Krhae et al., 2015). Just thinking about your partner during a stressful task can also serve as a stress moderator. For example, one study measured changes in blood pressure and heart rate while participants immersed one foot in ice water. One group of participants had their partner physically present, another group was told to call upon a mental representation of their partner during the ice water immersion, and the last group was told to think about their day during the ice water immersion. The participants in the first two groups had significantly lower blood pressure compared to the final group, suggesting that just thinking about your partner has a stress mitigating effect (Bourassa et al., 2019).

All relationships will have disagreements, but how you and your partner handle them can shed light on the kind of relationship you have. Do you work together to come up with solutions, or do you call each other names? Learning how to compromise and handle conflict can provide insight on how healthy a relationship truly is.

People in a healthy relationship value and make an effort to understand one another. Although it is impossible to split everything 50/50, a healthy relationship maintains a good balance of effort from each participant to meet the needs of the other. When you are in a healthy relationship, you feel comfortable sharing your feelings and opinions. This doesn't mean

**A healthy relationship supports mutual respect.**

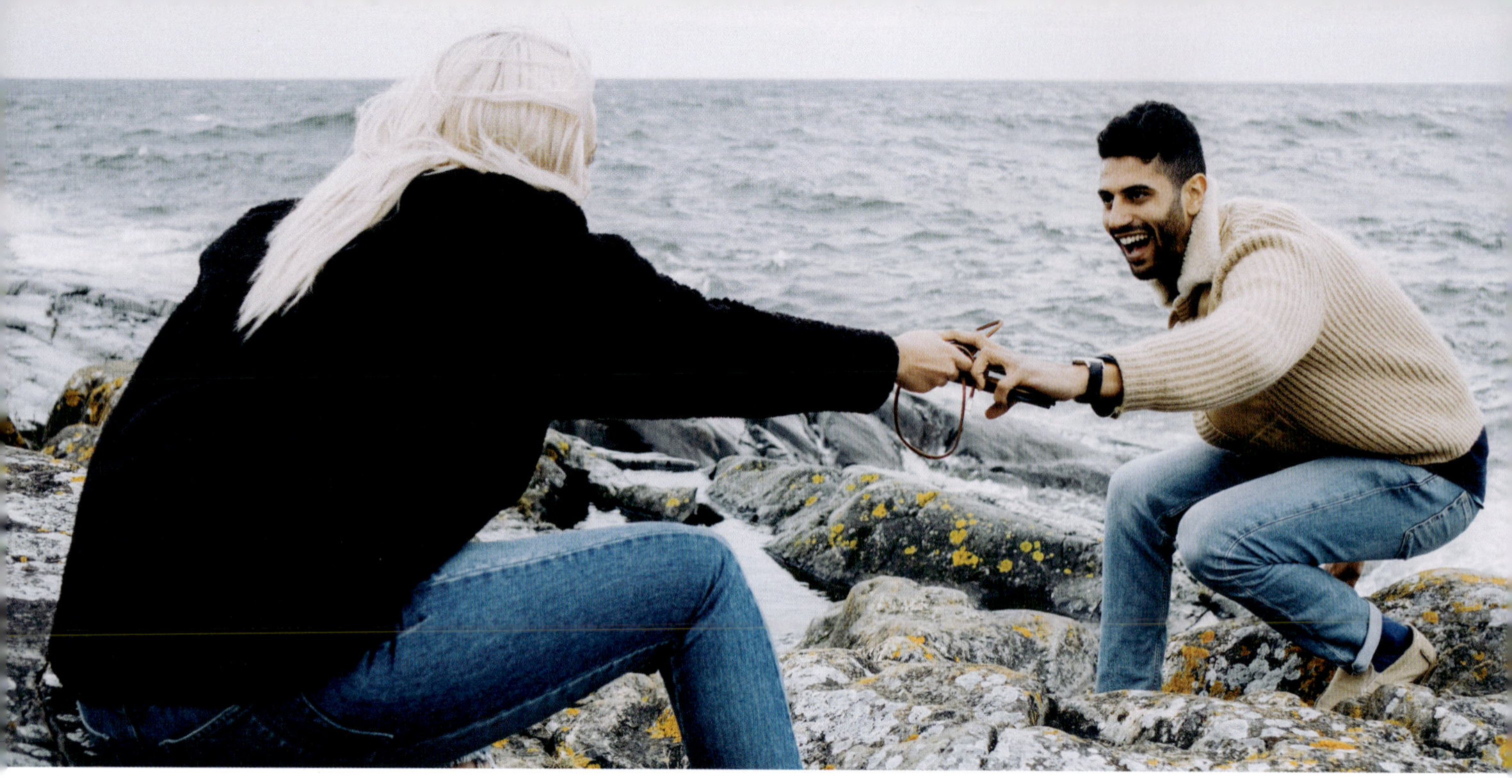

your partner has to agree with everything you say and do, but that you know your partner will accept you as you are.

On the other hand, an unhealthy relationship is one that you don't feel safe in or that lacks mutual respect and trust. Unhealthy relationships that do not have a basis of trust tend to have higher levels of jealousy. One person may hold power over the other and use that power to control them. It also may not be overtly obvious when a relationship is unhealthy. Refer to table 7.1 for some characteristics of healthy and unhealthy relationships.

## Setting Boundaries

To help support a healthy relationship, it is important to set boundaries with those around you. This can include your romantic partner as well as your friends. Boundaries are helpful in all types of relationships and can change as relationships change.

**Table 7.1** Healthy Versus Unhealthy Relationship Traits

| Healthy relationship | Unhealthy relationship |
|---|---|
| Equality: Both partners share decision making and responsibility. | Control: One partner makes all the decisions in the relationship. |
| Honesty: Both partners feel safe sharing feelings and thoughts with the other. | Dishonesty: One or both partners hide part of themselves or tell lies to avoid conflict or to manipulate the situation. |
| Trust: There is a sense of trust between partners. | Distrust: There is little trust in the relationship. It is characterized by jealousy. |
| Good communication: Both partners communicate well in the relationship. | Poor communication: One or both partners do not practice good communication skills. They make assumptions about each other and do not create a space for open communication. |
| Independence: Both partners enjoy spending time together as well as apart. | Dependence: One or both people feel as though they cannot live without the other. They feel lost without the other person and can't enjoy time away from them. |
| Consent: Both people ask for consent for engaging in any type of activities, including sexual activity. They feel safe to not give consent. | Nonconsent: Consent is assumed or not asked for. It feels uncomfortable to not give consent. |

## Breaking Boundaries

Brayden has been dating Sam for a few months. Sam has been following Brayden on social media and has asked Brayden to put a location tracking app on his phone and share access with Sam. Brayden doesn't feel comfortable doing so and tells Sam no. Sam complains that Brayden isn't committed to the relationship and says that if he doesn't do this, the relationship is over. Brayden gives in and puts the app on his phone. However, he hates that Sam knows where he is at all times and becomes unhappy in the relationship.

In this case, Sam used intimidation and threats to get Brayden put the app on his phone, pushing the boundaries too far for Brayden's liking. Setting healthy personal boundaries can help support relationships by setting the stage for relationship expectations. Everyone has different boundaries and expectations; what is right for one person doesn't mean it is right for another person. So, how can you tell if someone is crossing your boundary? The best way to tell is to reflect on your feelings. If you feel respected and comfortable with the request or behavior, then it is within your boundary. If you feel uncomfortable or disrespected, then you can consider it crossing your boundary.

Boundaries can also help promote healthy friendships. In most cases, boundaries are built as friendships are formed and maintained and often do not need to be communicated. However, there are times that clearly establishing and communicating boundaries can help maintain friendships. For example, let's say you and your best friend have a long-standing tradition of going out to eat and to see a movie every Sunday. One Sunday they bring someone they've been dating for a few weeks. You are upset because neither of you has ever brought another person on these outings, and you feel like a third wheel. Later that week your friend calls you to pick the next movie, and you tell them you would prefer it just be the two of you. You say that you would like to get to know their partner better, but not during your Sunday outings. Although this may be an uncomfortable conversation, it would avoid many problems and hurt feelings later. This example highlights the importance of setting boundaries within friendships.

Other examples that may warrant the need to set boundaries can include differing ideologies—for example, politics. If you and a friend constantly argue about politics, it may cause stress. You may even begin to experience stress before meeting up with your friend in anticipation of the uncomfortable dialogue that may occur. It is okay to disagree, but if the conversation continues to go in circles, it may be best to set a boundary of no political talk before the topic becomes a wedge between you and your friend. Many families have adopted similar boundaries that stipulate no talking about politics at the dinner table.

When you set boundaries, you create conditions that can help head off future problems, issues, and stressors. Here are some tips to help you set boundaries with others:

- *Get to the point.* It can sometimes be difficult to be direct, but this often works best when you are trying to set boundaries. If a friend asks to borrow money, saying, "I just don't loan money to other people, sorry—it is a personal thing" is more effective than saying, "I don't have any money right now." The first response stops the behavior now and in the future. The second response may stop the behavior right now, but you leave an opening for them to ask you the same question later.
- *Offer different solutions.* Instead of saying no and leaving it at that, offer alternative options. If a friend is asking to borrow money, you could say, "I don't loan out money, sorry. Is there something else I can help you with?" In this response, you are being clear about boundaries regarding money but still trying to offer support. However, do not offer support or another option if you are not willing to follow through.
- *Compromise.* There may be times when you must compromise your boundaries. It is important to be flexible. For example, your friend from the scenario presented above asks to borrow money again. This time your friend has a medical emergency and needs \$100 to help pay their rent. Due to

## A Note About Sharing Passwords

A recent trend in relationships is password sharing: About 70 percent of people in a relationship report sharing their password with their partner (Howard, 2018). Many people believe sharing PINs, passwords, or fingerprint and facial recognition keys to each other's devices displays a deep level of trust and intimacy in the relationship.

However, sharing passwords with your partner may not be a good idea. If a breakup were to occur, you are placing yourself at considerable risk. One study found that 21 percent of people admitted to spying on an ex-partner and 12 percent said they publicly shared their partner's personal information as an act of revenge (Howard, 2018). An ex-partner could also use your passwords to make purchases against your account, placing you at financial risk. Imagine the stress you would feel if your ex-partner had all your passwords to your social media accounts, bank accounts, and subscription services. To avoid the risk, don't share your passwords.

the unique circumstance, you may feel you want to compromise your boundaries and budget to include this unexpected expense. So you make an exception and loan your friend the money.

You can determine the strength of your relationship by how well you and your partner manage stress. Stress can derive from outside the relationship or from within. For example, Lily has a date with her partner after a stressful day at work. She really feels like she needs some time to decompress, but decides to keep her date because she doesn't want to hurt her partner's feelings. Unfortunately, Lily feels resentment that she didn't get to go home to spend some much-needed time alone, and she is a bit short tempered with her partner. They end up getting in an argument, and Lily ends the date early. In this case, stress came into the relationship and was not handled well.

The next day, Lily wakes up feeling better and calls her partner to apologize. She explains how stressed she felt and vows to share her feelings with her partner next time. In return, her partner promises she won't get upset if Lily cancels a date when she needs some time alone. Although this example highlights how stress can hurt a relationship, it also highlights how relationships can grow when the partners learn how to cope with stress.

**All people encounter stress; all relationships will also experience stress.**

When you encounter stress in a relationship, it is important to work with the other person to manage that stress. It shouldn't be an all *you* or *them* problem, but a *we* problem. Working with your partner to combat stress can help you grow stronger in your relationship. Research suggests that romantic partners who communicate with each other about their stressors are better able to manage their own stress (Lau, Randall, Duran, & Tao, 2018). Additionally, being in a positive, healthy relationship with another person can also serve as a stress management tool (Brauer, Proyer, & Chick, 2021).

## Interpersonal Communication

The way you communicate with others can help you develop positive, healthy relationships. **Interpersonal communication** is the way you exchange information with other people and includes both **verbal communication** (written and spoken language) and **nonverbal communication** (posture, dress, facial expressions, hand gestures, etc.). It occurs anytime two or more people are in the same space and are aware of each other's presence. Whether through words or actions, people read your cues to gather information.

Your ability to communicate can impact how you perceive the stressors in your life. Research suggests that effective interpersonal communication can significantly reduce psychosocial stressors (Mathews & Shajan, 2018). On the other hand, poor interpersonal communication skills can greatly hinder your relationships and may even be linked to dissatisfaction in relationships

## Stress Relief Through Animals

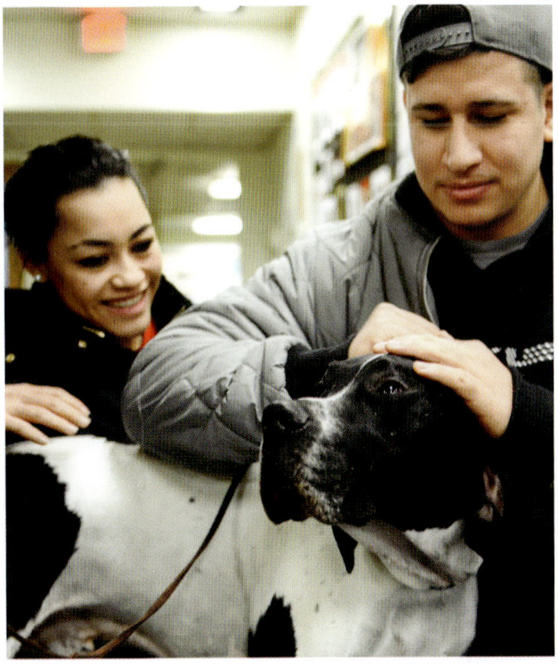

Humans and animals have existed together from the beginning. Research suggests that these human–animal interactions provide benefits for both (Young, Pritchard, Nottle, & Banwell, 2020). Therapy dogs can help reduce stress physiologically (measured by a reduction in cortisol levels) and improve overall feelings of happiness (Kline et al., 2020). Animal-assisted activities have been shown to reduce stress and promote wellness in humans (Ein, Li, & Vickers, 2018); studies show spending just 10 minutes with an animal can provide a significant reduction in stress (Pendry & Vandagriff, 2019). Colleges have taken notice, and many now utilize dogs to help students de-stress with events such as Doggie De-Stress or Pause With Some Paws. A group called PAWS (Pet Away Worry and Stress) also works to bring dogs, cats, bunnies, guinea pigs, mini horses, llamas, and even chickens to college campuses for students to visit and play with (Orellana, 2019).

Because stress can reduce the brain's memory and functioning, animal visits on campus during midterms and final exams can help students feel more relaxed and improve performance. The act of petting an animal can serve as a mindfulness activity that promotes an "in the moment" mindset, help reduce anxiety, improve feelings of love, increase feelings of self-worth, and serve as a distraction from a stressful situation (Brkjacic, Sucic, Lucic, Tkalic, & Lipovcan, 2020; Ein et al., 2018; Kalenkoski & Korankye, 2021). Does your campus offer similar programs? If not, consider asking your student affairs or engagement office to bring in animals during final exam week.

(Zemp, Nussbeck, Cummings, & Bodenmann, 2017). This section will highlight different types of communication and provide ways to improve your own interpersonal communication skills.

One of the most important factors in good communication is the ability to listen. Have you ever been speaking with someone and felt you were not being heard? **Reflective listening** is a technique that involves actively trying to understand the speaker's idea and checking back to ensure you have understood and interpreted their words correctly. Some methods for practicing reflective listening involve being quiet and listening to the speaker without interrupting, taking time to think about what the speaker has said, and repeating or offering your interpretation of their words to check for proper understanding. Reflective listening allows the speaker to confirm their message was heard and to make corrections about any misunderstandings or misinterpretations. Figure 7.1 shows the steps in reflective listening.

**Communication is key in developing and maintaining healthy relationships.**

### Verbal and Nonverbal Communication

Verbal communication is using language—spoken, written, or signed—to convey information. It is one way you can express your ideas, thoughts, and feelings to others. The standardized or literal definition of a word is considered its **denotative meaning**. For example, the definition of *love* found in the dictionary is "an intense feeling of deep affection."

Words, however, can take on different meanings based on context and lived experience; this is **connotative meaning**. For example, what does *love* specifically mean to you? Some may use it as a term of endearment: "Hello, love." You may

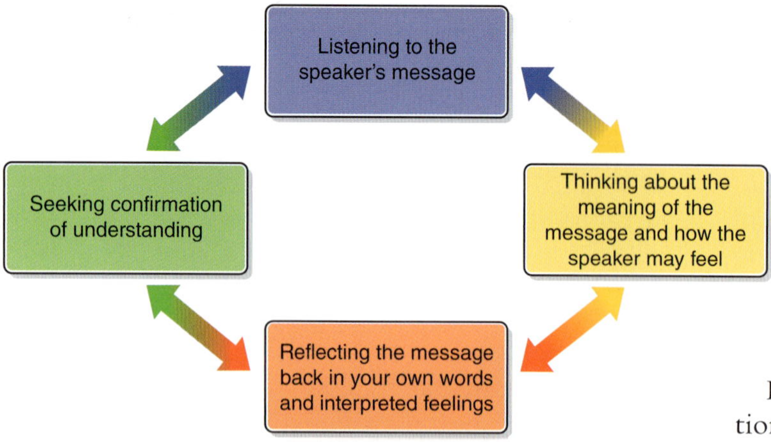


**Figure 7.1** Steps in reflective listening.

sometimes use it to express a liking of something ("I love ice cream") and other times to express deep feelings to another person ("I love you"). This can sometimes cause confusion when communicating: Two people may be using the same word with different connotative meanings. For example, you may say "love ya" to a friend at the end of an outing. In your mind, you are saying it to express a nice feeling you have for your friend. However, if your friend believes you are expressing a deep emotion for them, this may cause quite a predicament. It is important to think about the words you use and how you are using them.

Additionally, many people use **euphemisms**, which are words or phrases used as a substitute for ones that are socially awkward or negative. For example, when you sell your car, it is not *used*, but *preowned*. A couple who has sex without being in a relationship may call themselves *friends with benefits*. You might prefer being *in-between jobs* to *unemployed*. Sometimes, euphemisms can get in the way of communication because they can be a disguise to what you are truly trying to say.

Learning how to positively employ your communication skills can help you professionally and personally. Here are some tips to help you improve your verbal communication skills:

- *Think before you speak*. This may be something a parent or teacher has told you, but it is great advice. When tensions are high, the emotional center of the brain takes over, leaving little space for the frontal lobe (logical brain). When you take a few seconds (or minutes) to think about what you are going to say, you will make better choices in the type of words you use.
- *Use direct language*. As mentioned earlier, words can have different meanings for another person based on their lived experiences. Try to be forthcoming and direct.
- *Be open and honest*. Express your emotions. If you are unsure about your feelings, say so. It will help develop trust as you show the other person your real self.

It may surprise you to learn most communication is conducted nonverbally (Baroona, 2019). This type of communication generally occurs without conscious thought and is considered innate. For example, when you are speaking with someone, are you aware of your posture, hand gestures, and facial expressions? Do you tell yourself when to smile or frown during a conversation? Most people do not think about their nonverbal communication skills as they occur.

It may be easy to interpret basic nonverbal communication. In almost all parts of the world, a smile and a frown are universally recognized expressions. However, when it comes to more complex gestures, confusion can arise. Nonverbal communication is often culturally based—for example, giving someone the thumbs-up sign in the United States is typically interpreted to mean *good job* or *OK*. However, in many Middle Eastern cultures, this sign is a rude gesture with a meaning similar to a raised middle finger in the United States.

Nonverbal communication can be either positive or negative (see figure 7.2). Unlike verbal communication, which occurs one word at a time, multiple mechanisms of nonverbal communication can occur simultaneously. For example, you can change your tone of voice and facial expression at the same time. The following are modes of nonverbal communication:

- *Kinesics (body movement and facial expression)*. Facial expressions are a primary method for expressing emotions. Imagine sitting across the class from a good friend. Every so often, you both look at each other and smile. Without using words, you are communicating with each other.
- *Haptics (touch)*. Touch is the first type of communication you are exposed to. Infants

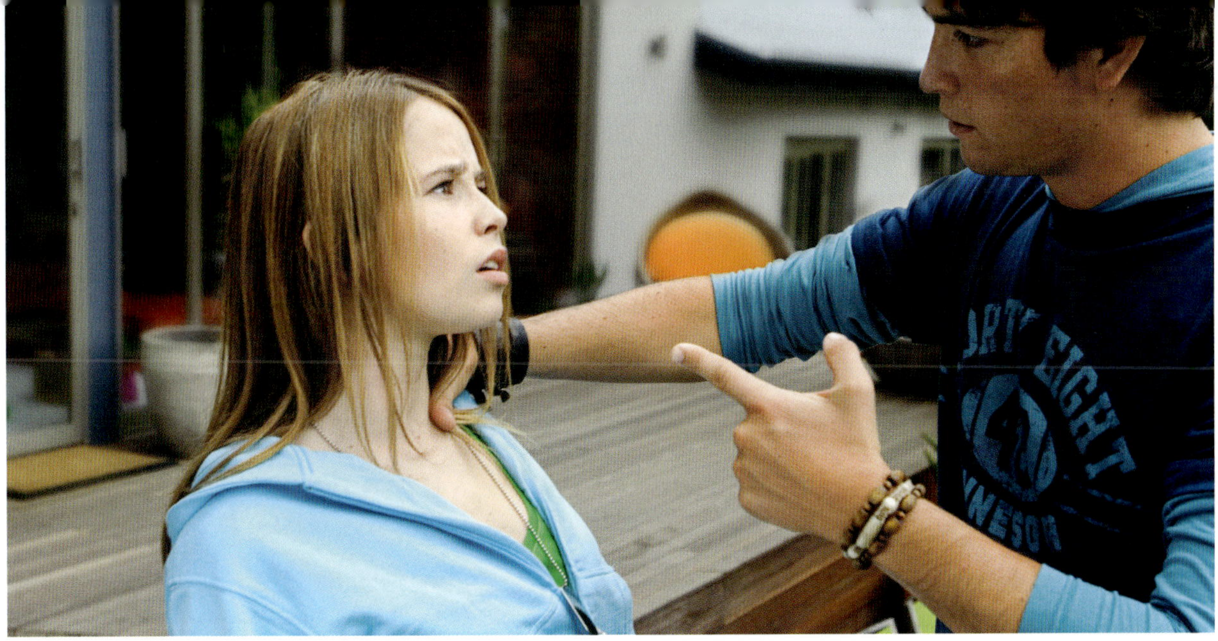

learn about love and trust through being touched. As you age, touch can be used to express emotions or offer support. Studies have shown that touch and hugs can reduce the cortisol response to stress. Self-touch, such as placing your hand on your heart or giving yourself a hug, can also have similar stress-reducing effects (Dreisoerner et al., 2021)

- *Personal appearance*. How you present yourself to others conveys meaning. For example, if your job requires business attire and you were to show up in sweatpants and a T-shirt, it may give the impression that you do not care about your job. Some professions use a uniform to help signal a position of authority—consider a police officer's uniform or doctor's lab coat. Personal appearance can also change based on the situation. For example, what you wear to work may be different from what you wear with your friends.
- *Proxemics (space)*. The space that people maintain around one another can have an influence on relationships. Have you ever been in an elevator with someone who infringed on your personal space? When your personal space is invaded, it can cause discomfort and stress, and you may start to shift or even move away. We have different space requirements depending on how close we feel with others; these preferences differ by culture. In the United States, proxemics generally reflect the following rules

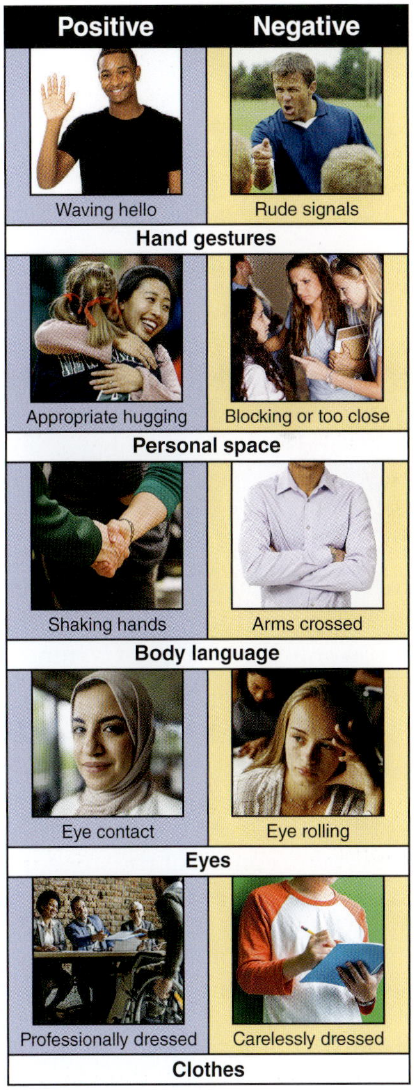


**Figure 7.2** Nonverbal communication can be either positive or negative.

(Department of Communication, Indiana State University, 2016):
  - Intimate space: 18 inches
  - Personal space: 18 inches to 4 feet
  - Social space: 4 to 12 feet
  - Public space: 12 feet or more
- *Paralanguage (vocal effects)*. Vocal qualities such as tone, pitch, speed, and volume can emphasize greater meaning. For example, the use of speed can indicate excitement—if you've ever listened to a teenager speak excitedly about their favorite band, it may be hard to follow. Speed can also indicate nervousness. Many people giving a public speech will talk very quickly as a result of nerves (and perhaps a hope to get the speech over with).

Since this study, COVID-19 changed the world and may have shifted expectations in the amount of space.

### Stress Communication

The way you communicate can help you better manage your stress. There are three categories of stress communication (Lau et al., 2018). The first is general explanation: With this type, you are neutrally and factually describing the stressor. The second category is emotion-focused communication, which describes how the stress made you feel. The third category, problem-focused communication, highlights solutions to the stressor or solicits solutions from others.

When you only use one type of communication to describe your stress, you are not disclosing the full issue, which may do little to help reduce or manage your stress. However, when you utilize all three categories, you are better able to express yourself, define the stress, and work on a solution. This places you in control of the stressor and not the stressor in control of you. For example:

- *Okay*. School is stressing me out.
- *Better*. I am struggling with one of my classes, which is stressing me out. I am worried about not getting a good grade.
- *Best*. I am struggling with one of my classes, which is stressing me out. I am worried about not getting a good grade. What are some resources I can use to help me raise my grade?

Learning how to communicate about your stress can help you better describe your feelings and experiences to others and ask for support when needed.

## Managing and Resolving Conflict

When managed effectively, conflict can help a relationship grow stronger. Unresolved conflict, on the other hand, can cause additional strain on a relationship. There are some types of conflict that have been shown to seriously damage a relationship (Rueda, Yndo, Williams, & Shorey, 2018). These communication styles, dubbed *the four horsemen*, can predict the end of a relationship (Gottman, 1994).

1. *Criticism*. No one enjoys being criticized. It makes the listener feel hurt, rejected, or bad about themselves. When you criticize your partner, you are essentially attacking their character, and if it is done often, it may lead to contempt. Can you see the difference between these two examples?
   - You always forget to take out the garbage. You are so lazy!
   - When you forget to take out the garbage, I get frustrated because the garbage in the house can attract bugs.

   In the first example, criticism is used to attack the person and call them names. The only response available is a defensive one. In the second example, a complaint is used to express feelings and explaining the reason for concern. It is offered in a way that shows there is room for improvement.
2. *Contempt*. In this style of communication (which can arise from criticism), you are mean to your partner and assume a position of superiority. You mock them, call them names, roll your eyes, and show general disrespect. Contempt is fueled by long-standing negative thoughts about your partner. Research has found that cou-

ples who communicate using contempt get sick more often compared to couples who use better forms of communication (Hysi, 2015). Contempt can wear you down and place additional stress on your body. It is the single greatest predictor of divorce.

3. *Defensiveness.* This is a typical response to criticism. Rather than working on the conflict, you feel attacked—and the best way to manage an attack is to shore up your defenses. When we become defensive, we tend to make excuses about our behavior and refuse to take any responsibility. As a result, the initial conflict is ignored.
4. *Stonewalling.* This is generally a response to contempt. Stonewalling occurs when you just shut down and no longer listen or respond to your partner. At this point, you are psychologically flooded and can no longer function in a productive state.

If any of these horsemen show up in your relationship, kick them out! The next section will provide you will ways to manage conflict.

## Communicating While Stressed

Conflict is associated with heightened emotions, which can impair your ability to communicate (Zemp et al., 2017). The areas of the brain associated with problem solving and creative thinking have reduced functioning to allow blood to flow to more primitive areas of the brain, and you are more likely to miss an important message or misunderstand the message being communicated. For these reasons, it is difficult to communicate effectively when stressed. Here are some tips to help you communicate during a conflict:

- *Wait or take a time-out.* Your body needs time to return to a nonstressed state. Tell your partner you are upset and want to talk, but you need a minute (or a lot of them) to calm down and think about what you are going to say. Waiting gives your body the time needed to return to normal functioning.
- *Prepare for the conversation by preparing a list of topics.* If it is a long list, understand that it may take more than one conversation to resolve the conflict.
- *Listen.* When the other person is talking, many people will only be thinking of what to say next. This makes it difficult to really listen to the other person. If you find yourself doing this, take a moment and refocus on what the other person is saying. You cannot effectively communicate if you are not willing to listen.
- *Take a different perspective.* Try to imagine what it would be like to be in the other person's shoes. Even if you don't agree with their perspective, this allows you to better understand their position.
- *If the conversation begins to turn negative, stop.* You may need to take a few minutes to return to a nonstressed state. Or perhaps the conversation needs to take a break for a day or two before you return to the topic.

One of the best ways to begin a conversation about conflict is to use *I* statements. *I* statements identify the conflict and allow you to share your feelings in a manner that doesn't disrespect or attack the other person. Here is the formula for using an *I* statement.

- "I feel . . . " (insert emotion or feeling)
- "When you . . . " (insert the behavior or action)
- "Because . . . " (describe why the behavior or action makes you feel that way)

After you have shared your concern, allow time for your partner to process what you said. Ask them for their perspective. They may have a perspective that you didn't consider, or they may not have realized that particular action had such an effect on you.

**Not all conflict can be resolved, but having a better understanding of the core issue can help you better manage it.**

There may be times when you feel you and the other person are repeatedly having the same argument. When this occurs, it may be a result of a fundamental difference in beliefs or core values. In this case, the issue may not be resolvable. However, if you take the time to consider the core issue and understand it from your partner's perspective, it may help you know where they are coming from and accept it.

## Conflict Management Approaches

There are different ways to handle conflict depending on the situation. You may tend to rely on one preferred method when encountering conflict, but this may not always be the best approach. Multiple strategies for dealing with conflict can be appropriate for a given situation, and having a menu of different conflict resolution styles to choose from can help you better match the resolution to the conflict, resulting in a better outcome (Mosadeghrad & Mojbafan, 2019). There are five styles of conflict management (Thomas & Kilmann, 1976; Ionut, 2020); try practicing each to become more familiar with the process.

1. *Accommodating.* With this approach, you give in to the conflict. This works best in situations where you do not have a strong opinion or the other person's solution is the best fit. This also works best when preserving the other person's feelings or the relationship is more important to you than the conflict.
2. *Collaborating.* This approach finds a solution where the needs of both parties are met with a win–win solution. This approach requires trust and a lot of time, but solutions tend to be long lasting.
3. *Avoiding.* This common strategy occurs when everyone pretends there is no problem. It is a good approach to use in situations where the conflict is temporary or will resolve itself on its own. It is not effective when the conflict will not go away on its own because conflict tends to bubble back up to the surface.
4. *Competing.* This approach is best when you have a strong opinion on the solution and you do not have a relationship to preserve with the other person. This approach is also known as the win–lose approach.
5. *Compromising.* In this approach, both sides give up something to work together for a solution, sometimes called the lose–lose approach. This requires a lot of cooperation from both sides and works well when both sides have equally important goals or tasks. In the end, neither side is completely happy with the solution, nor are they offended.

## Conflict Resolution

Conflict is unavoidable. However, there are steps to help you better understand the cause of the conflict and work together to come up with the best solution.

1. *Define the problem.* This provides an opportunity for each side to present their perspective on the problem. Express how you view the conflict and how it has impacted you. Listen to the other person with an open mind, and try to see the conflict from their perspective.
2. *Identify the cause of the conflict.* Now that the conflict has been defined, you want to discover what led to it. What happened to cause the conflict? What other factors might have contributed?
3. *Agree on a common goal.* How does each party think the conflict should be solved? What would make things better? Identify a goal each party wants to work toward.
4. *Brainstorm solutions.* Create a list of possible solutions. After a list is created, analyze the positive and negative aspects of each solution. Discuss how each solution would impact each party and which would be the best fit for solving the conflict.
5. *Come to an agreement.* Both sides agree on a final solution to resolve the conflict and agree to do their part in enacting it.
6. *Reflect.* After the solution has been implemented, reflect on the conflict resolution process and have each party share their perspective. Did they feel heard? What could have been done differently? Have each side identify how well the solution worked to resolve the conflict. Are there any lingering problems? Did the solution cause more conflict, or was it effective?

This method for resolving conflict encourages collaboration and cooperation to ensure all parties are involved in the solution. Even if the solution is not ideal, you will feel better about it if you feel heard and included in the resolution process.

Conflict is a source of stress, but it can be seen as an opportunity to work together to ultimately make the relationship stronger. This is true of both business and personal relationships. As you begin to practice your conflict resolution skills, you will become more confident and feel better equipped to manage disagreement. Although it will not eliminate stress from your life, these skills will help you better manage your stress and work better with others.

## Summary

Social wellness is the ability to form and maintain relationships. Having a strong social support network is important to help you cope with stress. Even simply knowing you have the support of others is enough to give you the fortitude to manage your stress. To help maintain positive relationships, interpersonal communication is key. Learning how to better communicate with others promotes relationships and can help reduce stress by avoiding miscommunication errors. Conflict in relationships is unavoidable, but having the tools to manage conflict in a healthy way can strengthen your relationships and help you feel more confident.

## WWW ONLINE RESOURCES

Visit HK*Propel* to access audio supplements, worksheets, and vocabulary flash cards for this chapter.

## DISCUSSION QUESTIONS

1. How would you rate your own social wellness? In what areas do you feel you have a high level of social wellness? In what areas do you feel there is a need for improvement? How can you improve your overall social wellness?
2. Explain the importance of a social support network. If you don't have a strong social support network, how can you develop one?
3. Some say social media can serve as a mechanism for social support, whereas others believe social media is harmful and can increase stress. What are your thoughts on social media? Do you consider it friend or foe? Justify your answer.
4. How can setting boundaries in a relationship minimize future conflict and stress? What boundaries have you set with your friends or partner? How have they helped you maintain positive relationships?

# 8

# Spiritual Wellness

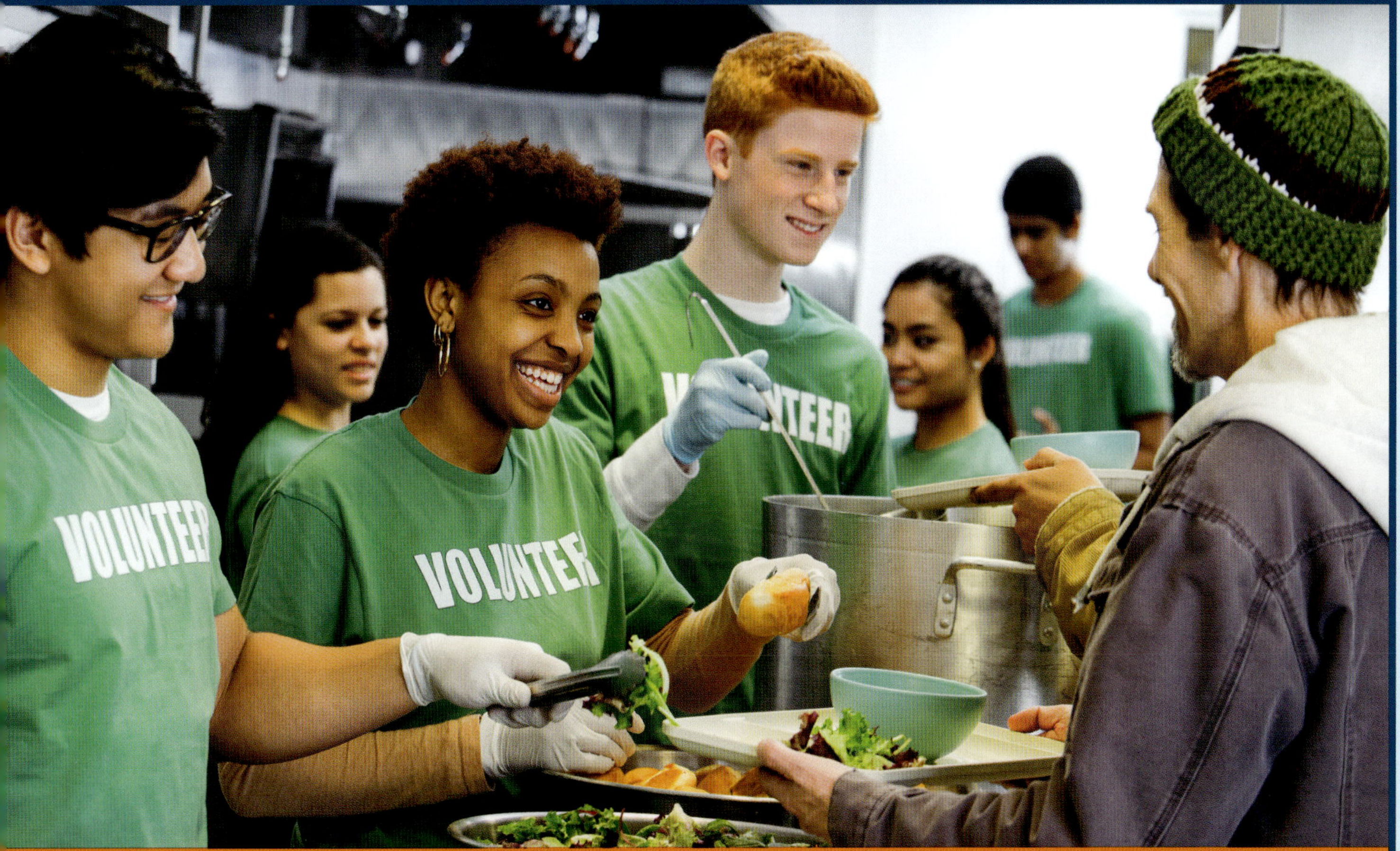


## LEARNING OBJECTIVES

After reading this chapter, you will be able to do the following:

- Describe how spiritual wellness plays a role in overall wellness
- Explain the different components of spiritual wellness
- Compare and contrast spirituality and religiosity
- Identify the link between spirituality and stress
- Examine ways altruism, gratitude, empathy, and compassion can increase spiritual wellness

# KEY TERMS

altruism
compassion
dispositional gratitude
empathy
gratitude
mentalization
religiosity
self-compassion
spirituality

Spiritual wellness is having meaning and purpose in your life. It is understanding your connection to the greater world and having beliefs and values that help guide your decisions. Spiritual wellness also means having harmony with your surroundings. Spiritual wellness can incorporate religion, but this is not a necessary component.

People who have high levels of spiritual wellness report being happier and having greater satisfaction in life (Deb, Thomas, Bose, & Aswathi, 2020). Another study found that students who reported high levels of spiritual wellness also had better interpersonal relationships and higher levels of concentration, persistence, self-confidence, and self-discipline, all of which have been positively associated with academic success (Pong, 2017).

Spiritual wellness has also been associated with positive health behavior. Having a higher sense of spirituality is associated with decreased levels of risky behaviors such as substance use and abuse (Odrovakavula & Mohammadnezhad, 2022). One study found a similar association between spiritual wellness and lower rates of substance abuse among undergraduate students in medical school (Raghuveer, Bhatia, & Sachith, 2022). This study also discovered lower levels of burnout and psychological distress among students who rated high levels of spiritual wellness. Having spiritual wellness may help you appreciate life and give you a stronger desire to make healthy decisions. For instance, if you feel you are in this world for an important reason, you are more likely to avoid trouble that might keep you from achieving your purpose.

**Spiritual wellness has been shown to help enhance your quality of life.**

Spiritual wellness has also been shown to improve outcomes for people with chronic conditions. One study of people with kidney disease found spiritual wellness to be associated with better disease acceptance. This is significant because those with better acceptance generally have better physical function and have higher levels of treatment compliance, both of which result in better outcomes (Zhang, Xue, Chen, An, & Chen, 2020). Spiritual wellness has also been associated with better end-of-life outcomes, whereas low levels of spiritual wellness has been associated with poorer quality of life (Balboni et al., 2022).

> Spirituality is recognizing and celebrating that we are all inextricably connected to each other by a power greater than all of us, and that our connection to that power and to one another is grounded in love and compassion. Practicing spirituality brings a sense of perspective, meaning and purpose in our lives.
>
> **Brené Brown**

Your journey to spiritual wellness is a personal one. For each person, the journey will look different. This chapter will therefore present the four main concepts of spiritual wellness—altruism, gratitude, empathy, and compassion—and provide you with ways to improve these traits to help guide your own journey.

## Spirituality and Religion

Many people believe spirituality and religion are the same thing. Though related, they hold separate and distinct meanings. **Religiosity** is a common construct used to measure a person's devotion and commitment to a formal religion and its beliefs and practices (Villani, Sorgente, Iannello, & Antonietii, 2019). **Spirituality** is more personal in nature and is identified as a human's desire for interconnectedness and quest for meaning (Villani et al., 2019). Having a strong sense of religiosity is correlated with high levels of spirituality, but people with high levels of spirituality may or may not identify with or participate in formalized religion.

Some view religion as extrinsic (from without) and spirituality as intrinsic (from within) (Park, 2021). Many think of religion in terms of a place of worship (a church, mosque, or temple) or a religious text (Bible, Torah, or Koran). However, these extrinsic things are meant to promote an intrinsic experience. Religion is a common set of values and symbols to help explain the world and our place within it, and research suggests that solely depending on the extrinsic component (attending worship, celebrating holidays, etc.) without reflecting on the intrinsic component—that is, just going through the motions without fully committing to the act—has little to no benefit (Han, Sun, Cheng, Chung, & Kao, 2022; Park, 2021). It is possible to belong to a religious group and fully subscribe to its intrinsic spiritual components—one of the goals of religion is to help people become closer to God, one another, and society. However, for many, religious practice and spirituality are separate and have not been fully developed. See table 8.1 for a comparison between the extrinsic and intrinsic components of religiosity.

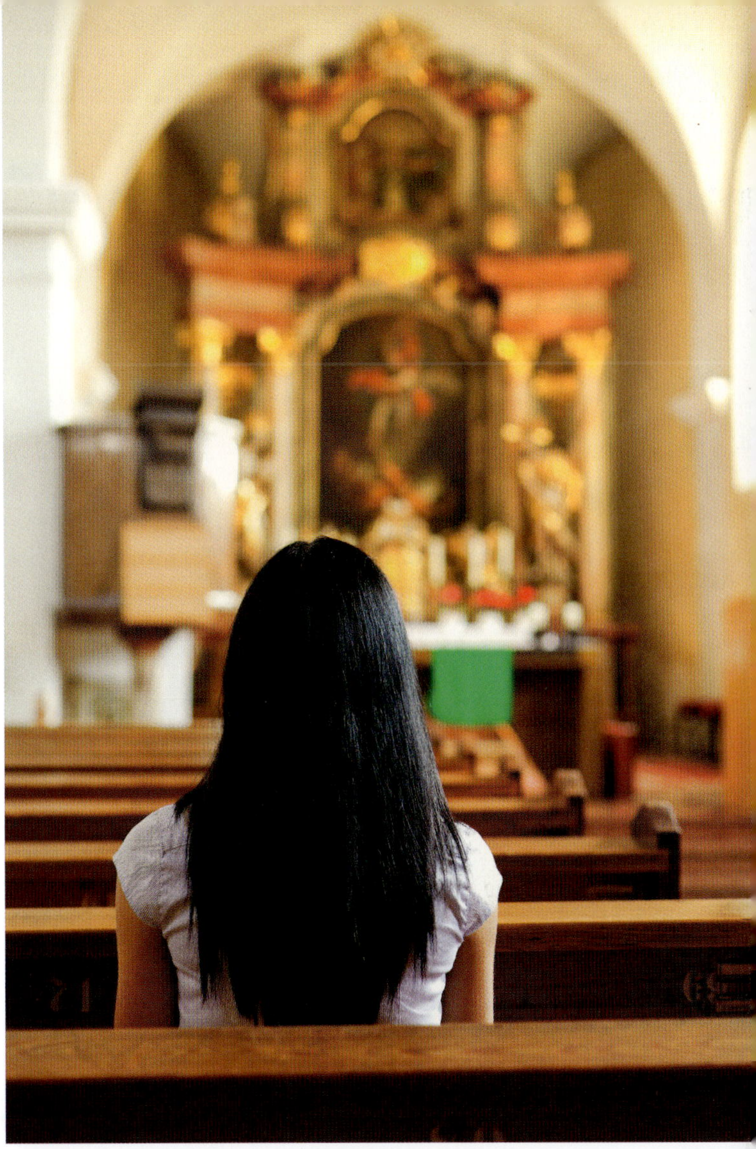

Both religiosity and spirituality are associated with better health outcomes and an increase in life satisfaction. To explain this association, it is believed that people with high levels of spirituality or religiosity maintain a more positive evaluation of their own life, even in the face of adversity (Ramsay, Tong, Chowdhury, & Ho, 2019). For example, when going through hard times, they may tell themselves, "God will not give me more than I can handle" or "this too will pass." Acknowledging that stress is only temporary and that you can handle it will make life more manageable and help you maintain optimism.

**Knowing you can handle hard situations can help you develop a better mindset in life.**

**Table 8.1** Intrinsic Versus Extrinsic Religiosity

| Intrinsic | Extrinsic |
|---|---|
| Motivated by core beliefs | Motivated by group norms |
| Deeply personal | Impersonal and structural |
| Not subject to social pressures or conformity | Subject to social pressures and conformity |

## Components of Spiritual Wellness

Spiritual wellness has been defined as the "glue that brings all pieces together" (Heyn, 2018). It is the thread the links all living things together and helps us make meaning of the world. As such, there are four tenets that serve as the underlying principles of spiritual wellness (Banks, 1980):

1. *Spiritual wellness acts as a unifying force that integrates the other dimensions of wellness (physical, emotional, intellectual, social, and environmental).* The elements of wellness are not separate, but united components that make up your whole self. When one aspect is suffering, it will negatively impact the others, and when you work on improving one aspect of health, it will also improve the others. For example, a study conducted on patients with chronic kidney disease found that those who had higher levels of spirituality were better able to cope with pain and had fewer signs of depression, lower risk of suicide, and better renal function after transplantation (components of mental, emotional, and physical wellness) compared to those who rates lower levels of spirituality (Bravin, Dos Santos Trettene, Andrade, & Popim, 2019).
2. *Spiritual wellness helps bring meaning to life.* This serves as an inner drive to contribute to life and make progress toward your goals. What drives you? How do you fit within the bigger picture? Having higher levels of spirituality can help you be more effective and happier at work. One study found that workplace spirituality is associated with more positive feelings about working and higher levels of self-efficacy and engagement at work (Corso, Carlo, Carluccio, Colledani, & Falco, 2020). In short, having higher levels of spirituality can help you enjoy your job more and be better at it.
3. *Spiritual wellness transcends the individual.* Spiritual wellness unites all individuals. This bond among humans allows you to make sacrifices to serve the needs of others. People with higher levels of spirituality are more likely to contribute to the public good: One study found people with higher levels of spirituality volunteered more compared to people with lower levels of spirituality (Hughes, 2021). When you help others, it makes you feel good about yourself.
4. *Spiritual wellness acknowledges that there is some higher power at work.* Regardless of what religion or higher power you worship, this aspect understands that there is some force behind the workings of the universe.

These tenets can be understood as the core beliefs that serve as the foundation of spiritual wellness. Four domains were then developed to describe how different types of relationships help serve these tenets of spiritual wellness (Fisher, 2011):

- *Personal domain* refers to the relationship with oneself. This domain includes self-awareness and self-worth. Having a meaning and purpose in life are factors associated with the personal domain.
- *Communal domain* refers to the relationship between the self and others as it relates to morality. This domain includes trust, forgiveness, and love.
- *Environmental domain* refers to the relationship between the self and the environment. It also includes the sense of awe one has with nature and the world around them.
- *Transcendental domain* refers to the relationship between the self and a higher being. This domain has many different meanings, but one commonality among them all is the sense of something beyond the human element. Religion, meditation, and prayer would all fall under this domain.

These spiritual domains show how the dimensions of wellness are interconnected. The focus of the personal domain—having a better understanding of yourself—can be seen as a facet of emotional wellness. In the communal domain, your focus is the relationships you have with others, a component of social wellness. The environmental domain's focus on respecting nature and your surroundings will improve your environmental wellness. Together with the transcendental domain, these reflect the interconnectedness that is often used to describe spiritual wellness (figure 8.1). It is the sense of peace and respect with yourself, others, and the world.

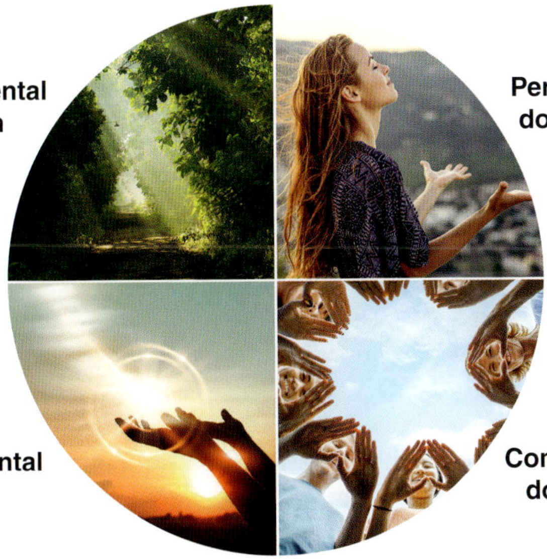


**Figure 8.1** Spiritual wellness is a set of relationships among different domains.

Research Spotlight

## Praying to Reduce Stress

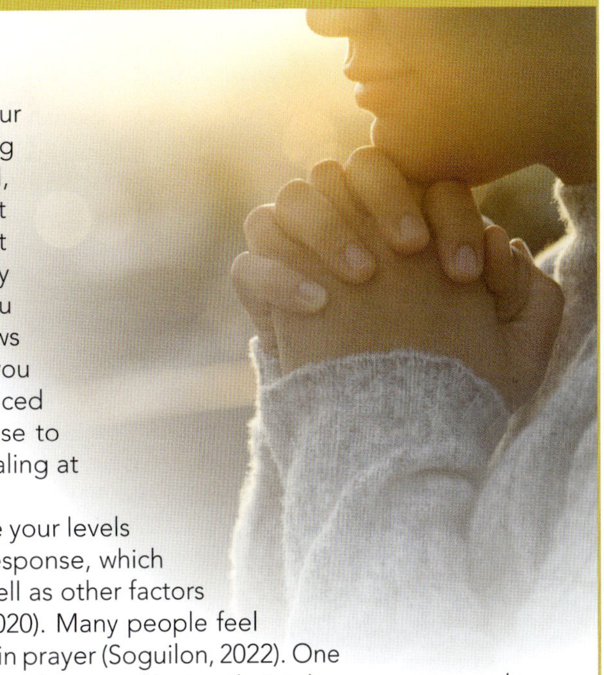

Prayer is a dedicated time for you to focus on your thoughts and concerns and release them by giving them to a higher power (LaBarbera & Hetzel, 2016). Let's say you are stressed about a test result from your doctor, which has been making it difficult to focus. You decide to pray and mentally give that stressor to God. When you pray, you give yourself permission to let it go, which allows you to focus on other things—hopefully, things you have control over. Prayer is the most widely practiced healing modality in the United States, with close to 80 percent of people resorting to prayer for healing at some point in their lives (Levin, 2016).

Studies suggest that praying can help reduce your levels of stress. Prayer can help elicit the relaxation response, which lowers your blood pressure and heart rate as well as other factors affected by stress (May, Cooper, & Fincham, 2020). Many people feel better emotionally and mentally after engaging in prayer (Soguilon, 2022). One study discovered that teachers who prayed more often rated loving their job more compared to those who prayed less often (LaBarbera & Hetzel, 2016). In a similar study conducted on Muslim nurses, job stress was correlated with life dissatisfaction, but among nurses who regularly practiced salat (prayer in Islam), job stress was reduced and there were higher levels of life satisfaction (Anchour, Muhamad, Syihab, Nor, & Yusoff, 2021).

Prayer can also reduce anxiety and sorrow. In a qualitative study on the effects of prayer, participants said they experienced more emotional stability and peace and a better connection with a higher power (Stockigy et al., 2021). Additionally, many felt prayer helped them better cope with negative life events (e.g., death, chronic illness).

Focusing on helping others is part of spiritual wellness that can be aided by prayer. It allows you to understand the suffering of others and ask for their suffering to be taken away. Many religions have special prayers to ask for help with healing another person. Lastly, many prayers focus on gratitude, which acknowledge and give thanks for all you have. This helps you focus on the positive things in your life and pay less attention to the negative things.

## Spiritual Wellness and Stress

Studies have shown that having high levels of spirituality may help you better manage your stress and reduce the physical symptoms associated with stress (McClintock et al., 2019). This may be partly a result of the way you think about stress and the control you have over it. When you believe you can control stress in your life, you are better able to follow through with actions that manage the stressor. When you encounter stress that is out of your control, spirituality allows you to place faith and trust in something greater than yourself. Figure 8.2 shows symptoms of spiritual stress versus spiritual wellness.

There are many opportunities for students to develop their spiritual wellness, including church groups, Bible studies, Hillel, meditation rooms, and Muslim centers. Many colleges have religious centers or meetings on or near their campuses to help students practice their faith or introduce them to new religious experiences. Check with your campus to see what types of opportunities are available for you.

Spirituality may also contribute to an increased level of resilience against stress. One study suggests that individuals with higher levels of spirituality tend to be better at handling stress because their brains allow more time to process the stressor before reacting (McClintock et al., 2019). Additionally, among those with higher levels of spirituality, their brain is better able to regulate emotions during stress, which also reduces the physical stress response. Imagine taking a test that will automatically shut down once a timer goes off. You know there is not enough time to complete the test, so you rush through it, not giving yourself any time to think about the answers. You would probably feel stressed and not perform very well. Now, consider taking a test with an unlimited amount of time. In this case, you would feel more relaxed, spend time considering your answers, and likely perform much better. Spirituality works in a similar way with stress: It provides your brain with additional time to analyze the stressor and respond in the most effective manner.

**Prayer has been shown to help reduce stress by providing an outlet for that stress.**

## Altruism

Have you ever purchased a present for someone and felt excited to give it to them? This is an example of **altruism**, a selfless concern for others. People who are altruistic are motivated to help others and receive pleasure from doing so. Altruism is associated with spirituality: Many religions around the world stress the importance of helping others, particularly strangers. Research suggests that people who are religious or spiritual or who live in religious areas are more likely to help strangers compared to those who are not religious or spiritual (Bennett & Einolf, 2017). One study also found the brain scans of people who rated themselves as highly altruistic to show

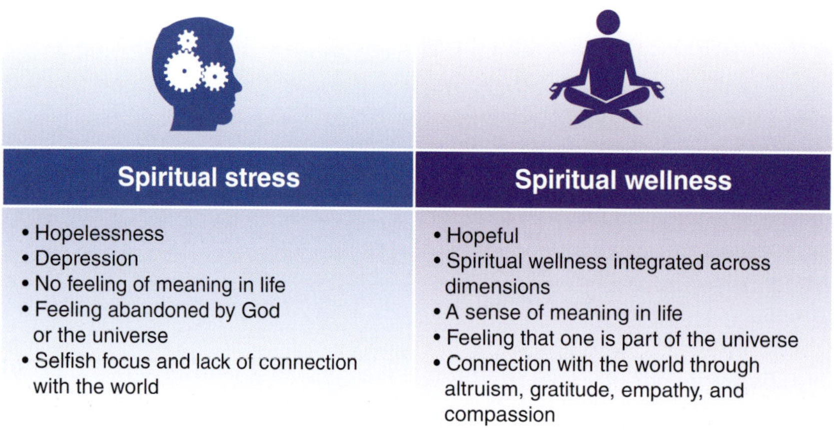


**Figure 8.2** Spiritual stress versus spiritual wellness.

## Let It Go

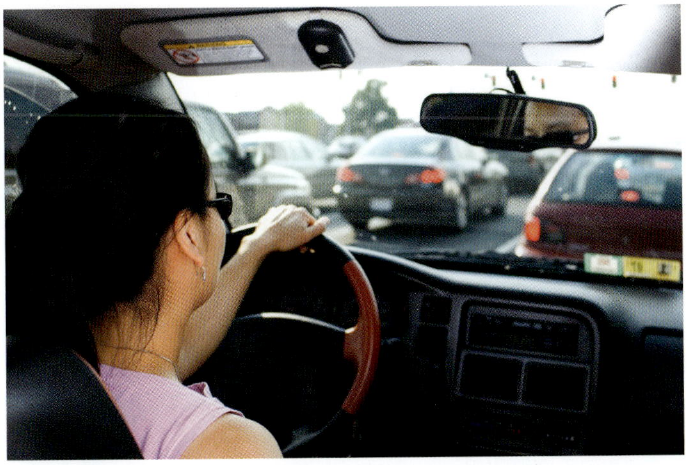

Jasmine is driving to class and gets stuck in traffic. It soon becomes evident that she will be late to class, and there is nothing she can do about it. Jasmine hates being late, especially to class, and feels increasingly angry and stressed the longer she is stuck. By the time Jasmine makes it to class, she feels so upset she cannot even concentrate on what is going on in class.

Jasmine's classmate Israel, who considers himself to have a high level of spirituality, is also stuck in traffic. Israel understands there is nothing to be done and that he might as well accept that he will be late to class. The ability to accept the situation and let it go makes it easier for Israel to cope. Instead of getting angry and upset, Israel decides to sing along to music to help pass the time. When Israel eventually gets to class, he can focus and participate.

These two scenarios exemplify the power you have in a stressful situation that you are unable to control—when you are able to acknowledge this and let it go, you will find a feeling of relief. Those with high levels of spirituality can mentally release uncontrollable situations into the hands of a higher power. Next time you encounter a stressful situation that is out of your control, give yourself permission to let it go. See if it helps reduce your stress and allow you to return to peace.

---

**The act of helping others promotes feelings of worthiness and prosocial behavior.**

greater cortical thickness in regions that were previously only associated with higher levels of personal spirituality (Miller et al., 2021).

Altruism can have greater benefits for the person offering help than the person receiving the help. One study conducted on people with physical disabilities found that those who volunteered had higher levels of self-esteem than those who didn't (Kulik, 2018). People with higher levels of altruism also rate their subjective well-being more highly (Ashwini & Indumathy, 2018; Huang, Shi, & Lui, 2018). Altruism has also been found to serve as protection against the development of major depressive disorder, even among people with a strong familial history of depression (Miller et al., 2021). People who help others generally have higher levels of emotional wellness.

Being altruistic can help promote a positive perspective on life (Ghiglieri, McAndrew, Baum, & Taff, 2021). It is common to compare what you have to others who have more and feel you are lacking. When you help others less fortunate than yourself, you can develop a new perspective. For example, if you live in a home that seems shabby, and you help someone without a home, you may begin to appreciate the home you have.

Finally, when you engage in the act of giving, it leaves you with a positive feeling about yourself. These positive feelings can help alleviate the symptoms of stress (Kuswartanti, 2020). When you behave altruistically, your brain releases neurotransmitters associated with feeling good (dopamine, oxytocin, and endorphins), which are part of the reward pathway that increases the likelihood of your repeating a behavior–in this case, giving or helping others (De Silva, 2022). This makes you more resilient against stress by promoting a positive outlook in life.

Some people are more naturally altruistic, whereas others must work on fostering behaviors that promote altruism. Some ways to foster altruism include the following:

- *Social interactions*. Surround yourself with people who help others. When you see the altruistic actions of others, it makes you want to engage in altruism.

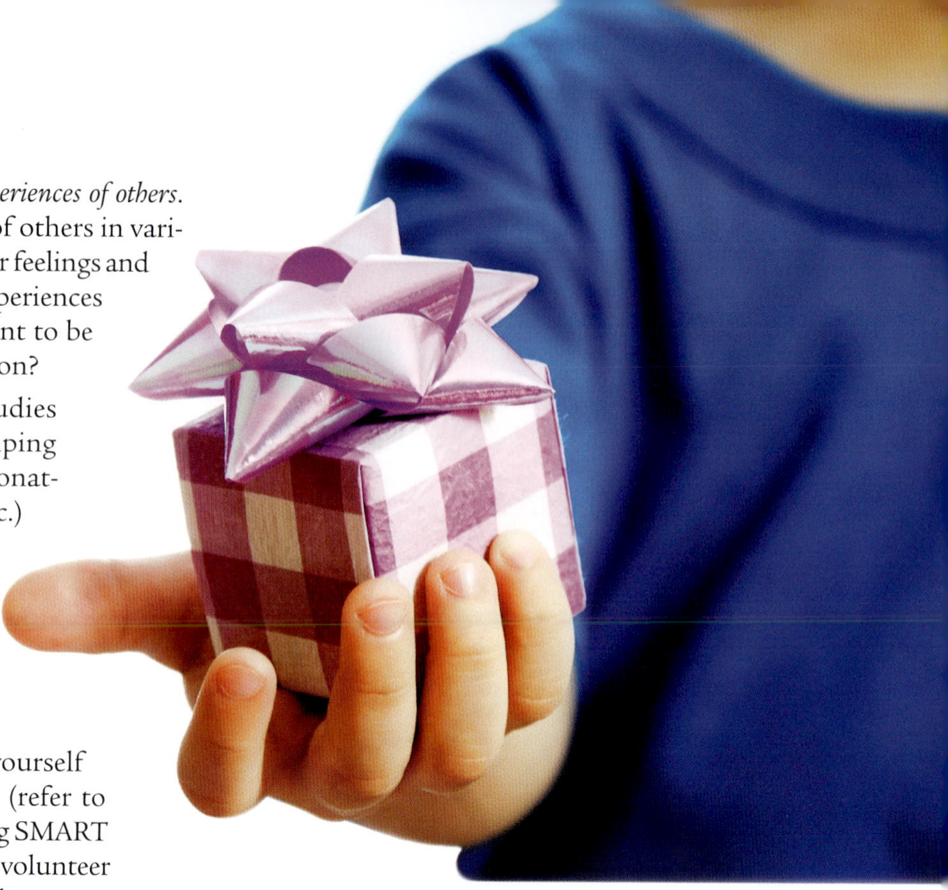

- *Consider the feelings and experiences of others.* Think about the feelings of others in various situations. How do your feelings and interpretations of those experiences differ? How might you want to be treated in the same situation?
- *Volunteer to help others.* Studies show that any type of helping behavior (volunteering, donating blood, food sharing, etc.) results in improved positive emotions (Aknin & Whillans, 2020). These positive emotions will reinforce your desire to continue helping others.
- *Set goals.* Create goals for yourself to become more altruistic (refer to chapter 6 for tips on writing SMART goals). Perhaps you want to volunteer once a month at a local shelter or go to an animal shelter to play with animals. Setting a goal for yourself improves your chances of following through with the behavior.

## Gratitude

**Gratitude** is an approach to life that comes from being thankful and acknowledging the good in your life. You can be thankful for both the tangible (a gift) or intangible (a beautiful sunset). Being grateful may also help connect you to other people, nature, or a higher power. In this way, gratitude is a part of spiritual wellness.

This idea of gratitude is embedded into many world religions. For example, gratitude to God is a core Christian tenet, and there are many phrases within the Bible that mention giving thanks for what you have (Knabb, Vazquez, Wang, & Pate, 2021). In Judaism, followers of Yahweh are encouraged to start each day with being grateful for waking up (Joseph, 2021). In Islam, people are asked to pray five times each day to thank and show gratitude to Allah (Joseph, 2021). In these religions and others, gratitude is a centralized theme that asks people to identify the things in their lives that they are grateful for.

If asked, you could probably come up with a long list of things you wish you had. However, always wishing for more places the focus on what you don't have, or a lacking perspective. On the other hand, if you were asked to come up with a list of all the great things in your life, you may have a harder time getting started, but once you start to acknowledge all you have, you will begin to gain a better appreciation for life. This allows you to change your viewpoint from one of lacking to one of appreciation.

**Dispositional gratitude** is defined as your general orientation to perceiving and appreciating the positives in life (Hartanto, Lee, & Yong, 2018). It is a conscious desire to interpret your experiences, even negative ones, in a positive light—for example, doing poorly on a test can be seen as feedback that you need to spend more time studying for that class. Research suggests that dispositional gratitude can help those with chronic pain. Living with chronic pain is physically and mentally draining, but those who practice dispositional gratitude have better outcomes, including less suffering, greater satisfaction in life, and lower levels of depression (Dillane, Murphy, O'Sullivan, & Di Blasi, 2021). Research suggests that the longer gratitude is practiced, the more pain is reduced. For example, someone who practices 20 minutes of gratitude per day will experience a greater reduction in pain compared to someone who only practices gratitude for 10 minutes a day (Carson et al., 2005).

Having higher levels of gratitude may help you better manage your daily life. People with higher levels of gratitude have lower levels of perceived stress, higher levels of self-esteem, and lower levels of anxiety and general worry (Nezlek, Krejtz, Rusanowka, & Holas, 2019). Gratitude can help you better manage your stress by giving you a positive mindset (Nezlek et al., 2019). In a study conducted on college students, researchers found that students who had higher levels of gratitude had lower levels of psychological distress (Huang, Qui, Alizadeh, & Wu, 2020). When you feel stressed about an upcoming exam, take a few minutes to remind yourself how grateful you are to be able to experience college and all that comes along with being a college student. Think about how finishing college will improve your life and about all the people who don't have this opportunity. Although you will still experience academic stress, it may feel more manageable to remind yourself that each test brings you one step closer to completing college.

**When you begin to pay attention to the positive things in your day, you will find you start paying less attention to the negative ones.**

It is important to remember the threat and challenge response is tied to your perception of the stressor (see chapter 2). Gratitude can enhance your ability to perceive stressors as challenging rather than threatening. One study found that when classmates engaged in gratitude expressions before a stressful task, the task was more likely to be viewed as a challenge (Gu, Ocampo, Algoe, & Oveis, 2022). They also found that giving expressions of gratitude helped reduce the negative physiological responses to stress and decrease perceptions of stress over time. The next time you work on a group project, consider what it would feel like to have each group member share a gratitude expression before beginning. It may change the dynamics of the group to make the work less stressful and more productive for all.

You can practice ways to show your gratitude and see how it impacts other areas of your life. Ways to improve your own gratitude include the following (Allen, 2018; Murphy & Rafie, 2021):

- *Gratitude journaling.* Keep a journal or notes about things you are grateful for. Think about your day's experiences and acknowledge the things that went well. If you are struggling, be grateful you are breathing or can move freely. There is always something you can find to be grateful for.
- *Gratitude letter.* Write a letter to someone in your life you are grateful for. In your letter, tell the person how they have positively impacted your life.
- *Three good things exercise.* At the end of each day, think of three good things that happened. As you begin to see things more graciously, you will notice your mindset changing to be more optimistic.
- *Mental subtraction.* Imagine what your life would look like if a positive event hadn't happened. What if you didn't meet your partner, graduate high school, or attend college? Where you would be in life? How did that positive event lead you to where you are now? Looking back at the positive events in your life and appreciating them for helping you get where you are today can help increase your feelings of gratitude.
- *Find gratitude in your challenges.* Even when you are faced with challenges, look for the good in those experiences. You may have to think creatively, but you can find ways that experience can help you in the long run. For example, going through a work, home, or family crisis can be draining and difficult when you are in the midst of it. However, with the gift of time you can reflect on the support that you had, any positive changes that the crisis led to, or simply express gratitude for having passed through the most difficult stages.
- *Death reflection.* In this exercise, imagine your death. It can be either very specific or general. Reflecting on your own death may help you gain more appreciation for life.
- *Experiential consumption.* Studies suggest people feel more gratitude after spending

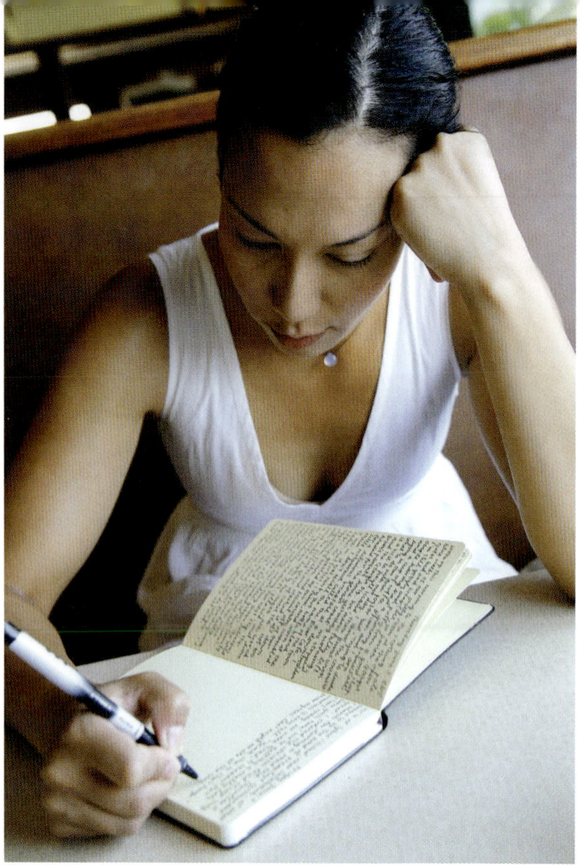

money on an experience (such as a concert or vacation) compared to purchasing a material item (such as a necklace or jeans). Spending money on experiences instead of things may help you be more grateful.

- *Volunteer*. For many, volunteering can expose you to others who are less fortunate than you. It can help you appreciate what you have.
- *Commit to at least one day a week where you will not complain about anything.* Start your day with the intention to view events through a positive lens.

## Empathy

**Empathy** is placing yourself into another's perspective to understand their viewpoint, feelings, and experiences. It involves listening to concerns and feelings without trying to solve or minimize them—the very act of acknowledging someone else's feelings can feel healing. Empathy and spirituality show high levels of correlation (Stewart, Whitworth, & Lawrence, 2022). Empathy is the part of spirituality that supports making meaningful and authentic connections through a deeper awareness of others and is related to having stronger social support and more satisfying relationships, which is associated with improved wellness. Additionally, having relationships that support empathy have been shown to reduce the negative effects of stress (Hunt, Denieffe, & Gooney, 2019).

**Being listened to can help release pent-up emotions and stress.**

Empathy is a multifaceted idea that consists of three constructs (Raine & Chen, 2018):

1. Affective empathy: The ability to appropriately respond to other people's emotions
2. Somatic empathy: The ability to feel what another person is feeling
3. Cognitive empathy: The ability to understand someone's response to a situation

Humans may be hardwired to experience empathy. The human brain contains mirror neurons, which are activated in the same way when you watch someone else perform an action as when you perform the action yourself. These neurons, originally discovered in the brains of macaque monkeys, are believed to play a role in social interaction and empathy by creating an emotional response to the feelings and behaviors others are experiencing (Bonini, Rotunno, Arcuri, & Gallese, 2022; Kilner & Lemon, 2013; Simpson, Murray, Paukner, & Ferrari, 2014).

For example, when you see someone get hurt, the mirror neurons will respond as if you were hurt yourself. Recent research suggests that mirror neurons do not play as large of a role as initially thought; it is now believed that an area in the brain called the *mirror neuron system* is responsible for observation and actions, not just mirror neurons acting in isolation (Heyes & Catmur, 2022).

Increased levels of empathy are associated with decreased levels of perceived stress and serve as moderator to workplace stress. For example, a decrease in empathy among doctors and nurses was correlated with an increase in perceived stress and workplace burnout (van Vliet, Jong, & Jong, 2017). Clinical empathy is a particularly important skill in the field of health care because it improves communication and helps strengthen the relationship between the patient and health care provider (van Vliet et al., 2017).

Case Study

## The Me Generation

Empathy is a valuable and desired skill by employers because it supports social interactions within the workplace and within the professional context (Hess, Strobel, & Pan, 2016). However, current college students show a 40 percent decline in empathy compared to 20 years ago (Konrath, O'Brien, & Hsing, 2010). At the same time, there has been an increase in narcissism.

Modern media and how you engage with it can have an impact on your level of empathy. Also known as the app generation, today's college students grew up with social media and created networks of online friends. However, these relationships are different from face-to-face friendships and may lack the real engagement that promotes empathetic behavior—when online friends become too burdensome, there is a tendency to tune out. Another contributor may be the rise in first-person shooter games, which may numb people to the pain of others (Shoshani, Braverman, & Meirow, 2021).

The way we engage with our phones may also deter us from fully engaging with others in person. For example, 89 percent of cell phone owners admitted to using their phone during their last social engagement (Raine & Page, 2015). Most of the people surveyed also believed their phone decreased their level of social engagement and took away from the conversation (Raine & Page, 2015).

Some suggestions for improving empathy include being deliberate about when you disconnect from your phone. Take some time each day to turn off your phone and be in the present moment. Secondly, spend some quality face-to-face time with others, during which you put away the phone and enjoy the company. Lastly, practice uni-tasking. Our phones have made it easy to multitask, but this is not always the best option. Engage in one thing at a time and take time to focus on the task at hand.

### Discussion Questions

1. How would you characterize your own cell phone use? Do you consider it healthy or problematic?
2. How would you encourage your friends to adopt healthier cell phone habits?
3. Do you feel your generation is empathetic? Justify your answer.

Relationships that have higher levels of cognitive empathy also have lower levels of perceived stress. In a study conducted on new parents, there was a strong relationship between the mother's parenting stress and marital satisfaction (Dong, Dong, & Chen, 2022). However, in relationships where the father showed high levels of cognitive empathy toward the mother, the mother experienced less parenting stress compared to relationships where the father did not show cognitive empathy.

**Your capacity for empathy is subject to change under different conditions of stress.**

In times of low stress, your capacity for empathy is at its peak (Karakilic et al., 2018). However, when under high amounts of stress, your capacity for empathy is decreased. It has been suggested that the neural pathway for empathy and the stress response are very similar; thus, perhaps when the pathway is being used to deal with high amounts of stress, the empathetic pathway is blocked or not functioning as it should (Karakilic et al., 2018). In other words, when your brain is busy managing stress, it doesn't have the ability to effectively pursue empathetic responses. When you can cope with your stress, you will also find your empathetic responses are heightened, allowing you to better connect with others.

Increasing your empathy can serve as a buffer against stress and increase your levels of wellness. One way to improve your own levels of empathy is to practice mentalization. **Mentalization** is the ability to understand your mental state, intentions, and actions, as well as those of others. When you mentalize, you are constantly aware of your own feelings and the feelings of those you are interacting with. Mentalization is considered both an inborn trait and a skill that can be practiced (Luyten, Campbell, Allison, & Fonagy, 2020). It is usually developed through infant-parent bonding but can also be developed later in life (Chovanec, 2020).

Mentalization is an automatic process. However, in people with a lack of empathy, this process is sometimes deficient and may need to be further developed. Some ways to practice mentalization include the following (Hagelquist, 2017):

- *Emotional thermometer*. Think about your current emotional state. On a scale of 1 to 10, what is your emotional temperature? If you have a high emotional temperature, take some time reflect on your emotions and identify ways to bring them down. When your emotional temperature is high, it is likely that your level of empathy will be low. This practice allows you to be self-reflective to help you better manage your emotions so that you can view things from multiple perspectives.
- *Model mentalization*. Think about a conversation you had with another person. Reflect on the emotions, feelings, needs, goals, reasons, or thoughts you experienced during the conversation. Then reflect on what you think the other person's emotions, feelings, needs, goals, reasons, or thoughts may have been. Share what you learned with the other person to determine your accuracy.

Another way to practice empathy is to actively pay attention to the other person when talking. Focus on their facial expressions and body language for additional clues about their emotions. Share your observations with the other person—for example, "It sounds like that is really stressing you out and you are worried about handling it." In this response, you are making an educated guess about how the person is feeling and checking to see if you are accurately interpreting their emotional state. This is similar to the reflective listening technique presented in chapter 7.

Finally, allow yourself to be vulnerable. Sharing your own experiences and how they made you feel can deepen your relationship with others. As you learn to share your own emotions, you become more able to feel empathy toward yourself and others (Thonhauser, 2022).

## Compassion

**Compassion** refers to the feeling of understanding another person's suffering and wanting to do something to reduce that suffering. Some scientists believe compassion is a trait that is vital to the survival of our species (Gilbert, 2019). Charles Darwin's work supports the idea that compassion is the main reason behind our evolutionary success, and that communities with the greatest number of sympathetic members would best flourish and have the most offspring (Ekman, 2010).

**Self-compassion** is the practice of being kind and understanding to yourself when you are confronted with what you deem as personal failings. Recognize that no one is perfect, including yourself, and accept that you are human. Self-compassion consists of three tenets (Mahurin-Smith & Beck, 2021):

1. *Treat yourself kindly.* We tend to be kind to others but have a difficult time being kind to ourselves. When you do poorly on a test, you might tell yourself you are stupid and you will never learn the material. Instead, talk to yourself as if talking to a friend. Tell yourself it is okay and that you will change how you study to do better next time.

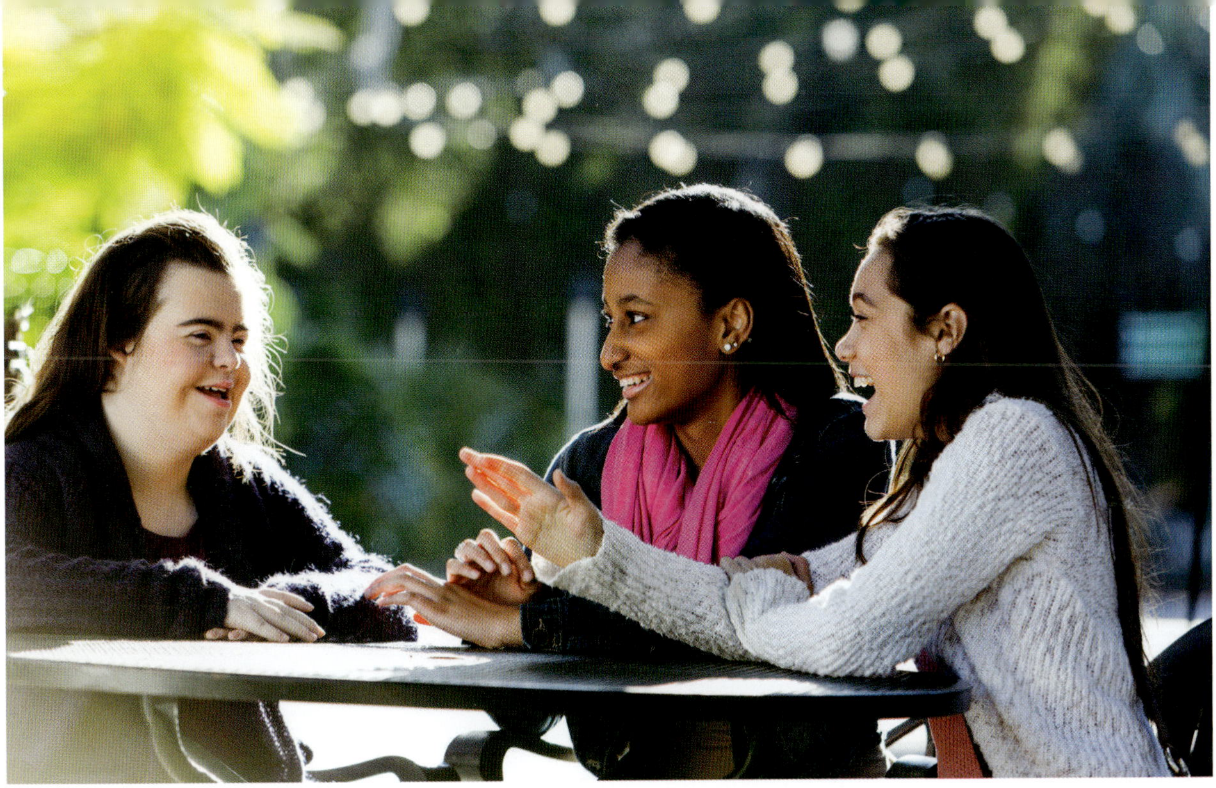

2. *Understand that suffering is part of the human condition.* You do not have to be alone in your suffering. Share your experience with others to help reduce your own burden. It is part of being human and helps unite us.
3. *Be mindful of your emotions and respond to them appropriately.* Think about your emotions from a nonjudgmental perspective. Observe what you are feeling and compare it to the suffering of others to gain clarity and a larger perspective.

Studies show when you practice self-compassion, your levels of perceived stress go down (Mahurin-Smith & Beck, 2021). People with high levels of self-compassion understand that all people face stressful situations. Moreover, they tend to view stress from a challenge perspective rather than a threat perspective, increasing their ability to cope (Chishima, Mizuno, Sugawara, & Miyagawa, 2018). Self-compassion has also been associated with decreased social anxiety and increased health-promoting behaviors (Bates, Elphinstone, & Whitehead, 2021; Li, Deng, Lou, Wang, & Wang, 2019).

**Having compassion has been shown to reduce stress.**

Compassion for others can also improve your overall wellness. First, when you are compassionate, it activates and strengthens the pleasure circuits in your brain, leading to an overall increase in feelings of pleasure and happiness (Esch & Stefano, 2004). Compassion may also lead to a reduced response to stress by lowering cortisol levels. Finally, practicing compassion can help strengthen your relationships with others—friends who are compassionate with each other tend to experience greater satisfaction in the relationship.

## Summary

Spiritual wellness is your connection to a higher power and to others. It is how you see yourself as part of the greater world. It is deeply personal and helps guide your beliefs and values and how you act on them. It reduces stress by helping you focus on the good in your life and the goodness you bring to others. Supporting others is a way of connecting to them and to the larger universe and helps you gain a better perspective on your own life, ultimately improving your spiritual wellness.

## ONLINE RESOURCES

Visit HK*Propel* to access audio supplements, worksheets, and vocabulary flash cards for this chapter.

## DISCUSSION QUESTIONS

1. Describe your personal spiritual wellness.
2. Compare and contrast spirituality and religiosity.
3. Many religions focus on helping others. In what ways does helping others help you? Describe a time when you helped someone else. How did it impact you?
4. How does having spiritual wellness help manage stress?

9

# Environmental Wellness

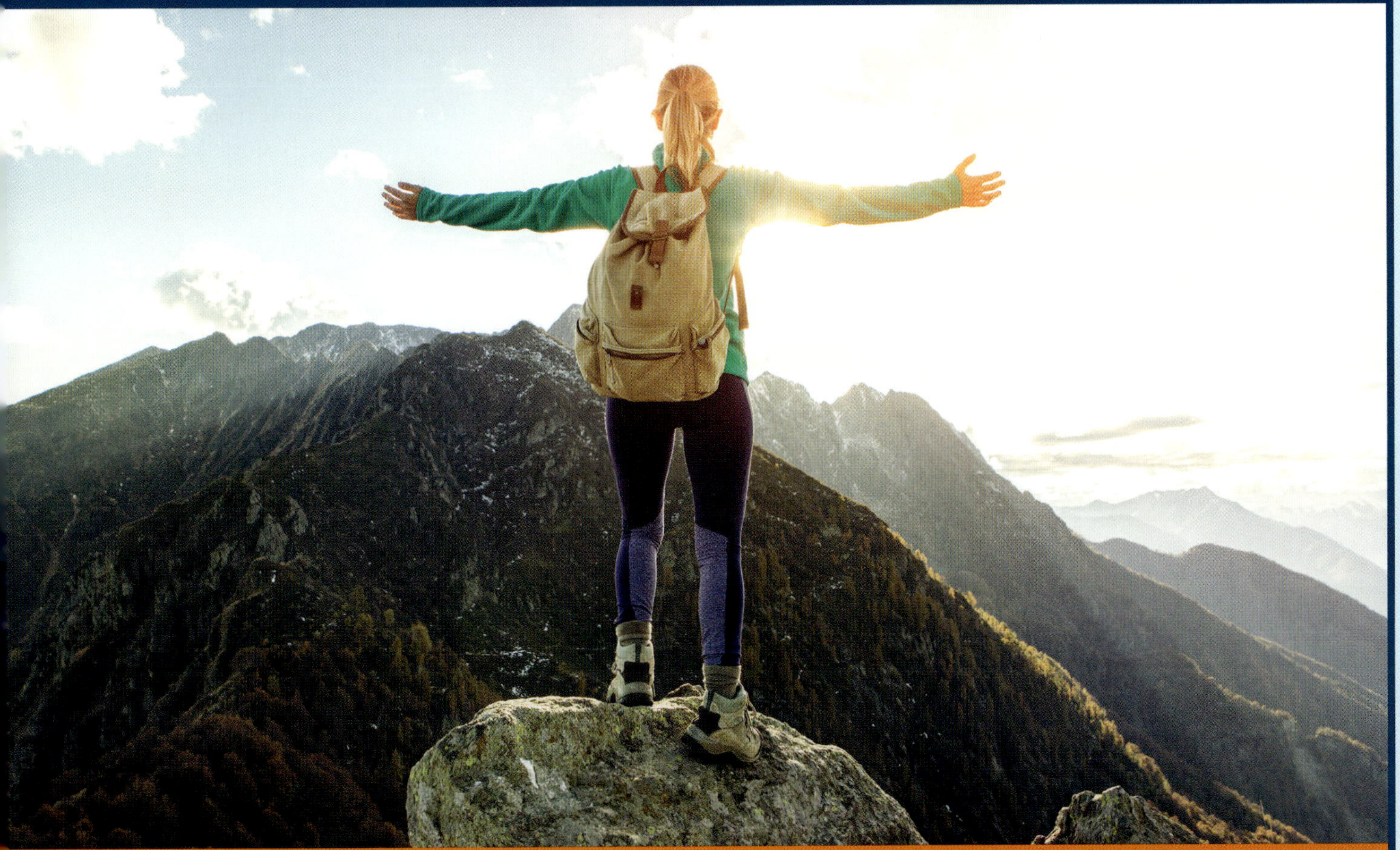

## LEARNING OBJECTIVES

After reading this chapter, you will be able to do the following:

- Evaluate the impact of the environment on stress
- Identify ways to improve your environment to help better manage stress
- Defend the argument that nature promotes reduced stress
- Describe components of the built environment that contribute to and reduce stress
- Discuss how stress levels are influenced by environmental factors such as light, temperature, air quality, noise, and color

# KEY TERMS

air quality
biophilia
blue light
built environment
chromotherapy
environmental noise
food desert
food insecurity
forest bathing
light pollution
melatonin
plant parenting
stress recovery theory

Environmental wellness is your connection between yourself and everything that surrounds you, including your home, your workplace, your community, and nature. Whereas spiritual health describes your connection with the metaphysical world, environmental wellness describes your connection with the physical world.

When you focus on your environmental wellness, you begin to understand how your daily surroundings impact your personal and work life and how your own habits impact the natural environment. When you begin to take notice of your actions and adjust them to improve your environment, you will feel a sense of accomplishment and deeper respect for your surroundings, which helps reduce stress. This chapter will explore the components of environmental wellness, which include your personal surroundings, nature, and the built environment. This chapter will also discuss the ways light, temperature, air quality, noise, and color can impact your environmental wellness and ways to improve your environmental wellness.

## Environmental Wellness and Stress

Your environment can either help reduce your stress or be a source of stress. For example, the housing market is part of your environment. Having access to affordable housing would be a stress reducer for many people. On the other hand, there are some areas in the United States where housing is scarce or unaffordable, causing significant stress. One study found that housing disadvantage is associated with poor mental health later in life (Singh, Daniel, Baker, & Bentley, 2019). Those not living in stable housing also find it more difficult to access health care (Aidala et al., 2016).

The quality or safety of your neighborhood can have a large impact on your health. For example, alcohol use disorder is higher for those living in neighborhoods that experience high rates of foreclosure (Sandel et al., 2016). One possible contributing factor is that people use alcohol to manage the stress of living in a neighborhood in flux (Frone, 2016). People living in low-income neighborhoods tend to have poorer health outcomes compared to people living in high-income neighborhoods. This may partly be explained by the combination of being exposed to multiple environmental hazards and poor housing quality, both of which are more frequently found in low-income neighborhoods (Morello-Frosch, Zuk, Jerrett, Shamasunder, & Kyle, 2011).

**Affordable housing is a health concern and impacts communities across the country.**

It is important to be aware of what you can do to improve your environment and therefore your stress levels. For example, what can you do to improve affordable housing options? Educate yourself on affordable housing issues in your own neighborhood. Identify policies that can impact affordable housing (e.g., rent assistance, home ownership assistance, zoning restrictions). Finally, be active as a voter and identify politicians who promote affordable housing policies and practices. More examples of the impact of environmental wellness on stress will be discussed throughout this chapter.

## Personal Surroundings

Environmental health includes your personal space, such as your bedroom, study space, and car. It refers to how you feel in those spaces and how you can adjust them to promote wellness. How would you describe your personal space? It is cluttered, neat, or somewhere in between? Does clutter make you feel flustered, or are you the type of person who knows where everything is despite the appearance of disorganization?

How you organize your space can promote or distract from your wellness journey. Your personal surroundings are also completely under your control. Being intentional about how you design the space around you can better help you focus and feel a sense of calm. Some people feel calm (or stressed) when they are around a particular color or scent.

Your personal space can provide some insight on your level of stress. Studies have found a correlation between clutter in a person's workspace and their stress at work (Dao & Ferrari, 2020; Roster & Ferrari, 2019). Clutter at home has a similar impact; it has been associated with poorer psychological health, impacting older adults more intensely than younger ones (Swanson & Ferrari, 2022).

How you design and maintain your personal space can also give others insight on your mental and emotional state. For example, consider Gabriella, whose bedroom is a complete mess. She has dirty clothes on the floor, clean clothes in a laundry basket, an unmade bed, and various old food containers lying around. What impression would you have of Gabriella's mental state? Based on how she maintains her personal space, you would probably assume it is in disarray. In this case, you are correct: Gabriella is a part-time student and often works overtime to help keep herself afloat. She is under a lot of stress and doesn't have much time to clean because she uses most of her free time to study. Take note, however, that this assumption is not always correct. For some, the state of their personal space doesn't give a strong indication of their wellness.

One of the best ways to promote a calm environment is to declutter your space. This can help change your mindset from "more is better" to "enough." This mindset helps support wellness by encouraging you to practice gratitude for what you have (see chapter 8) and to focus less on needing more things to make you happy (Khamis, 2019). For some, the act of decluttering is associated with released stress—as each excess item is taken away, so is a certain level of stress (Chameberlin & Callmer, 2021). The same study found that after decluttering, many people reported improved mental health.

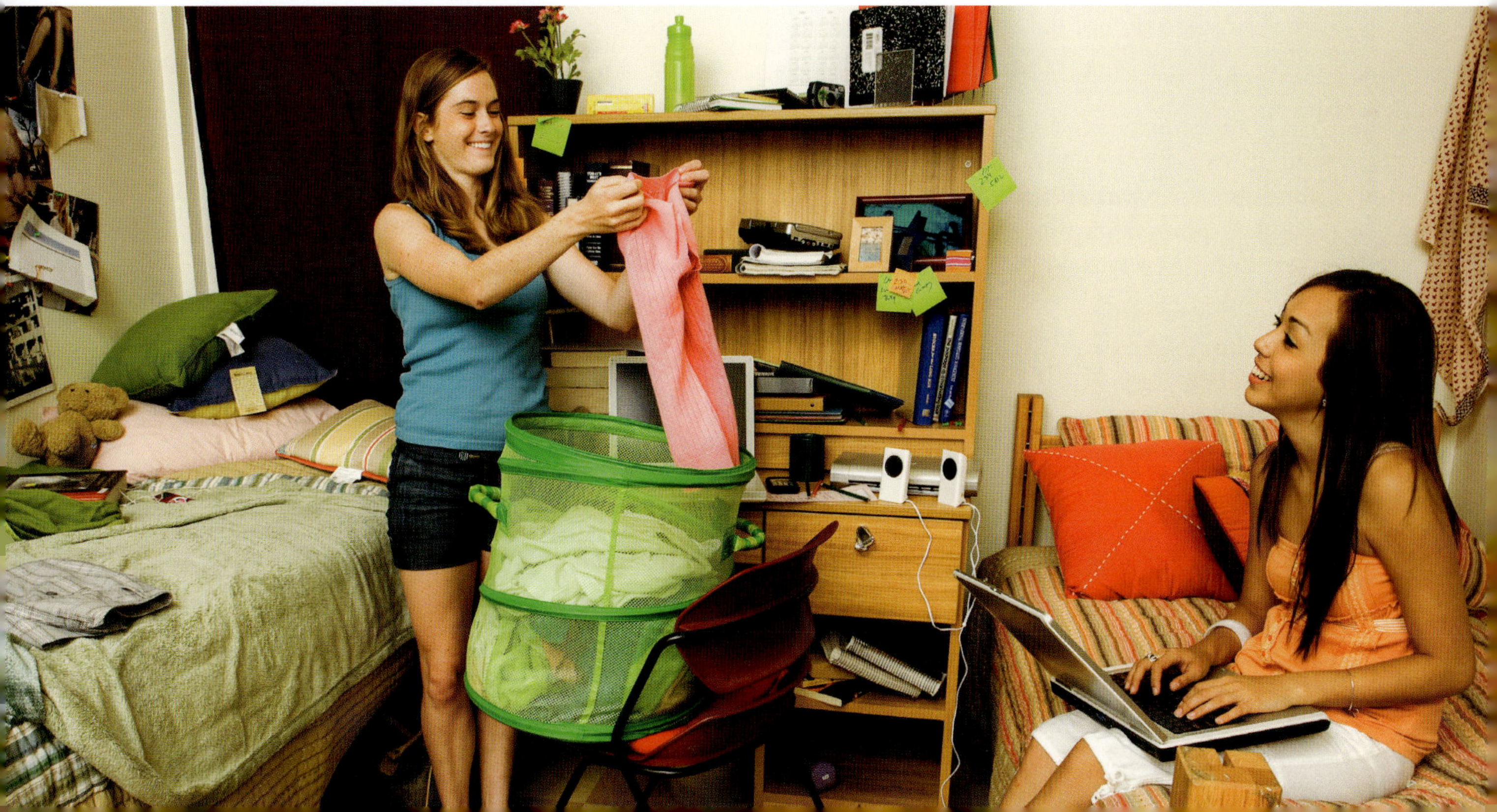

## Decluttering Your Space

Being organized can help you better focus and manage stress. For some, knowing how to start the decluttering or organizational process is difficult. There are many different techniques for decluttering your space. One popular one was created by Marie Kondo (2014), who describes decluttering as a Japanese art using the following steps:

- *Remember that decluttering is a marathon, not a sprint.* It will not be completed in a day. Be ready to spend time decluttering, and remember that the benefits of having a tidy space are worth it.
- *Tidy up by category, not by room.* Begin with clothes. Find all your clothes and place them in one pile. Go through each item, one by one, and only keep those things that bring you joy or speak to the heart. For items that no longer bring you joy, thank them for their service and let them go.
- *Imagine how you want your space to look.* What do you want your space to look like? Create an image or cut out photos to help you imagine your perfect space, and then go about creating it.

Another way to improve your personal surroundings is to bring nature into your space. **Biophilia** describes the innate tendency humans have to love and connect with nature; the millennial generation even coined the term **plant parenting** to describe their affection for plants. Studies suggest that indoor environments that incorporate natural elements promote health, have restorative properties, and help reduce stress and anxiety (Yin et al., 2020). Indoor plants can help support overall wellness by providing pleasant aesthetics, improving air quality, and removing airborne pollutants (Kraus, Senitkova, & Juhasova, 2021).

Research shows that people who have more greenery at home, including indoor and outdoor plants, experience better mental health compared to those who do not have plants (Hall & Knuth, 2019). Having potted plants has been shown to improve positive emotions while reducing negative emotions, including stress (Han & Li-Wen, 2019). When you interact with plants, it suppresses your sympathetic nervous system, which reduces physical and psychological stress (Lee, Lee, Park, & Miyazaki, 2015). In a meta-analysis, the presence of indoor plants has been associated with enhanced cognition, reduced blood pressure, and improved academic achievement (Han, Ruan, & Liao, 2022).

**Tending indoor plants serves as a model of how to care for yourself.**

There are many options for inexpensive houseplants, with some requiring very little maintenance. There are plants for every type of indoor light condition and for beginners and experienced plant parents alike. Start small—if you have never cared for a plant before, get a hardy one and have it next to your bed. See if its presence positively impacts your stress levels and overall wellness.

In addition to the benefits of houseplants, studies have shown that gardening can reduce anxiety and stress in addition to many other health and wellness benefits, which are maximized when you garden at least two or three times per week (Chalmin-Pui, Griffiths, Roe, Heaton, & Cameron, 2021; Dzhambov et al., 2021). Many people have ranked their gardens highest, compared to their other spaces, in terms of perceived health restorative values. Being outside in the sun for more than one hour a day can help reduce stress; moreover, exposure to sunlight can naturally increase serotonin levels, which promotes happiness and helps regulate stress (Hwang, Choi, & Hong, 2023; Sansone & Sansone, 2013). The physical exercise of gardening also serves to help reduce stress (Scott, Masser, & Pachana, 2020). Finally, growing your own vegetables can help your diet: People are more likely to eat vegetables that they grew themselves (Palar et al., 2019).

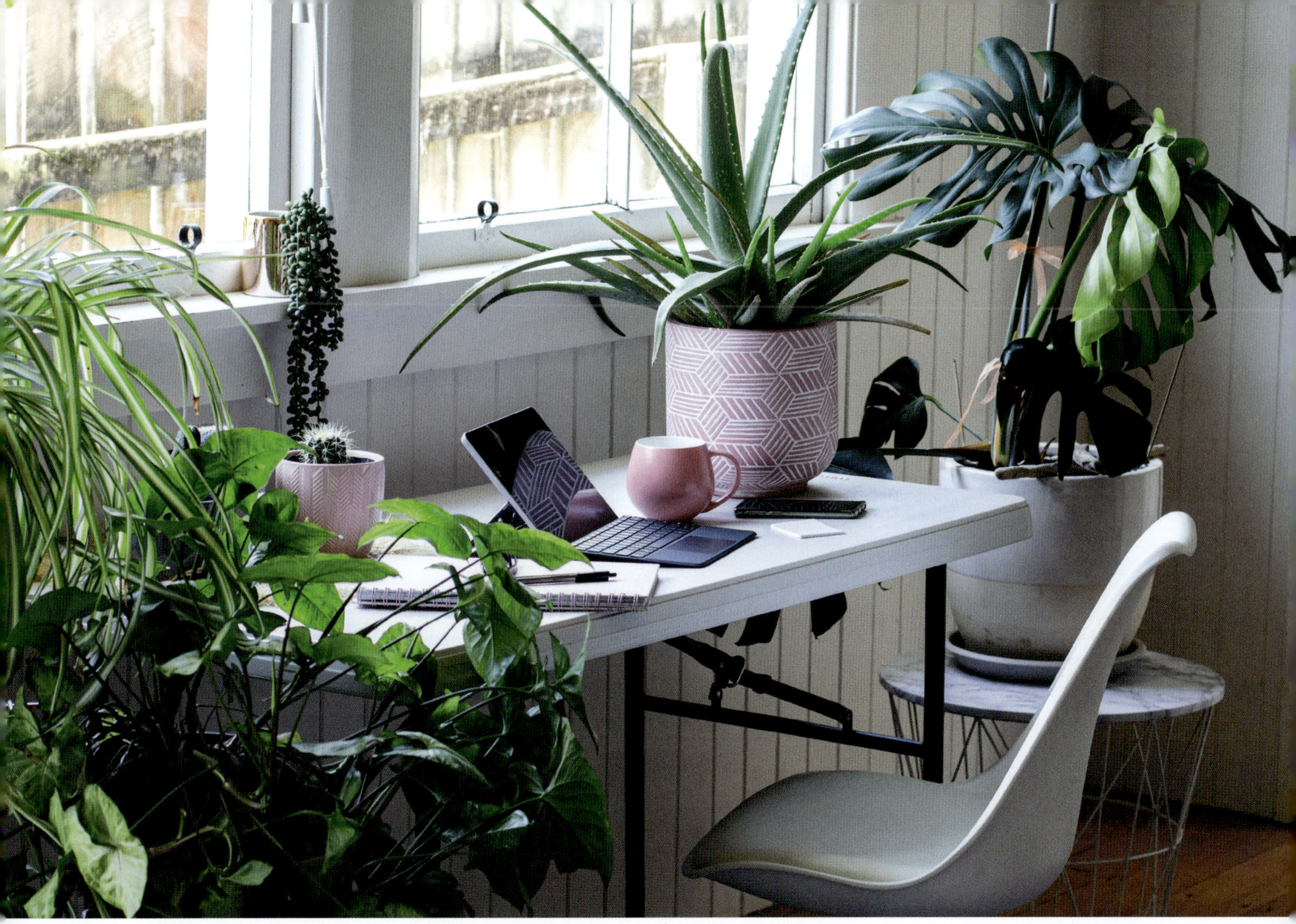

Research Spotlight

## Go Play in the Dirt: A Vaccine for Stress?

Years ago, scientists noted that as society became more modern, children were spending less time playing outside in the dirt but becoming sicker. They theorized that the lack of exposure to microorganisms in dirt led to an impaired immune system (Pfefferle, Keber, Cohen, & Garn, 2021). This exposure created more biodiversity in the gut microbiota, which may serve as a way to help train our immune system to better detect bacterial infections and lead to a more effective immune response (Yoo, Groer, Dutra, Sarkar, & McSkimming, 2020).

Scientists have been able to isolate a lipid from the bacterium Mycobacterium vaccae (MV), found in dirt, that has been shown to reduce symptoms associated with stress in mice (Bowers et al., 2021). A similar study on mice showed that MV exposure resulted in reduced inflammatory responses associated with stress (Smith et al., 2019). Perhaps future research may show that childhood exposure to MV may serve as a protective factor against stress and other mental disorders later in life. The good news for kids? Playing in dirt and getting dirty has health benefits that can last well into adulthood. It seems there were benefits to having your parents tell you to go play outside.

## Nature

Being outdoors in nature has shown to positively impact mental health and significantly reduce feelings of depression and anxiety (Haider et al., 2021; Young et al., 2022). **Stress recovery theory** describes these positive effects received when immersed in nature. You don't need a green thumb to enjoy the benefits—just spending time in natural settings can significantly reduce stress and anxiety, lower heart rate and cortisol levels, and improve concentration (Hall & Knuth, 2019). Simply taking a walk near greenery, such as a park or woods, may provide long-lasting benefits for your health and overall stress. One study found that spending at least 20 minutes outdoors near nature reduces cortisol levels (Hunter, Gillespie, & Chen, 2019). These lower perceived stress levels were observed regardless of the activity (walking, jogging, sitting), with the peak benefit occurring within 20 to 30 minutes.

**Allowing yourself time during the day to stop and be in the moment within nature can result in better overall wellness.**

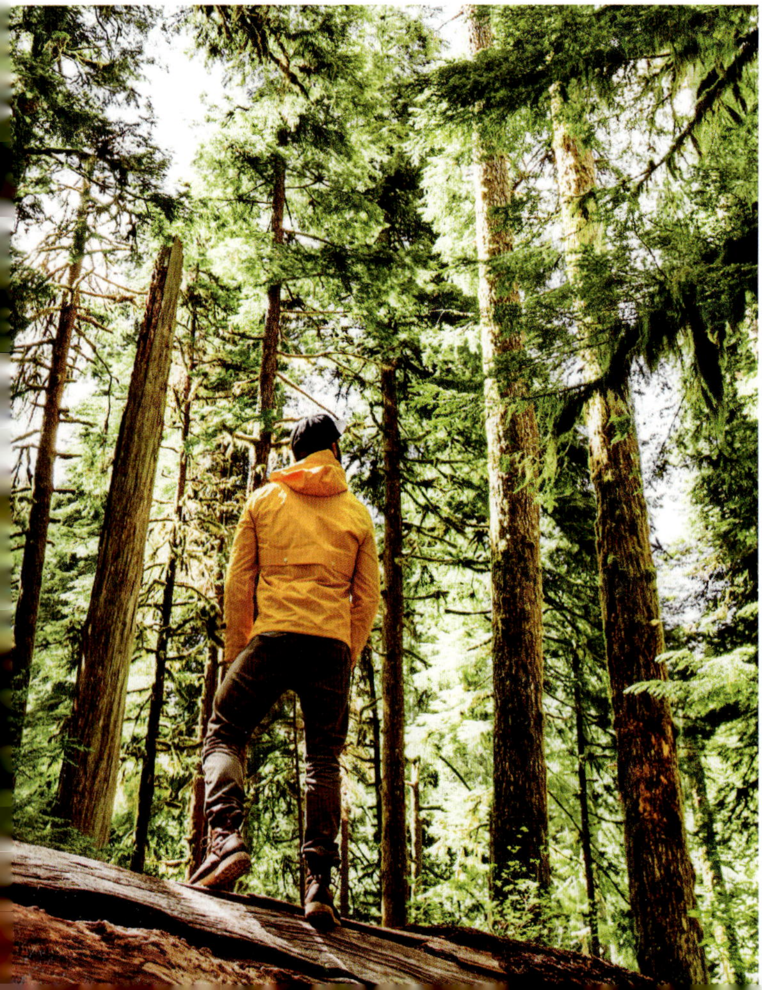

**Forest bathing** is a term that was coined in Japan in the 1980s to promote the act of walking in the forest to reduce stress and combat a rise in depression among working adults. The benefits of forest bathing may be attributed to the volatile organic compounds (VOCs) present in the trees, which have been shown to suppress the sympathetic nervous system—just the mere exposure to these compounds has been shown to reduce stress (Matsubara & Kawai, 2018). Other studies found forest bathing to help improve psychological functioning while improving positive mood states (Furuyashiki, Tabuchi, Norikoshi, Kobayashi, & Oriyama, 2019). Being in a forest and paying attention to your surroundings may help you be more present in the moment and can also bring a sense of peace and inner calm.

> Those who contemplate the beauty of the earth find reserves of strength that will endure as long as life lasts.
>
> **Rachel Carson**

If you do not live near a forest, don't worry. Research shows that any type of natural environment can help decrease perceived levels of stress, increase parasympathetic system activity, and decrease sympathetic nervous system activity (Wang, Shi, Zhang, & Chiang, 2019). What is important is that you expose yourself to nature and the natural environment (Ewert & Chang, 2018). Just spending time outside in a park, a forest preserve, or even your backyard can help reduce overall stress levels and help you recover from stress faster (Corazon, Sidenius, Poulsen, Gramkow, & Stigsdotter, 2019).

Even looking at posters of nature can provide some positive health benefits. Patients exposed to posters of plants reported lower levels of perceived stress compared to those who were not exposed to those posters (Beukeboom, Langeveld, & Tanja-Dijkstra, 2012). Another study found that murals of trees were most beneficial, in terms of perceived stress relief, among children in a pediatric hospital (Pearon et al., 2019). Consider choosing wall art with nature scenes to improve your personal environment.

## Built Environment

The **built environment** consists of all the man-made parts of where you live and work. It includes residential areas, commercial buildings, streets, parks, and any other community infrastructure. Your built environment can greatly impact your overall wellness. What image comes to mind when you think of a "bad neighborhood"? You may envision houses that are in disrepair, garbage piled up outside, and a general sense of overcrowding. These types of neighborhood characteristics have been associated with increased levels of stress. There has also been some evidence that neighborhoods with lower curb appeal—such as the presence of garbage, graffiti, and poor building conditions—increase levels of perceived stress among the residents who live in that area (Plascak et al., 2021). Another study found a strong association between the deterioration of the physical qualities of an environment and mental health problems (Nunez-Gonzalez et al., 2020). Additionally, these areas also tend to lack green space and parks, which have been shown to improve wellness and reduce stress.

Living in densely populated areas prone to overcrowding and noise can be detrimental to physical health (Frumkin et al., 2017). In ancient Rome, there were pleasure gardens available to the elite class to allow them to get away from the hustle and bustle of the big city (Hartswick, 2004); today, many cities include park areas and green spaces (e.g., Central Park in New York City, Millennium Park in Chicago, Topanga State Park in Los Angeles). These spaces can provide many health benefits—for example, those who live near parks and sidewalks are more likely to have higher levels of physical activity compared to those who do not. Studies show that when people have access to trails in their neighborhood, they are more likely to engage in physical activities, including walking and biking (Smiley, Ramos, Elliott, & Wolter, 2020). It was also shown that those who utilize the trails reported higher levels of health and wellness.

A community's resources, including availability of shopping and walkability, also have an impact on both physical and mental health. Neighborhoods that have access to health care, grocery stores, and green spaces support healthier lifestyles. However, many areas do not have these necessities. **Food deserts** are areas that do not have easy access to quality fresh foods. There is a relationship between food deserts and stress, which is even more pronounced among economically and socially vulnerable populations (Crowe, Lacy, & Columbus, 2018). A lack of grocery stores has been associated with higher prices for groceries, more time spent traveling to grocery stores, and lower fruit and vegetable consumption. In recent years, many grocery retailers have left big cities and urban areas to move to suburban areas, creating food deserts even in highly populated areas (Crowe, Lacy, & Columbus, 2018).

**Food insecurity** is not having access to sufficient food or food quality. Approximately 15 percent of college students have reported being food insecure, with another 16 percent being at risk for food insecurity (Payne-Sturges, Tjaden, Caldeira, Vincent, & Arria, 2017). Students who are experiencing food insecurity report high levels of stress, inability to develop meaningful social relationships, feelings of hopelessness, and disruption of their academic studies (Meza, Altman, Martinez, & Leung, 2018). Many colleges have responded by offering food pantries on campus. Student who utilize food pantries report improved performance and having more money to spend on other necessities, such as rent (McArthur, Fasczewski, Farris, & Petrone, 2020). Unfortunately, there are some stigmas associated with using food pantries, and many students who are food insecure do not utilize that option.

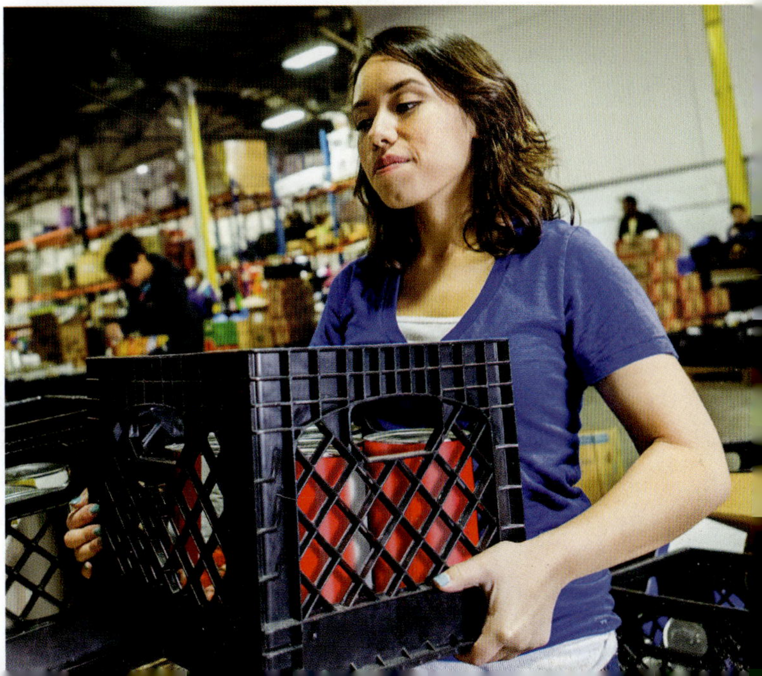

## Light

Humans respond to the natural cycles of day and night. During the day, when it is light, we are awake and active. At night, when it is dark, our body starts winding down to help us fall asleep. Before the invention of electric lights, humans were not exposed to much light at night, but the introduction of artificial light shifted the way we engaged with the night, ultimately extending our daytime hours. The excessive use of artificial light is now referred to as **light pollution** (figure 9.1). Light pollution consists of the following (International Dark Sky Association, n.d.):

- Sky glow: Brightening of the night sky over cities and towns
- Light trespass: Light falling in areas where it is not intended or needed
- Glare: Excessive brightness that is uncomfortable
- Clutter: Bright, confusing groupings of lighting

Light pollution impacts over 80 percent of the world's population (Bedrosian & Nelson, 2017). As a result, the Milky Way is no longer visible in most parts of the world. Light pollution is projected to continue to increase, affecting all life on Earth (Davies & Smyth, 2017). Figure 9.2 shows an example of recent changes in light pollution.

Although much light pollution is caused by things out of your control, such as street and city lights, there are things you can do to improve your own levels of light pollution. At your home, turn down indoor and outdoor lights at night. Consider using motion sensors for outdoor lighting so they only turn on when necessary. If you use decorative outdoor lighting for holidays, use timers or turn them off when you go to bed. Using warm-colored LED lights will also reduce energy use. Another option is to use colored lights, which may reduce the negative effects of artificial lighting.

Even indoors, our exposure to light at night is unprecedented in human history (Bedrosian & Nelson, 2017). The use of artificial light at nighttime, which is much brighter than natural night light, has been shown to disrupt physiology patterns that promote fitness and reduce stress and cortisol levels (Davies & Smyth, 2017; Grunt et al., 2020). Think about your own sources of light at night. Do you leave the television on as you sleep? Do you read on a tablet or play on your phone before going to bed? Are there lights on in your house or bedroom at night? Exposure to excessive nighttime light can impact your body's ability to differentiate between day and night and interfere with your sleep cycles. Exposure to artificial light at night has been linked to a variety of health disorders, including mood disorders and lowered sleep quality and quantity (Bedrosian & Nelson, 2017; Xiao et al., 2020). For example, one study found that people who read from an e-reader or tablet within four hours of bedtime

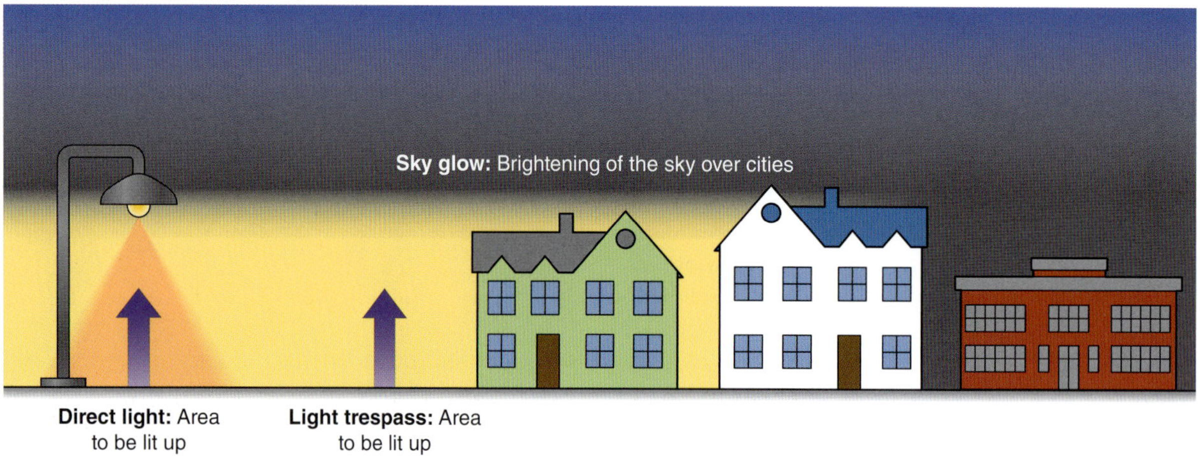


**Figure 9.1** Two common components of light pollution are sky glow and light trespass.

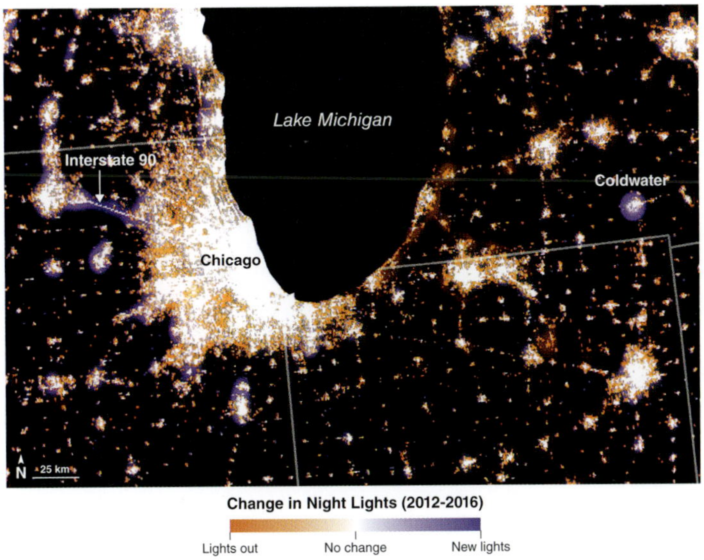


**Figure 9.2** Areas with light pollution. This image shows the increase (purple) and decrease (orange) in light pollution across a four-year span.
Image from NASA's Earth Observatory.

had a harder time falling asleep and were not as alert in the morning (Bedrosian & Nelson, 2017). Even having a small nightlight in your bedroom has the potential to interfere with your sleep. When your sleep is disrupted, you are more likely to feel stressed throughout the day, and your ability to recover from the day's stress is also reduced (Nollet, Wisden, & Franks, 2020). Think about the last time you didn't get enough sleep: How did you feel waking up in the morning? How did you feel throughout the day? How does this differ from when you have a good night's sleep?

**Exposure to artificial light at night may make it more difficult to fall asleep.**

Another way that artificial light impacts stress is through **melatonin**, a hormone produced by the body in response to darkness that is responsible for helping you fall asleep at night. Melatonin and stress have a complicated relationship. Melatonin influences the nervous system to act against stress by increasing the activity of the parasympathetic nervous system. However, stress increases the activity of the sympathetic nervous system, which can interfere with melatonin production at night and make it more difficult to fall asleep (Storoni, 2018). This is the mechanism that explains why high levels of stress can impair your sleep. At the same time, when you have insufficient melatonin production at night, your sympathetic nervous system increases its activity, making you more reactive to stress and continuing the cycle (Storoni, 2018). The production of melatonin can be blocked by nighttime exposure to **blue light**, increasing your risk for depression, stress, and anxiety (Repova et al., 2022). Most visible light contains some blue light, the shortest but highest-energy wavelength of the spectrum. However, humans are currently being exposed to more blue light than ever before through LED technology, such as television and personal electronic devices, which emit high amounts of blue light.

Blue light isn't all bad. There have been studies that suggest blue light can be effective in helping boost memory and cognitive function and improve symptoms associated with PTSD (Killgore et al., 2019). Thus, the goal should not be complete elimination of blue light, but rather a decrease in nighttime exposure to blue light. In recent years, blue-light blocking glasses have been marketed that claim to reduce exposure to blue light, alleviate eye strain when using electronic devices, and improve sleep quality. However, most studies have found no evidence supporting these claims (Lawrenson, Hull, & Downie, 2017). If you want to reduce the effects of blue light exposure, the American Academy of Ophthalmology (2022) recommends the following:

- Set your electronic devices to night or dark mode. This lowers the brightness of the light being emitted.
- Avoid using screens one to two hours before going to sleep.
- Using electronic devices at least an arm's length away from your eyes.
- Use a screen filter to reduce glare and brightness from screens.
- Dim the lights in your house or bedroom one to two hours before going to sleep.

## Temperature

With global climate change has come an increase in temperature, which has negative implications for human health. For example, excessive heat has been shown to impact the functioning of the nervous and circulatory systems and is related to negative birth outcomes (Li, Ferreira, & Smith, 2020). Globally, temperatures have already risen about 1.4 degrees Fahrenheit since recordkeeping began in 1880 (Li et al., 2020).

Being hot and uncomfortable can impact your mental health and lead to stress. It may feel harder to think and conduct work, and you are less likely to want to engage in any physical activity. Researchers found that temperatures over 80 degrees Fahrenheit lasting for longer than 10 days tend to impact people's moods and stress levels (Li et al., 2020). With an increase in the number and duration of heat waves, as shown in figure 9.3, actively working to manage your stress will be critical.

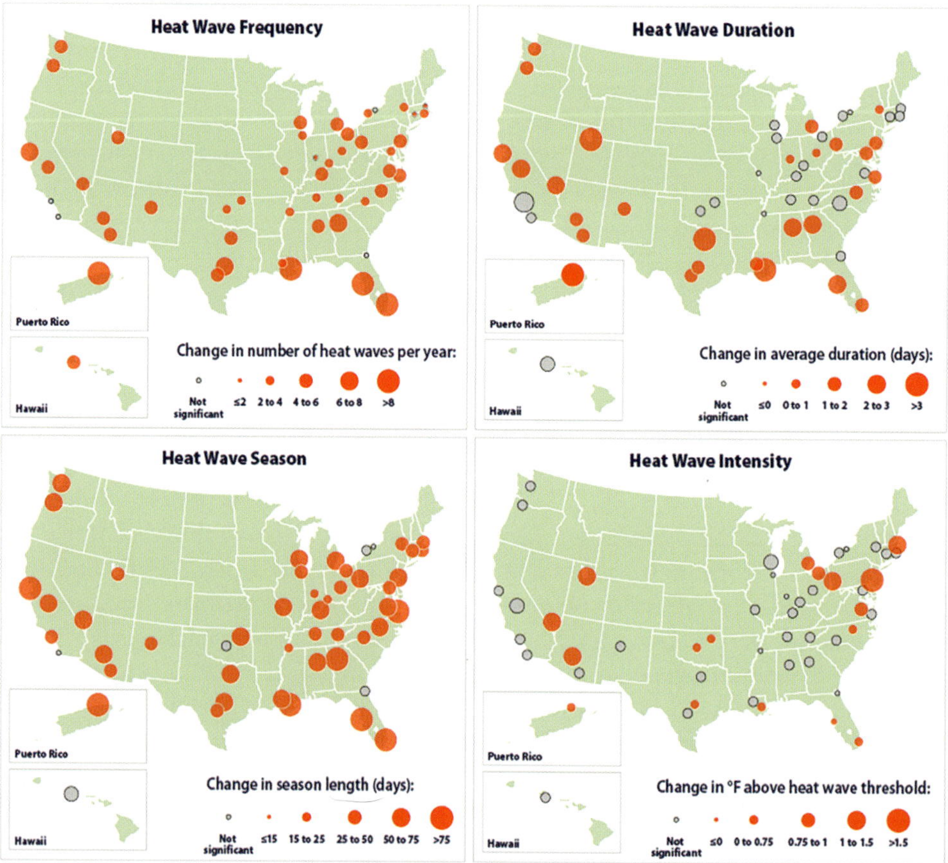


**Figure 9.3** Heat wave characteristics in 50 large U.S. cities, 1961-2021. Data show an increase in heat waves across the United States. What strategies can you implement to reduce the effects of heat stress?

From: NOAA (National Oceanic and Atmospheric Administration), Provided to EPA by NOAA (2022). Available: www.epa.gov/climate-indicators/climate-change-indicators-heat-waves.

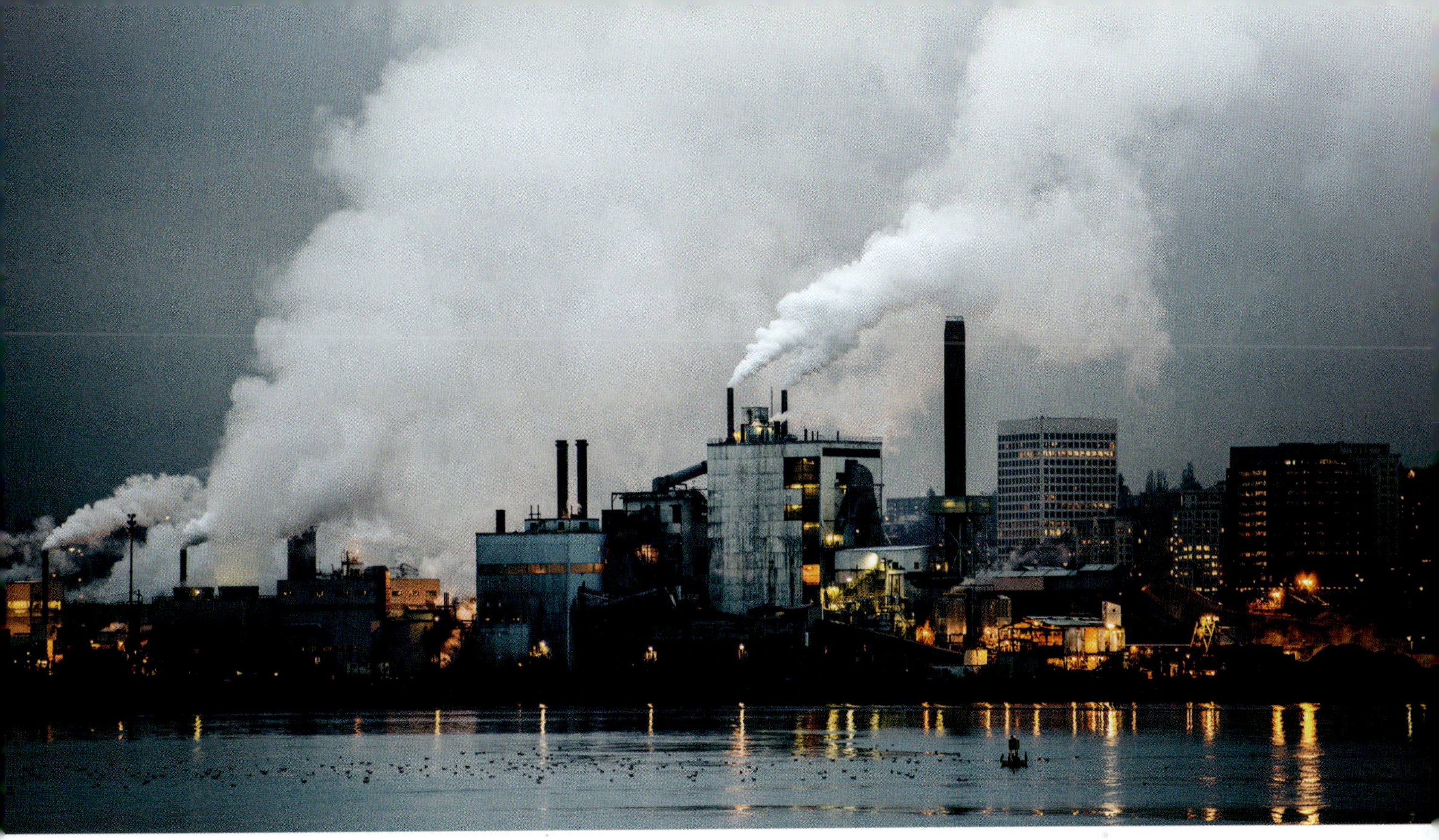

On the other hand, cooler days have immediate effects on your mental health—for every day the temperature ranges between 60 and 70 degrees Fahrenheit, there is a decrease in self-reported mental health difficulties (Li et al., 2020). It was also noted that cooler days do not negatively impact mental health compared to warmer days. Think about your own weather preference. Do you prefer hot, warm, cool, or cold days? Do you notice a change in your mood based on the temperature?

## Air Quality

The **air quality**, or the extent to which your ambient air is free of pollutants, can impact your mental health and self-perceived levels of stress. Growing up in an environment that contains high levels of air pollution, when coupled with stress, can impact children's development. Even being exposed prenatally to pollution and stress can cause an increase in psychiatric symptoms later in life (Pagliccio et al., 2020). Higher levels of stress are more common among areas of lower socioeconomic status. Other variables associated with living in those neighborhoods may also contribute to the higher levels of negative mental health outcomes.

Recent studies show that exposure to air pollution causes the brain to activate the hypothalamic-pituitary-adrenal (HPA) axis and release stress hormones (Thomson, 2019). Being chronically exposed to higher levels of air pollution can therefore cause chronic stress, which may contribute to an increased risk of hypertension, obesity, and depression (Thomson, 2019). Even perceived notions of air pollution can impact your levels of health. One study found that people rated their health as lower and had an increase in disease when they felt they were exposed to higher levels of air pollution (Orru, Nordin, Harzia, & Orru, 2018). Being exposed to air pollution may also impact your perception of stress. For example, one study found that people's stress levels increased on days they were exposed to higher levels of air pollution (Nuyts, Nawrot, Scheers, Nemery, & Casas, 2019). Similarly, when you are under stress, your body's ability to handle air pollution is decreased. Moreover, chronic stress can magnify the impact of air pollution, worsening the impact of air pollution on the lungs (Arthur et al., 2018).

There are some steps you can take to reduce your exposure to air pollution. The first and most effective way to reduce indoor air pollution is to manage it at its source. Some pollutants such as asbestos can be sealed or removed. Asbestos was a common product used in ceilings, drywall, cement, insulation materials, and paint prior to the 1980s and is generally safe until it gets disturbed or starts peeling, releasing particles in the air (Zhang et al., 2021). If you are living in a rental, contact your landlord or property owner for abatement of asbestos or similar harmful pollutants.

**If you are a renter and suspect asbestos, contact your landlord, who is required to have the substance tested and abated by a professional.**

Another way to improve indoor air quality is to improve ventilation. Use the vents in your bathroom and put on the ventilation fan when cooking on the stovetop to help filter out particulates and keep the air circulating. Open windows and doors to let in fresh air. However, avoid letting in outdoor air on high pollution days. You can also use air purifiers to help filter out pollutants. An effective air cleaner is one that can collect pollutants from indoor air (expressed as a percentage efficiency rate) and how much air draws through a filter (expressed in cubic feet per minute) (Environmental Protection Agency, 2022).

> If the environment is happy, people will laugh and your grief will go away.
>
> **Srinivas Mishra**

## Noise

In the beginning of the 20th century, Nobel Prize winner Robert Koch stated, "One day man will have to fight noise as fiercely as cholera and the plague" (Hahad, Prochaska, Daiber, & Munzel, 2019). A century later, Koch's prediction that noise would one day become a hazard to human health has largely proven true. Exposure to chronic noise makes it more difficult to focus and decreases your resistance to stress, and excessive **environmental noise**, or the sounds from external sources such as traffic, airports, and construction, has been attributed to an increase in poor mental health and cardiovascular disease (Rudolph et al., 2019). It is believed these problems arise because exposure to chronic noise activates the stress response cycle and its associated physiological changes, such as increased heart rate and blood pressure. For example, have you ever been woken up by a loud noise in the middle of the night and felt your heart racing? Being exposed to noise at night can also trigger the stress response cycle, promoting the release of cortisol and hindering sleep (Rudolph et al., 2019). Stress also reduces melatonin, which helps maintain sleep. People who live in areas that are loud and active at night—such as near major highways, railways, and airports—are prone to chronic stress and reduced levels of sleep.

There has been an association between chronic noise exposure and maladaptive stress coping mechanisms. For example, one study found that people who are exposed to chronic noise tend to engage in less physical activity, consume more alcohol, and smoke to manage stress. Although these may reduce the physical symptoms of stress in the short term, these behaviors will not mitigate the chronic effects of stress, and they also contribute to an increased risk of chronic health conditions (Hahad et al., 2019).

Chronic noise is more common in urban settings compared to rural areas (see figure 9.4). Larger cities tend to be closer to highways and populated roads that continue to be used throughout the day and night, contributing to noise pollution (Ma, Li, Kwan, & Chai, 2018). Additionally, there is a link between higher levels of noise pollution and low-income communities, which are more likely to be located near direct transportation routes, such as freeways (Science for Environmental Policy, 2016). One way to mitigate this problem is to build noise barriers, which have proven to be an effective way to protect affected neighborhoods from excessive noise (Pinsonnault-Skvarenina, Carrier, Bockstael, Gagne, & Leroux; Sun, Zhao, Zhang, Chen, & Zhang, 2021). However, lower-income areas tend to have fewer resources and less effective noise barriers, both between housing units (e.g., within apartment buildings) and between housing and major roads (e.g., road and railway noise barriers).

**When you are exposed to chronic stress, your stress response cycle is continually activated, which will eventually wear down your body.**

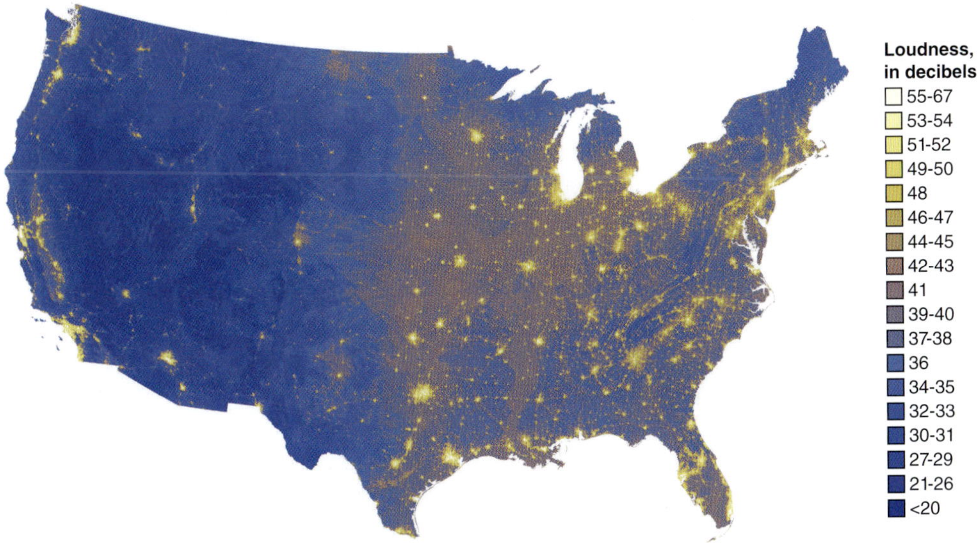


**Figure 9.4** Noise levels across the United States.
From: National Park Service, Natural Sounds and Night Skies and Inventory and Monitoring Divisions. Available: www.nps.gov/subjects/sound/soundmap.htm.

## Color

What are the colors of your bedroom, office, or main living space? Have you ever considered how those colors make you feel? Bright and vivid colors have been shown to enhance cognitive effort (as measured by a reading task) compared to dull and subdued colors (Al-Ayash, Kane, Smith, & Green-Armytage, 2016). Moreover, warm colors (red and yellow) have been found to increase the activity in the autonomic nervous system, whereas cool colors (blue and green) decrease that activity (Oh, Lee, & Park, 2021).

The colors that have the most impact on mood are red, yellow, green, and blue. Red symbolizes power and strength: Consider a fast red car or walking a red carpet. Red is also seen as a danger cue: Think of the color of blood, a stop sign, or a red light. The color red has been shown to promote the release of adrenaline, allowing you to act fast. As such, red is thought to increase stimulation, which may also increase your levels of stress (Perry et al., 2020). Being in a red room can increase your heart rate and activate the stress response system (Oh et al., 2021).

Yellow, like red, is a stimulating color; however, it is more associated with optimism, hope, and joy (Duyan & Rengin, 2016). Yellow is attention grabbing and energizing and can help place you in a positive state of mind. The colors red and yellow together have been known to increase your appetite; this is known as the ketchup and mustard theory and helps explain why many fast food companies use red and yellow as part of their marketing plan (Hambly, 2022). Yellow may also increase your metabolism. Many believe the color yellow can increase frustration and that a yellow nursery will cause a baby to cry more often. However, these notions about the color yellow have not been proven in repeatable scientific studies (O'Connor, 2011).

Green is considered a cool color and is found frequently in nature; the stress-relieving effect of green spaces was discussed previously in this chapter. Green also represents security and self-reliance (think money). Green is restful and comfortable on the eye, reducing eye strain. Some hospitals use green to promote healing; using green LED has been shown to promote wound healing (Fushimi et al., 2012). It has been shown that surrounding yourself with green can reduce your stress levels and promote a sense of calm (Gunes & Olgunturk, 2020; Manav, 2007). For

**Colors have an impact on our mood and can impact our levels of stress, particularly the colors that surround you in your indoor spaces.**

Case Study

## Color and Light Therapy

**Chromotherapy** is a form of treatment that uses color and light to treat certain mental and physical conditions. This technique has been traced back to ancient civilizations of Egypt, China, and India, when sun-filled rooms were used to help combat depression (Azeemi, Rafiq, Ismail, Kazmi, & Azeemi, 2019). Today, color therapists use color by either sight submersion or directing color onto different parts of the body (Azeemi et al., 2019). Each color has a different wavelength and frequency, which provides different outcomes. When light is absorbed through the skin, it can trigger changes in the cells (Azeemi et al., 2019).

The medical field has been using light therapy successfully to treat many conditions. Babies born with jaundice are treated with blue light therapy to help the body break down bilirubin and excrete it (Shirzadfar & Sheikhi, 2020). Red light therapy is being promoted to help with hair loss and acne and to improve wound healing (Zarei, Wikramanayake, Falto-Aizpurua, Schachner, & Jimenez, 2016). One study looked at different colors of LED lights and found that workers experienced greater stress reduction when using green or blue LED lights as compared to red or yellow (Lee, Oh, Kim, & Jang, 2018).

### Discussion Questions

1. List the colors in your main living space and identify whether they impact your mental health.
2. Which colors do you feel most impact your mental health?
3. If you could repaint one room you spend the most time in, what color would you choose and why?

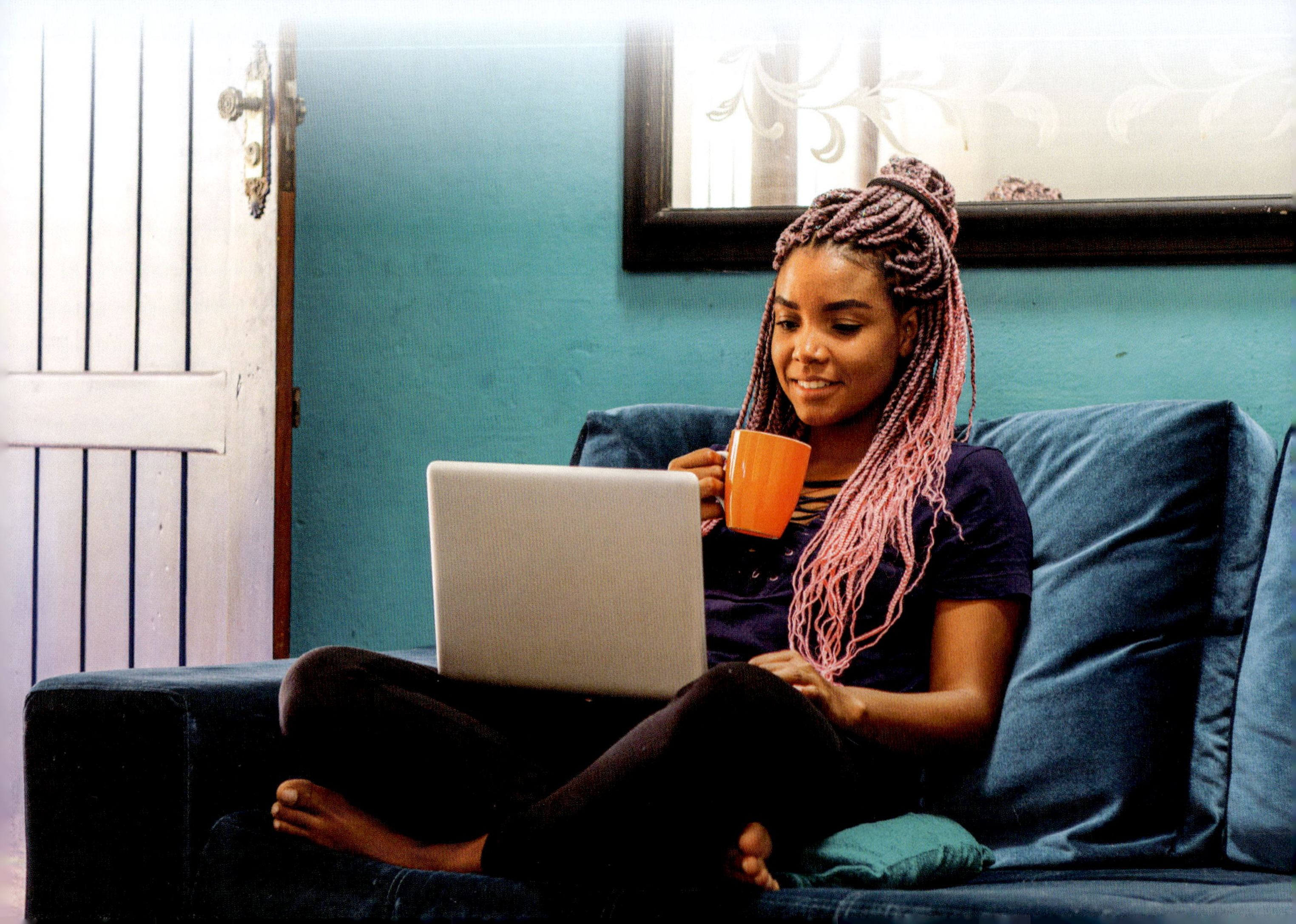

example, one study found that driving in a green landscape can improve your mood and reduce stress, whereas driving in barren or monochromatic scenery can lead to a negative mood state and increased stress (Jiang, He, Larsen, & Wang, 2020). Another study found that being exposed to the color green during a breathing exercise helped reduce levels of stress (as measured by heart rate, blood pressure, and cortisol levels) more than just using the breathing exercise alone (Suli, Aini, & Prasetyo, 2020). In the study, participants looked at a green cloth while they practiced deep breathing. They also were instructed to imagine they were inhaling and exhaling the green aura from the green cloth. Another study found that people who work in green spaces have less stress when compared to other colors (Lee, Oh, Kim, & Jang, 2018). The next time you feel your stress levels go up, try to find a green space to sit in.

Blue is another cool color that has been shown to promote calmness, improve mood, and reduce stress. It brings on a sense of trust, which is why many uniforms are blue, such as those of flight attendants and police officers (Manav, 2007). Blue has also been associated with feelings of neutrality because it doesn't elicit strong positive or negative emotions (Gunes & Olgunturk, 2020). Blue is associated with serenity and peace: Just being in a blue room can lower your heart rate (Oh et al., 2021). One study found that a blue environment lowered levels of salivary cortisol among workers more than any other colors except green (Lee et al., 2018). Living with a view of a lake, ocean, or any body of water has been shown to greatly decrease levels of psychological distress. If you don't have a waterfront view, don't worry—similar results were observed for people who have images of water in their living spaces.

## Summary

This chapter discussed how the environment in which you live, work, and play has an impact on your health and stress levels. Some components of your environment you have complete control over, such as the condition and arrangement of your study space and bedroom, whereas others you have less control over, such as your built environment and air quality. It is important to recognize the environmental factors that contribute to your stress levels so that you can make efforts to reduce those influences as well as to enhance the factors that help reduce your levels of stress.

## ONLINE RESOURCES

Visit HK*Propel* to access audio supplements, worksheets, and vocabulary flash cards for this chapter.

## DISCUSSION QUESTIONS

1. Because noise has a large impact on stress, do you feel landlords should be responsible for reducing noisy living conditions? Justify your answer.
2. Of all the environmental factors that impact stress, which do you feel has the greatest impact in your life? How does it increase or decrease your stress?
3. What are three changes you can make to your environment to help you reduce stress? Create a plan that identifies your environmental problem areas, what you will do to improve those problem areas, and the steps you will take to implement those changes.

PART III

# Practical Strategies for Managing Stress

# 10

# Mind–Body Approaches

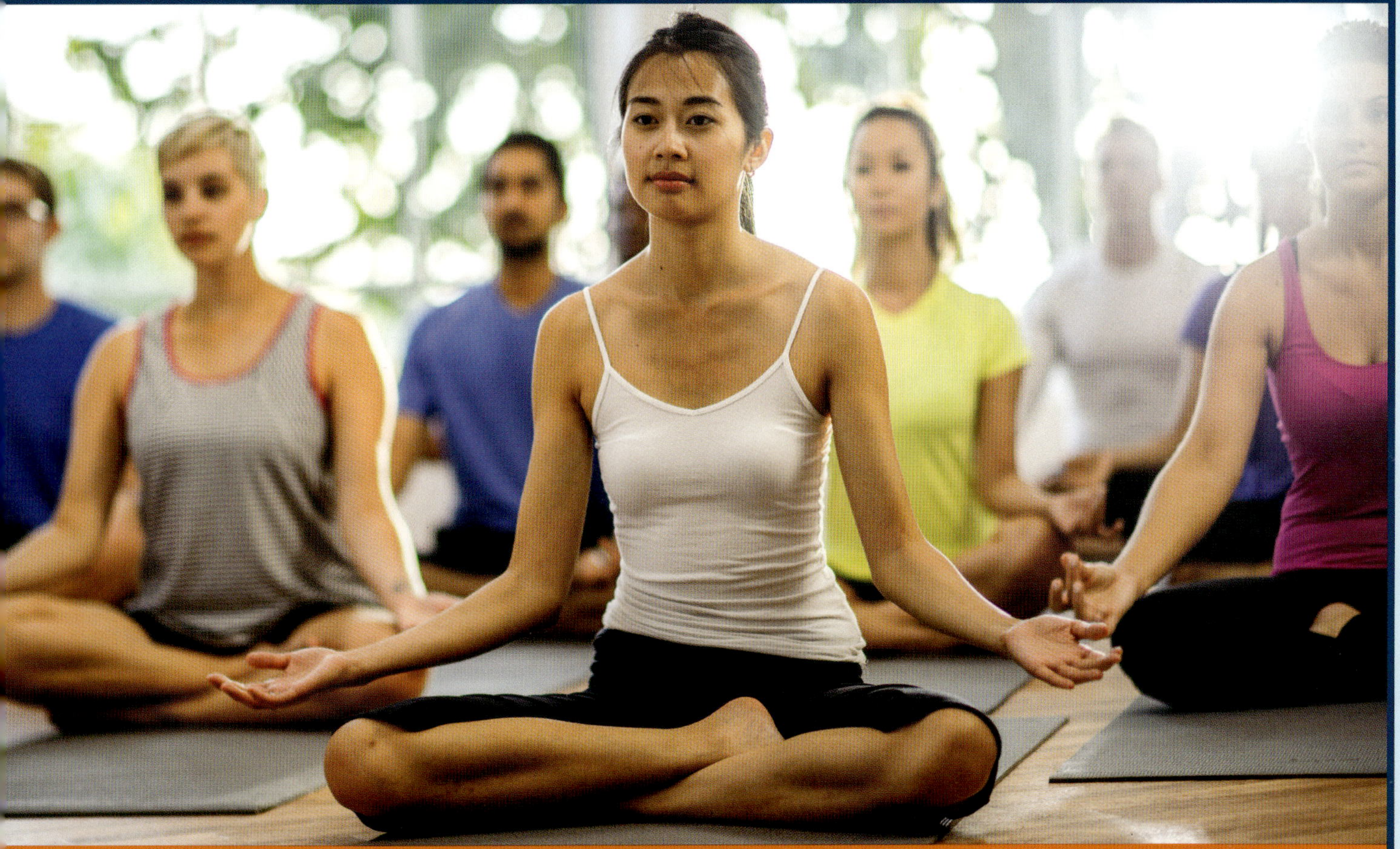

## LEARNING OBJECTIVES

After reading this chapter, you will be able to do the following:

- Examine the different types of breath work and their impact on stress
- Develop a plan to help better manage emotions
- List and describe types of yoga and how they can help manage stress
- Explain the practices of mindfulness and meditation and their role in managing stress
- Discuss how art therapy can help manage stress
- Understand how movement therapy can help manage stress

# KEY TERMS

- 4-7-8 breathing
- anchor breathing
- art therapy
- asana
- bhramari
- box breathing
- breath awareness
- breath work
- diaphragmatic breathing
- flow
- mantra
- meditation
- metacognition
- mindful breathing
- mindful breathing meditation
- mindfulness
- movement therapy
- nadi shodhana
- pranayama
- ujjayi
- yoga

Throughout this textbook, you have learned about the body's physiological response to stress and the ways the body adjusts to the presence of stress. You have explored notions of stress through the perspectives of the different dimensions of wellness and learned how stress affects and is affected by those dimensions. At this point, you may be feeling overwhelmed. Don't stress out. This chapter will provide you with a variety of mind-body approaches to stress management, including yoga, meditation and mindfulness, breath work, art therapy, and movement therapy. As you read through the chapter, pick one or two from each category to try.

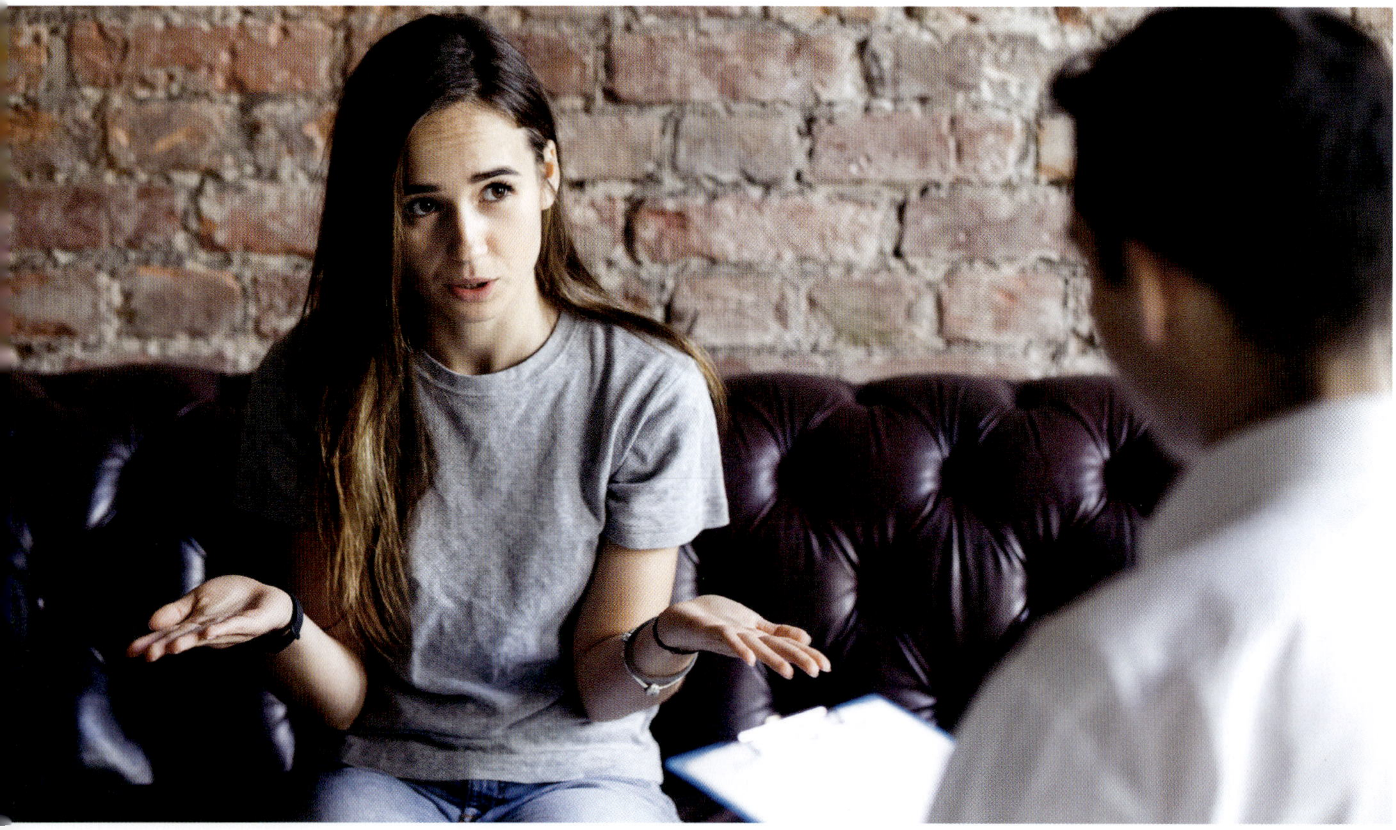

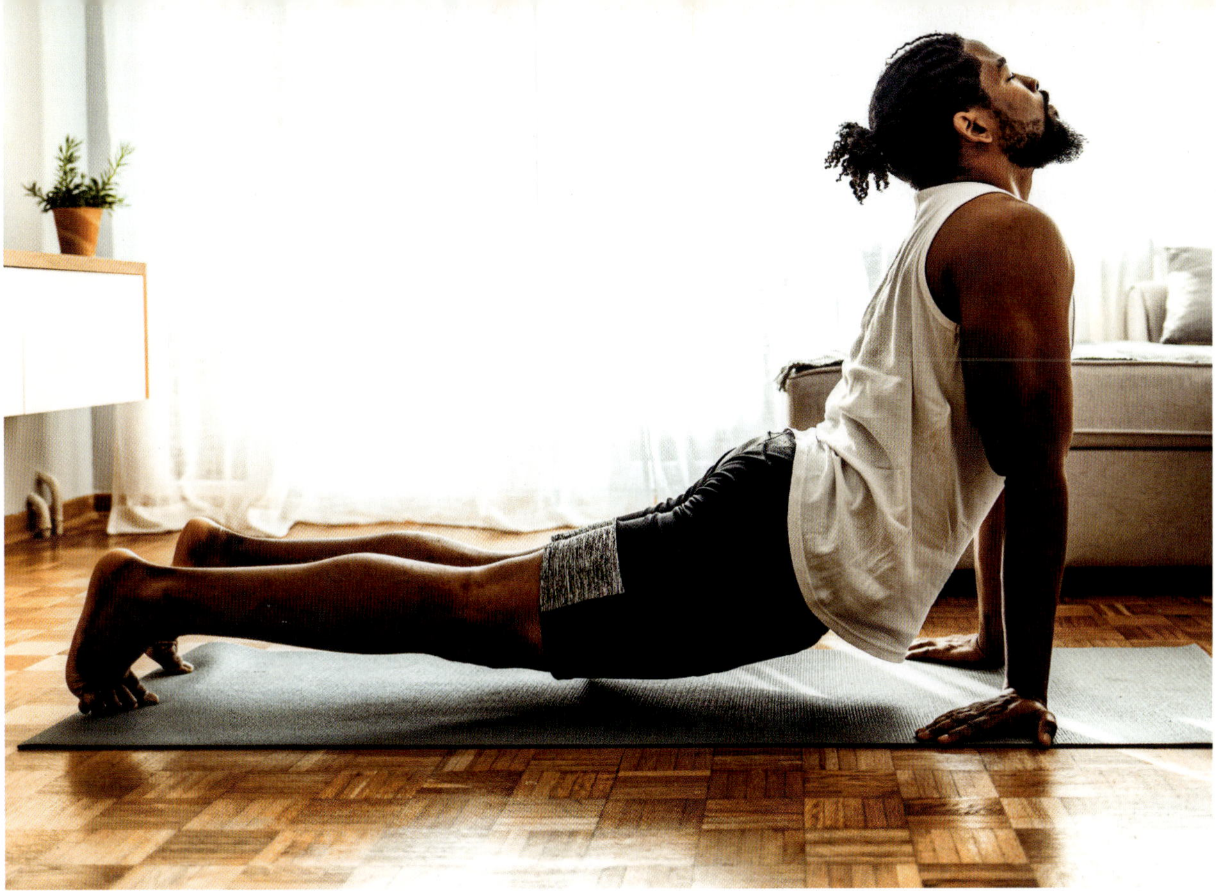

## Yoga

**Yoga** (from the Sanskrit word *yuj*, meaning "union" or "to join") is a type of complementary and integrative medicine that focuses on the mind-body-spirit connection. Yoga has been shown to help with a variety of conditions. Research has shown that adolescents who practice yoga have more enhanced emotional regulation skills (Janjhua, Chaudhary, Sharma, & Kumar, 2020). It also found that students who regularly practice yoga tend to rate themselves as happier, healthier, more energetic, and more focused compared to those who do not practice yoga. Similarly, research has shown that college students who practice yoga have better emotional regulation in areas of cognitive appraisal and self-compassion, and they show decreased negative affect as well as less suppression of negative emotions (Patel, Nivethitha, & Mooventhan, 2018).

Yoga reduces the activity of the sympathetic nervous system and increases the activity of the parasympathetic nervous system. This helps reduce the levels of stress hormones in the body and improve general sense of well-being (Tripathi, Kumari, & Ganpat, 2018). One study found that yoga helped decrease levels of stress and increase levels of attention and focus among college students (Tripathi et al., 2018). Other studies found similar positive benefits, including the reduction of stress and its symptoms, among a wider population of adults (Tong et al., 2020; Wang & Szabo, 2020).

**Yoga is an effective tool for managing stress.**

There are different branches of yoga, each representing a different focus and set of characteristics (Pankhania, 2005). All forms of yoga have stress-relieving properties, although some studies suggest that yoga practices incorporating meditation have the best outcomes in terms of stress-relieving properties (Marshall, McClanahan, Warren, Rogers, & Ballmann, 2020). Engaging in yoga practices can help reduce cortisol levels for both chronic and acute stress responses and may even reduce the severity of the stress response.

### Hatha Yoga

Hatha yoga is the most practiced type of yoga in the United States. It focuses on breath, body, and mind, with classes lasting between 45 and 90 minutes. This type of yoga is great for managing stress, improving emotional health, and easing back pain and arthritis (Neyaz, Sumila, Nanda, & Wadhwe, 2019; Wang & Szabo, 2020). It is considered a gentle yoga and is great for beginners. Classes consist of breathing, **asanas** (postures or poses), and meditation.

## Raja Yoga

Raja yoga focuses on meditation, energetics (a person's physical, mental, emotional, and spiritual energy), and a strict adherence to a series of disciplinary steps known as the eight limbs of yoga (Vivekananda, 2015):

1. Yamas: Five social observances (nonviolence, truthfulness, nonstealing, chastity, and nonpossessiveness)
2. Niyamas: Five moral observances (purity, contentment, self-discipline, self-study, devotion)
3. Asana: Yoga posture
4. Pranayama: Breathing technique
5. Pratyahara: Withdrawal of the senses
6. Dharana: Concentration
7. Dhyana: Meditation
8. Samadhi: Enlightenment or bliss

## Karma Yoga

Karma yoga focuses on creating a path of service to create a future free from negativity and selfishness. This is also considered the yoga of action (Pallathadka, Pallathadka, & Devi, 2022). It is the act of serving others—in this sense, providing for others (think volunteering). Ultimately, it is putting goodness, kindness, and compassion out into the world.

## Bhakti Yoga

Bhakti yoga focuses on creating a path of devotion, acceptance, and tolerance and encourages you to adopt a spirit of unconditional love (Bryant, 2017). It involves focusing your mind, emotions, and senses on the divine. The core practices include the following (Bryant, 2017):

- *Kirtan.* This is the practice of devotional chanting.
- *Japa.* This is the repetition of **mantras**. Common mantras include Namaste ("light within me salutes the light within you"), Om Namah Shivaya ("I bow to the self"), and Lokah Samastah Sukhino Bhavantu ("may all beings everywhere be happy and free"). You can do these in any language.
- *Devotion to the divine.* This can be devotion to a god, a guru, or yourself and others.

## Jnana Yoga

Jnana yoga is considered one of the most difficult forms of yoga. It is the practice of obtaining knowledge of reality through meditation and contemplation (Sruthi, Mishra, & Harti, 2022). To practice jnana, you practice self-inquiry to help remove your own biases and worldly influences on your thoughts and core beliefs. To put it more simply, jnana yoga refers to three processes: hearing the truth, contemplating or thinking about the truth, and living the truth (Om, 2020). The three core texts include the following (Om, 2020):

- *Sravana.* Hearing or experiencing the sacred knowledge of the ancient Vedic texts. This can also be interpreted as learning about your experience and being.
- *Manana.* Thinking and reflecting on nonduality. You can also think of this of reflecting on how the universe is interconnected and how you fit within the universe.
- *Nididhyasana.* Constant and profound meditation about your inner self. You can think of this as understanding your true self.

## Tantra Yoga

Tantra yoga focuses on the ritual, ceremony, or consummation of a relationship. Tantra means "to weave" in Sanskrit (Norian & McLaughlin, 2021). In this sense, it means to obtain spiritual enlightenment by connecting with your energy and those around you. It is further separated into red and white tantra. White tantra refers to solo practice, and red tantra refers to sexual practice (Norian & McLaughlin, 2021).

1. Quiet the mind.
2. Be comfortable with silence. It may take some time to get comfortable with silence, but stick with it. Yoga is often practiced with familiar music; however, this may take away from the meditative quality.
3. Don't think of flexibility or physical fitness as the end goal. Traditional tantra is focused on deep relaxation. Learn to relax

all parts of your body and mind to fully embrace tantra.

4. Lean into pleasure. This may include sex but can also include other types of pleasure.
5. Follow your own path. Access your own strength to discover your true self and what you truly derive pleasure from.

## Meditation and Mindfulness

Meditation and mindfulness are techniques designed to help you clear your mind and focus on the present. **Meditation** refers to the practice of spending time in contemplation to achieve a mentally clear state of mind. **Mindfulness** means fully paying attention to something to appreciate it with all senses. Although both are effective ways to manage and reduce stress, meditation is an exercise that you can practice to enhance your state of mind, whereas mindfulness is a state or quality of life that you can work toward.

### Meditation

Although some believe that meditation is the act of emptying your mind of thoughts, it is merely a way to help you see your thoughts more clearly (Reddy & Roy, 2019). We live in a time in which it is common to be bombarded by information from all directions. You may find it hard to concentrate, or you may feel overwhelmed or burdened by all the input. Meditation can help you create a mental barrier and stay in the present moment. Meditation can also help you build awareness of your feelings and thought processes, facilitating a better, more positive outlook on life. This practice also helps you build compassion for yourself and others, leading to healthier relationships (Luberto et al., 2018).

**We tend to be our own worst critics. Increasing our compassion for ourselves can help us lead more positive lives.**

Numerous studies have shown the benefits of meditation. One study found that individuals who meditate regularly have higher functioning antibody responses and can better fight off infections compared to those who do not meditate (Thibodeaux & Rossano, 2018). Meditation has been shown to reduce the severity of psychological disorders, including stress-related disorders (Thibodeaux & Rossano, 2018). One study found that practicing meditation can help reduce levels of perceived stress and improve well-being among medical students—a population with high rates of stress and depression compared to the general population (Yang, Schamber, Meyer, & Gold, 2018). Additionally, other studies found that those who regularly practiced meditation had lower cortisol levels compared to those who do not practice meditation (Koncz, Demetrovics, & Takacs, 2021). There are different types of meditation; all have stress-reducing benefits. A few of them will be discussed here.

#### *Om Meditation*

Om meditation, also called mantra meditation, is based on the mantra *om*, considered to be the sound of the universe, the name of the absolute. Om meditation is believed help you connect with your inner soul by combining your breath and sound (Harne, Tahseen, Hiwale, & Dhekekar, 2019). This technique has been shown to impact the parts of the brain, vagus nerve, and circulatory and respiratory systems that help you better manage stress (Harne et al., 2019).

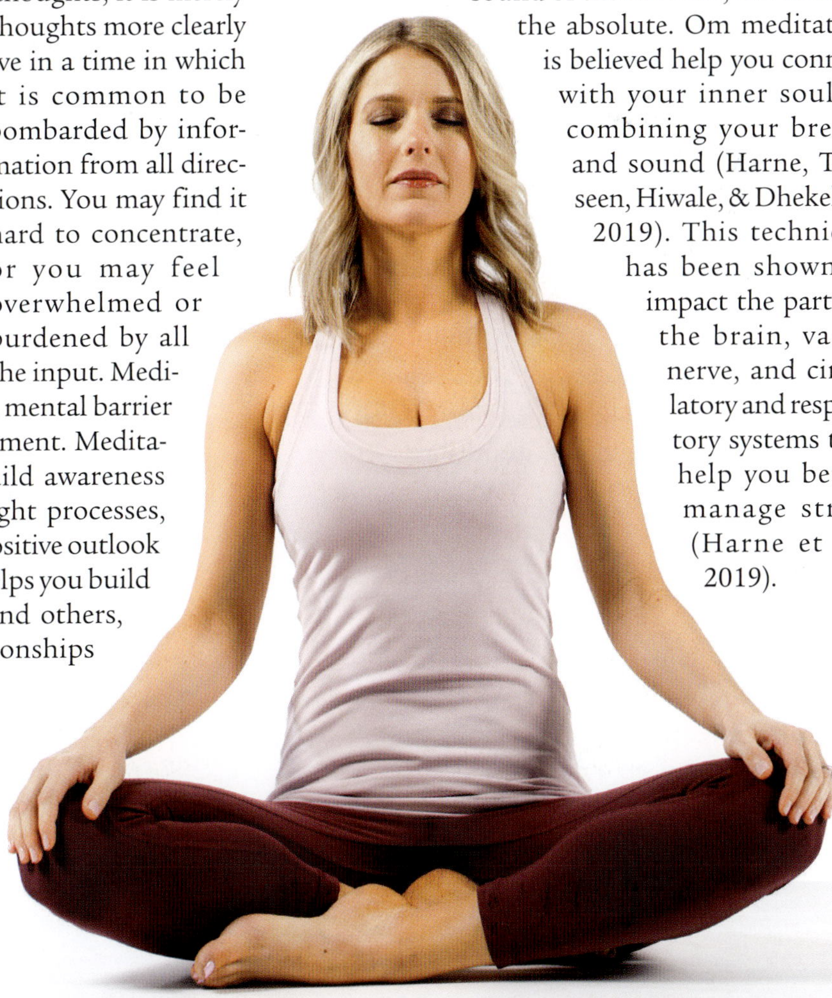

Here is how to practice om meditation (Ray, 2010).

1. Sit cross-legged on the floor with your back straight, or use a chair if you cannot sit on the floor. Keep your hands on your knees or thighs. Relax your facial muscles.
2. Gently close your eyes or glance downward.
3. Close your mouth and breathe naturally. Keep your face and jaw relaxed with your teeth slightly parted.
4. While you inhale and exhale, chant "om." Fit the chant to your breath. Break down the sound to "A-A-U-U-M." Say the first two syllables with your mouth open and the last two with your lips together. It should feel like a sound and vibration within your whole body.
5. Continue sitting and breathing while chanting "om," continuing to pay attention to the vibration in your body.

### Present Moment Meditation

Present moment meditation, also called mindfulness meditation, is the practice of paying attention to where you are and what you are doing without being overly sensitive to what's going on around you. With present moment meditation, you allow thoughts and feelings to pass through you without judging them. You acknowledge them and move on. You use your senses to place you in the present moment, not thinking about the past or future. Here are some tips to help you practice present moment meditation, which you can do almost anywhere:

1. Get into a comfortable position.
2. Start breathing slowly. Pay attention to the air entering your lungs.
3. Pay attention to the sounds and scents around you. Describe them in your mind.
4. If you have distracting thoughts, acknowledge them and move on. Imagine them as clouds passing overhead.
5. Focus on the position of your body.

### Spiritual Meditation

Spiritual meditation is used in many world religions. The focus is on obtaining a deeper understanding of spiritual or religious meaning and connecting with a higher power (see chapter 8). Examples of spiritual meditation in different religions include salat in Islam, contemplative prayer in Christianity, and Kabbalistic prayer in Judaism.

### Focused Meditation

Focused meditation uses any of the five senses to help you sharpen your concentration and attention. There are many ways to practice focused meditation, such as the following (Carpena, Souza Tavare, & Menezes, 2019):

- Counting mala beads
- Listening to a gong
- Staring at a candle flame
- Counting your breaths
- Moon gazing

### Transcendental Meditation

Transcendental meditation was developed by Maharishi Mahesh Yogi to help quiet the mind and induce a state of peace and calm (Joshi et al., 2022). In this type of meditation, an instructor teaches you the methods and works with you to create a personal mantra. For those not willing to commit to sessions with an instructor, you can work on your own and repeat a mantra for 20 minutes.

### Progressive Relaxation

Also known as body scan meditation, progressive relaxation is geared toward reducing tension in your body. One way to practice progressive relaxation is to slowly tighten and relax different muscle groups in your body one at a time (Bernstein, Borkovec, & Hazlett-Stevens, 2000).

### Loving-Kindness Meditation

Loving-kindness meditation, also known as metta meditation, is used to help strengthen feelings of compassion, kindness, and acceptance toward yourself and others. Loving-kindness meditation has been shown to improve mood and reduce symptoms of depression (Kearney, Malte, Storms, & Simpson, 2021). To practice this form of meditation, imagine a person (even one you don't like) and send loving thoughts to them. At the same time, open your mind to receiving kindness.

### Guided Meditation

In this type of meditation, sometimes called visualization or imagery meditation, you focus on mental pictures of images you find relaxing. Guided meditation is usually led by a teacher or guide and helps evoke feelings of calm. There are also many free videos and podcasts that you can use to practice guided meditation.

## Mindfulness

Mindfulness is a way of looking at the world with all your senses (see figure 10.1). It can be practiced formally or informally and can be adopted to be a way of life. To live a mindful life, participate in your everyday activities with the awareness of doing so, paying attention to your senses as you engage in these activities. There are many benefits to being more mindful in life: People who engage in mindful behavior have enhanced attention and executive control (Yakobi, Smilek, & Danckert, 2021). Mindfulness allows you to engage fully in life, free from distraction and judgment (Witkiewitz, Roos, Colgan, & Bowen, 2017). It helps reduce stress by focusing on the present which decreases negative or unpleasant thoughts. Lastly, it can help you better manage your emotions by giving yourself time to experience the present moment. This may also lead to a reduced stress reactivity when encountering stress.

Mindfulness can be practiced anywhere at any time. Once you begin to practice these behaviors, you may find it becomes habitual and you no longer need to actively engage in mindfulness exercises. Here are some ways to practice mindfulness in your daily life (Smalley & Winston, 2022):

- *Walking to a destination.* The next time you are walking from one place to another, pay attention to your steps. Notice how your feet feel in your shoes as they hit the ground. Listen to the sounds around you.

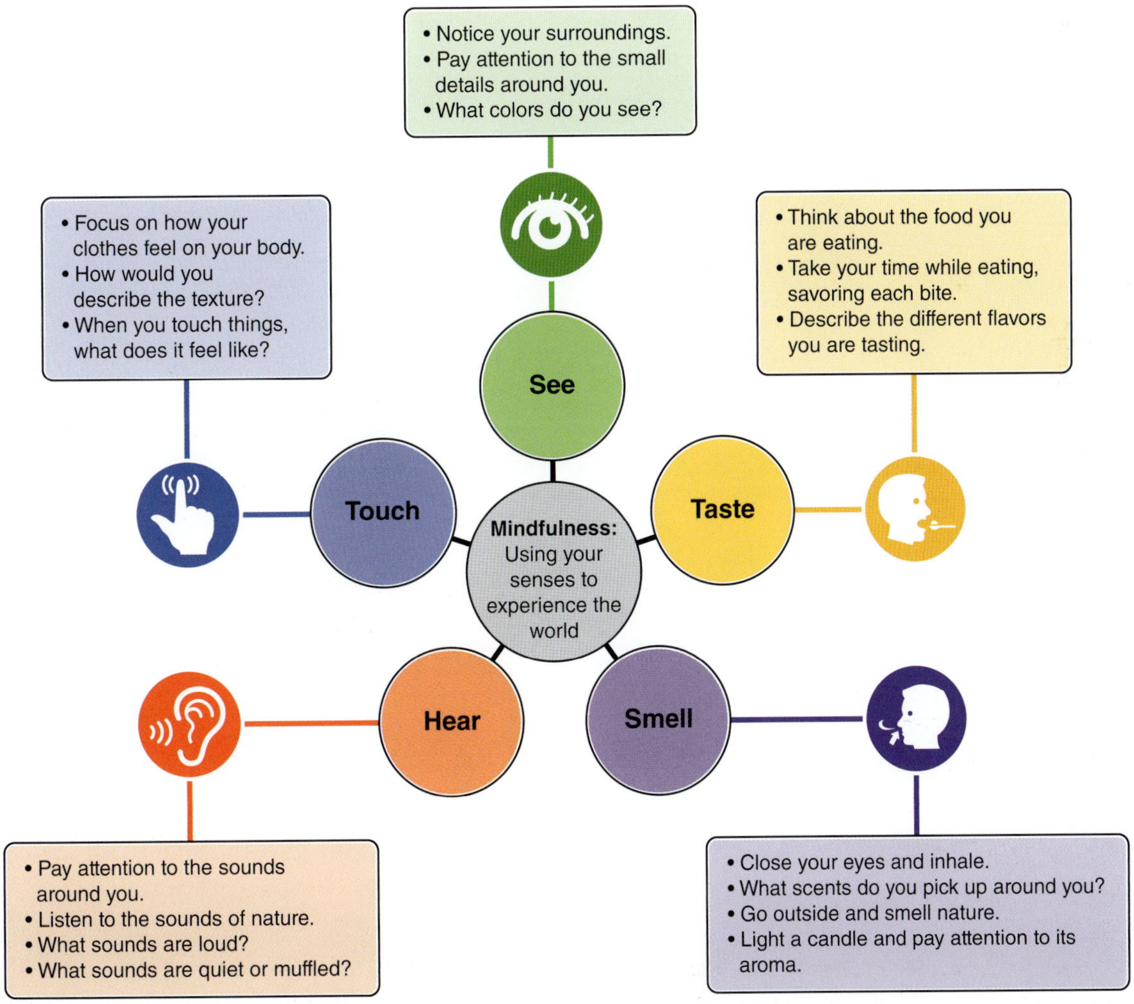


**Figure 10.1** Mindfulness approaches.

Research Spotlight

## Metacognition

Mindfulness has also been shown to increase your metacognition. **Metacognition** is your ability to understand how you learn and how to use strategies and tools to improve your understanding. Metacognition supports stress management by providing the cognitive knowledge to better understand your own behavior, the reasons behind your behavior, and how they relate to your emotions (Drigas & Mitsea, 2021). When you have a better understanding of your thoughts and actions, you feel more in control of the events in your life and tend to make better decisions. Metacognition also includes the ability to self-regulate your emotions and behavior, another important stress management skill. Studies have found that mindfulness can decrease patterns of negative thinking while increasing metacognitive awareness (Drigas & Karyotaki, 2018; Kudesia, 2019).

Pay attention to the breeze hitting your clothes, your hair, and your skin. Notice the temperature. Are you feeling hot? Cold? Are there any smells around you? How would you describe them?

- *During a conversation.* When you speak with another person, pay close attention to what they are saying. What do you think they are feeling? What does their body language tell you? Do not add to the conversation, just listen and ask questions.
- *Being quiet.* Take a few minutes each day and practice being quiet and still. Pay attention to your body and how you feel in the moment. Use your senses to identify how you feel.

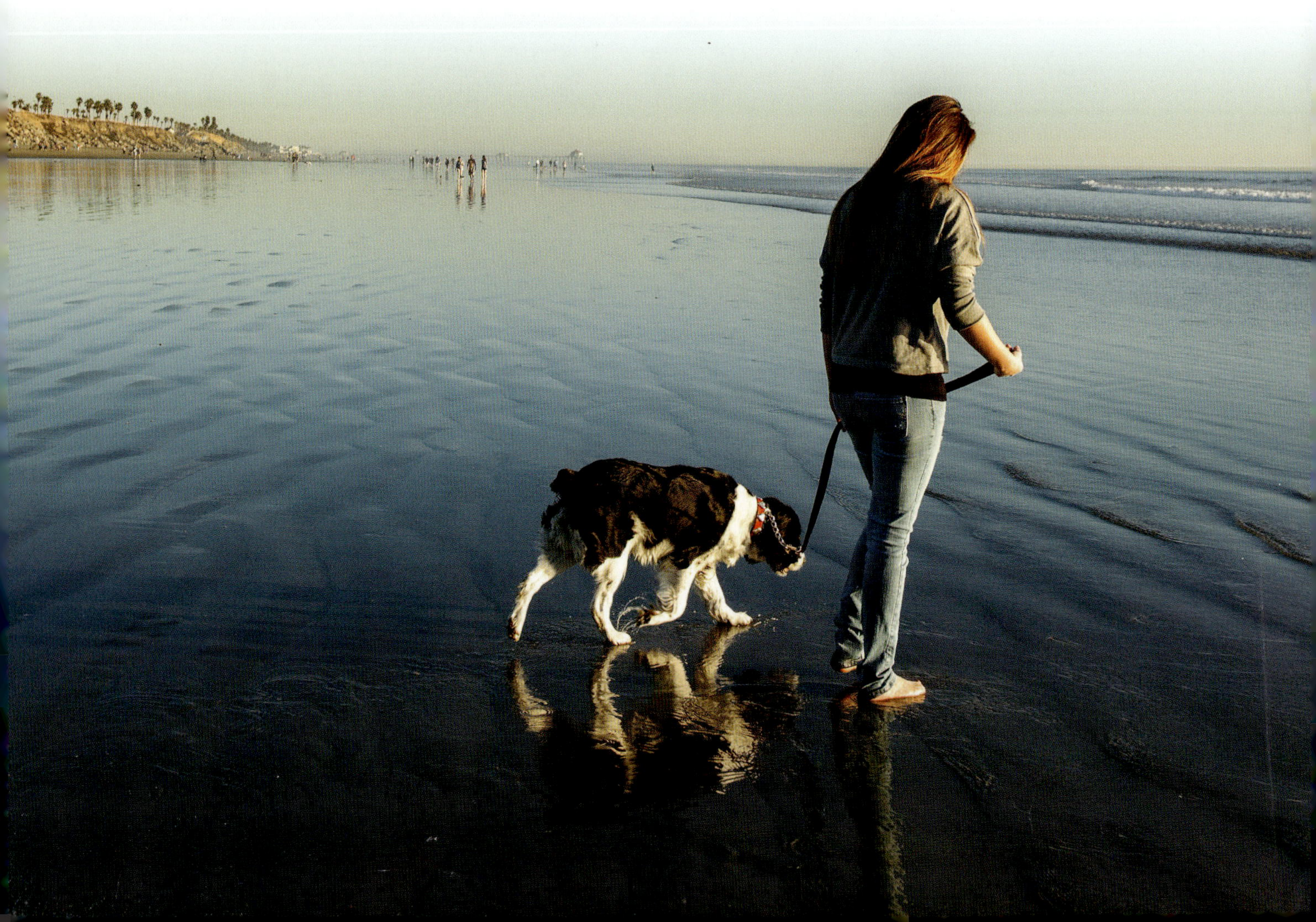

## Breath Work

Have you ever had someone tell you to "just breathe"? Obviously, you do not need to be told to breathe; however, **breath work**, or breathing in a meaningful and purposeful way, has been shown to be an effective stress management tool and to improve physical and mental wellness (Goldstein, Lewin, & Allen, 2019; Ma et al., 2017). Short and shallow breathing only fills the base of the lungs, but deep breathing fills all parts of the lungs, activating the parasympathetic nervous system and reducing stress and anxiety (Naik, Gaur, & Pal, 2018). The following breathing techniques can be practiced to reduce stress.

**Practicing breath work can activate your parasympathetic nervous system.**

### Pranayama

**Pranayama** is an ancient Indian tradition that refers to the practice of breathing. It is often practiced alongside yoga, but it can also be practiced on its own. It involves controlling the breath for different durations while focusing on different aspects of breathing. Pranayama consists of three phases:

- Puraka: Inhalation
- Kumbhaka: Retention
- Rechaka: Exhalation

One study conducted on men found that practicing pranayama for 12 weeks significantly decreased heart rate and blood pressure (Naik et al., 2018). The most significant effect of practicing pranayama was the reduction of perceived stress among the participants. There are many different types of pranayama, each with their own benefits. A few are discussed next.

#### Nadi Shodhana

**Nadi shodhana**, or alternative nostril breathing, is an exercise believed to help purify the body's energy. It has been shown to increase the activity of the parasympathetic nervous system (Kaur, 2021). The following steps highlight the practice of nadi shodhana.

1. *Inhalation*. Block your right nostril with your right thumb and inhale for six seconds.
2. *Breath hold*. Use your right index finger to block your left nostril and hold your breath for six seconds (both nostrils are blocked).
3. *Exhalation*. Release your thumb from your right nostril and breathe out for six seconds (left nostril is now blocked).
4. *Inhalation*. With the left nostril still blocked, breathe in for six seconds.
5. *Breath hold*. Use your right thumb to block your right nostril and hold for six seconds (both nostrils are blocked).
6. *Exhalation*. Release your index finger from your left nostril and breathe out for six seconds (right nostril still blocked).
7. *Repeat*. Repeat this cycle nine times from the start.

#### Bhramari

The **bhramari** (bee) breath is named after a black bee that is known for its buzzing. This exercise is good for reducing stress, anxiety, agitation, and anger (Kuppusamy, Kamaldeen, Pitani, Amaldas, & Shanmugam, 2018). This technique is particularly good for beginners because the humming sound helps block out distractions. Here are the steps to practice bhramari:

1. Sit in a comfortable position.
2. Close your eyes or lower your gaze. Pay attention to the feeling of sitting on the ground or chair with your back straight. Breathe in and out through your nose.
3. Press your pointer fingers on the cartilage of your ears to block out external sound.
4. Keeping your ears blocked, take a deep breath in through your nose. On the exhale, make a humming sound. Repeat as often as you like.

When practicing bhramari, pay attention to the vibration you are creating in your face. If you do not feel the vibration, try humming louder or at a different pitch. It is this vibration that promotes relaxation and calm.

#### Ujjayi

**Ujjayi** (also known as conqueror's yoga) is the most common breathing technique used with yoga. Both inhaling and exhaling are done through the nose, using sound to help block distractions, synchronize your senses, and control your thoughts. You may feel like you are not getting enough air at first, but with practice, it will become easier. Here are the steps (Rosen & Fraley, 2002):

1. Keeping your mouth closed, breathe in. Constrict your throat a bit so that your breathing makes a rushing sound, almost like snoring. Use this for both inhalations and exhalations.
2. Use your diaphragm to control your breathing.
3. Keep your inhalations and exhalations equal in duration.

## Diaphragmatic Breathing

**Diaphragmatic breathing** is a slow and deep breathing exercise that uses the diaphragm, the large dome-shaped muscle located at the base of the lungs, to control air movement. When you inhale, the diaphragm pulls down, opening the lungs and filling them with air, and when you exhale, the diaphragm pushes up, forcing air out of the lungs (figure 10.2). All breathing involves the diaphragm, but you can control how effectively you utilize your diaphragm to help you breathe more efficiently. When breathing normally, your lungs do not fill to capacity, but diaphragmatic breathing allows you to use 100 percent of your lung capacity. As such, this technique can help you strengthen your diaphragm, decrease oxygen demand, and use less effort and energy to breathe (Cleveland Clinic, 2022). This is important because the diaphragm is a key element in your body's functioning; for example, diaphragmatic functioning is associated with cardiac and lymphatic health (Kocjan, Adamek, Gzik-Zroska, Czyzewski, & Rydel, 2017).

When you encounter stress, whether a jump scare at a movie or a looming deadline, your body responds by activating the stress response system. Diaphragmatic breathing can help activate the parasympathetic nervous system and lower levels of the stress hormone cortisol, returning the body to a prestressed state (Hamasaki, 2020; Hopper, Murray, Ferrara, & Singleton, 2019). Diaphragmatic breathing can help people modulate their emotions and has also been shown to help manage conditions such as chronic obstructive pulmonary disease (COPD), asthma, postoperative respiratory function, and cardiorespiratory performance (Hamasaki, 2020).

You can control how effectively you utilize your diaphragm to help you breathe more efficiently. For example, if you have poor posture and sit with your back hunched over, you create less space in your ribcage to fully expand when inhaling. This may result in your body adopting an adaptive breathing strategy to compensate for the decreased

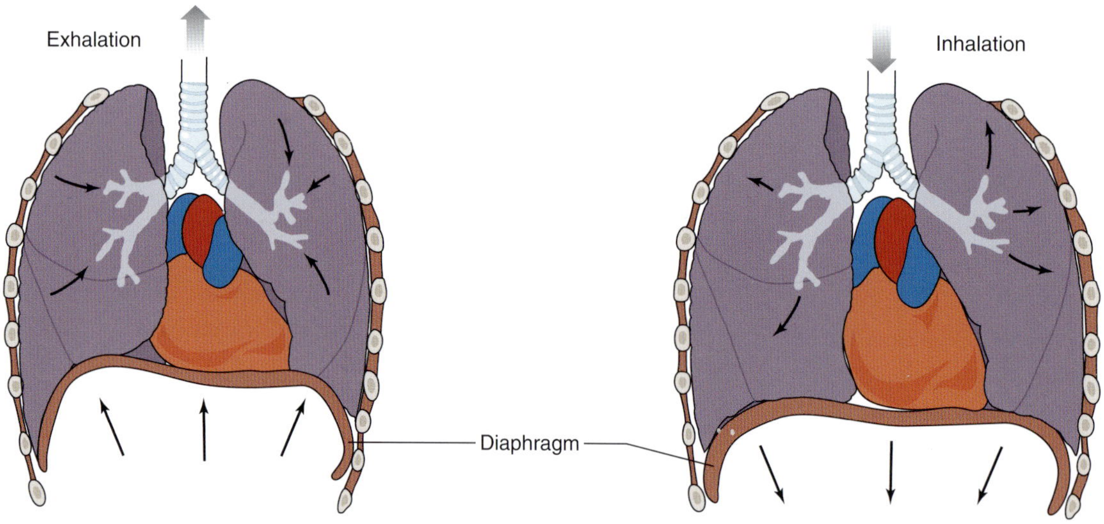


**Figure 10.2** Anatomy of breathing: The diaphragm moves upward during exhalation (left) and down during inhalation (right).
Reprinted by permission from L.A. Cartwright and K.S. Peer, *Fundamentals of Athletic Training*, 4th ed. (Champaign, IL: Human Kinetics, 2019), 124.

space in the rib cage. As such, it can lead to decreased respiratory efficiency, shortness of breath, increased lumbar discomfort (back pain), increased pelvic instability, and headaches (Kocjan, Adamek, Gzik-Zroska, Czyzewski, & Rydel, 2017).

**When practicing any type of breathing exercise, it is important to maintain proper posture to ensure the diaphragm and rib cage can fully engage in the breathing process.**

Diaphragmatic breathing involves the stomach, abdominal muscles, and diaphragm. Try practicing for 5 to 10 minutes at a time, three or four times a day. Use the following steps (Liu, Wiedman, Lovelace-Chandler, Gong, & Salem, 2023).

1. *Start lying down*. It is best to start practicing diaphragmatic breathing while lying down so that you can better focus on the movement of your chest and abdomen. Once you have more experience, you can try to engage in diaphragmatic breathing while sitting up.
2. *Make yourself comfortable*. You may want to place a pillow under your head and knees. Place one hand in the middle of your chest. Place your other hand just beneath your rib cage.
3. *Inhale*. Slowly breathe in through the nose, concentrating on bringing the air toward your stomach. You should feel your hand on your stomach rise up; your hand on your chest should remain still.
4. *Exhale*. When you exhale, tighten your abdominal muscles and let your stomach fall downward while exhaling through pursed lips. Your hand on your chest should remain still.

It's not the stress that kills us; it is our reaction to it.

**Hans Selye**

## Mindful Breathing

**Mindful breathing** links diaphragmatic breathing and mindfulness to help you remain in the present; as such, it is considered both a breathing exercise and a meditation practice. It has been shown to help reduce stress and increase feelings of calm (Schwind et al., 2017). Mindful breathing can be coupled with other therapies such as cognitive behavioral therapy.

Studies show that mindful breathing can help you feel a better sense of control, which helps you make better, less impulsive decisions. Imagine you are driving very fast when a deer comes out in front of you. In this scenario, you only have a fraction of a second to think and will likely react from instinct or fear. On the other hand, let's say you are driving slowly and see the deer come onto the road 50 yards ahead of you. In this scenario, you have plenty of time to think about how to react and make the safest choice. Mindful breathing is like the second scenario, allowing you to slow your thinking and calm your emotions while remaining in the present. This sense of control can also help improve metacognitive processes, which support making positive health-related choices (Pozuelos, Mead, Rueda, & Malinowski, 2019). Studies have found when mindfulness and self-control are increased, levels of stress go down significantly (Song & Park, 2019). Mindful breathing has also been shown to help reduce chronic pain, which also provides relief from stress (Zeidan & Vago, 2016).

There are many different techniques for mindful breathing. Consider trying out a couple on your own. Start small and spend five minutes per day on mindful breathing. Research shows just five minutes a day can decrease stress and improve mindfulness (Chui, Wai, Lai, See, & Tan, 2021).

### *Mindful Breathing Meditation*

Use the following steps for **mindful breathing meditation**:

1. Find a comfortable position and relax.
2. Take a deep breath in, hold it for a few seconds, and slowly let it go. Start to focus on your breathing: Think about the air entering your lungs, filling them, and leaving.
3. As you breathe in, envision how the air travels through your nose and mouth, through your trachea, and into your lungs. Imagine it filling the empty space in your lungs. As you breathe in, say "Breathing in, I know I am breathing in."

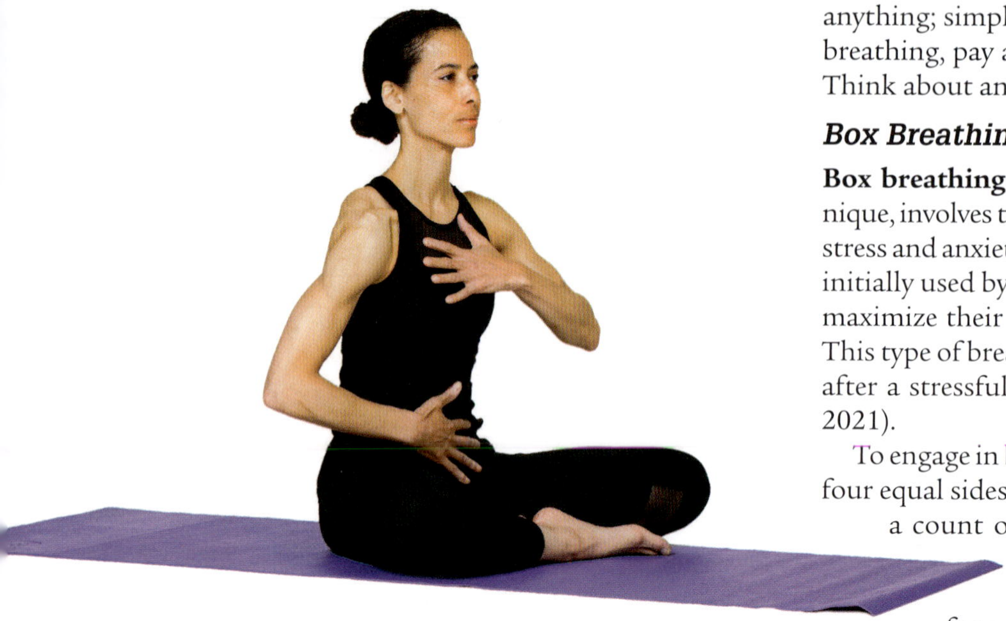

4. As you exhale, imagine the carbon dioxide and other waste flowing out of your lungs, through your trachea, and out of your nose and mouth. As you exhale, say "Breathing out, I know I am breathing out."

If thoughts enter your mind (and they will), acknowledge the thoughts and move on. Think of them as clouds passing by. You notice the clouds but do not give them all of your attention. During your breathing, you can say, "Dwelling in the present moment, I know this is a peaceful moment."

### Anchor Breathing

Another mindful breathing technique you can try is **anchor breathing**. Imagine yourself on a boat. The boat—your body—is anchored exactly where you want to be. You feel safe, happy, and calm on the boat. It is a beautiful day, and the world feels at peace. With your hands on your chest, take a deep breath in. Breathe out slowly. Think about your ribs moving up and down like a gently swaying boat as you take in each breath. When your mind wanders, bring it back to your anchor. Think about distracting thoughts as leaves in the wind. You see them, but let the wind take them away.

### Breath Awareness

**Breath awareness** is one of the easiest mindful breathing techniques to practice. For this exercise, sit or lie down in a comfortable position. Focus on your breathing. You do not need to change anything; simply be aware of it. As you continue breathing, pay attention to how your body feels. Think about any tension you have and release it.

### Box Breathing

**Box breathing**, also known as the square technique, involves taking slow, deep breaths to reduce stress and anxiety (figure 10.3). Box breathing was initially used by Navy Seals and police officers to maximize their performance when under stress. This type of breathing is useful before, during, or after a stressful event (Norelli, Long, & Krepps, 2021).

To engage in box breathing, imagine a box with four equal sides. Breathe in through the nose for a count of four, hold breath for a count of four, breathe out for a count of four, and hold breath for a count of four, imagining moving around the sides of the box with each step. This example utilizes four seconds at each step but can be customized to your needs (Norelli et al., 2021).

### 4-7-8 Breathing

**4-7-8 breathing**, also known as the relaxing breath, is based on the pranayama breathing exercise mentioned earlier in this chapter. It has been shown to reduce oxygen consumption, heart rate, and blood pressure. Additionally, it increases parasympathetic nervous system activity (mea-

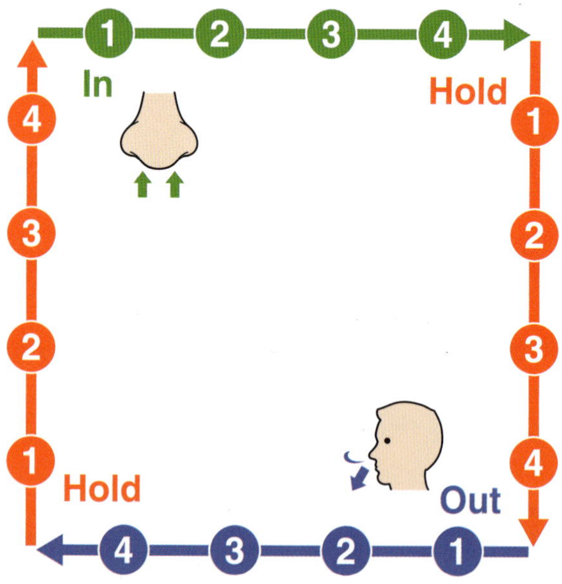


**Figure 10.3** Box breathing.

sured by an increase in theta and delta waves) and decreases sympathetic nervous system activity (Vierra, Boonla, & Prasertsri, 2022). This breathing method was found to increase the activity of the GABA neurotransmitter, which helps reduce levels of cortisol and adrenaline in the body (Pandekar & Thangavelu, 2019). As such, studies found the 4-7-8 breathing method may help reduce stress and anxiety and help with falling asleep (Russo, Santarelli, & O'Rourke, 2017). It can also help reduce tension, exhaustion, and fatigue (McNair, 2020).

**4-7-8 breathing gets easier with practice.**

When you first start to practice this technique, you may feel lightheaded. It is recommended that you start with only three or four repetitions and do not get up for a few minutes after you finish (figure 10.4). To practice this technique, sit or lie down, place the tip of your tongue on the tissue right behind your top front teeth, and follow this pattern (Vierra et al., 2022):

1. Empty your lungs of air.
2. Breathe in through the nose for four seconds.
3. Hold your breath for seven seconds.
4. Exhale forcefully through the mouth by pursing your lips and making a "whoosh" sound for eight seconds.
5. Repeat the cycle up to four times.

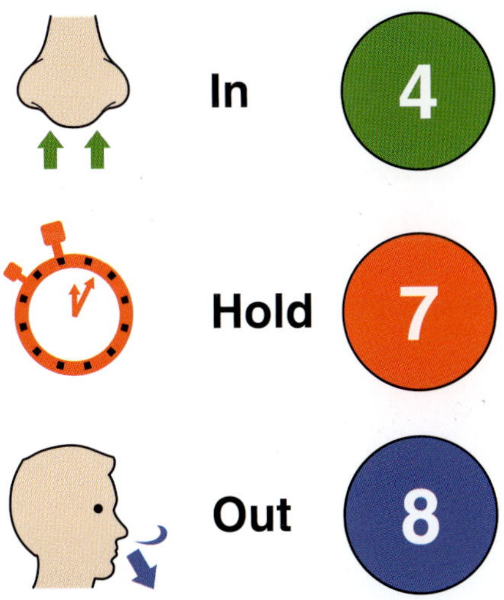


**Figure 10.4** 4-7-8 breathing.

## Art Therapy

**Art therapy** is the use of creative expression to enhance mental health. Whereas an art class focuses on teaching specific skills and techniques to create a finished piece of art, art therapy directs the client to create art that is an expression of their perceptions, feelings, and thoughts (Vaartio-Rajalin, Santamaki-Fischer, Jokisalo, & Fagerstrom, 2021).

Kids are usually great at utilizing art to express themselves. Many adults, on the other hand, have lost this skill. Adults tend to be more critical of their work and place too much emphasis on the product being perfect rather than on the process of creating. However, like riding a bike, you do not need a formal lesson to re-engage your creative side. You just need some encouragement.

Art therapy has been shown to be a great stress relief tool (Kaimal, Ray, & Muniz, 2016). Studies show that engaging in some type of art for just 45 minutes can significantly reduce your stress, regardless of the type of art or medium you are working with (Lith, 2016). It is time for you to spend with yourself, forget about the pressures of life, and focus on being in the moment—much like mindfulness. Art can also help you get into a state of **flow**, the state of mind when you are fully engrossed in an activity. Research shows that flow can improve performance and help lower stress levels. Lastly, art therapy can help you relax (Kaimal et al., 2019). When you are ruminating about a problem, art therapy can allow you to free your mind.

**Art can be a form of self-care.**

Art therapy can be done alone, but it may be best to start with a professional who can guide you through the process. Art therapists are trained professionals who hold a degree in psychotherapy or art therapy. There are many different media options, including the following:

- Painting
- Collage
- Drawing
- Poetry
- Coloring
- Playing or composing music
- Sculpting
- Photography
- Creating textiles

Case Study

## Engaging in Art to Reduce Stress

People under stress may find it difficult to allow their mind to relax. Art therapy can help reduce stress by encouraging you to slow down and get your mind off your stressor. Even if you are not an artist, the act of creating something allows your mind to drift, which promotes relaxation. Creating art has been shown to reduce cortisol levels and improve overall mood (Kaimal et al., 2016).

Art therapy does not have to include formal sessions that take place with a professional, nor does it require a lot of preparation and materials. It is also a relatively inexpensive activity and can be as long or short as you want it to be (Braus & Morton, 2020). Art therapy is not a lesson on how to create art; it is an experience that allows your emotions to come through (Farokhi, 2011). There are many different forms of art you can practice, including ceramics, paint, music, drawing, or photography. What's important is that you allow your mind to wander and feel present in the moment.

### Discussion Questions

1. How can creating art help you manage stress?
2. What type of art would you consider trying? How can you make time to include art in your schedule?
3. Your friend says she is bad at art and doesn't think art therapy will work for her. How would you try to convince your friend to create art as a stress management technique?

## Movement Therapy

**Movement therapy** refers to any type of mindful movement practices used to treat the mind, body, and spirit. Movement is believed to be the first language we learn, and as we grow older, much of our communication is done through body movement, facial expression, and the use of space. As such, movement therapy helps promote health and wellness by encouraging proactive participation in your own health (Phuphanich, Droessler, Altman, & Eapen, 2020). Studies have found movement therapy to be effective in reducing stress and psychological distress (Brauninger, 2012; Martin et al., 2018). Like art therapy, movement therapy doesn't need to be formal, but it may be best to start with a movement therapist to help you learn how to engage in the practice.

## Summary

Stress is in our lives and all around us. This chapter discussed many methods to help you better manage your stress. Yoga is a great tool to help focus your mind and emotions that also can be combined with a variety of breathing exercises to ignite the parasympathetic nervous system and invoke feelings of relaxation. Some forms of yoga may also include postures or asanas. Meditation can help build awareness and compassion by helping focus your thoughts. Mindfulness is another practice to increase your awareness and experience the world with all your senses. Finally, creative expression through art or movement can help you better define and express your emotions. The next chapter will focus on ways to prevent stress by being proactive in your decision making.

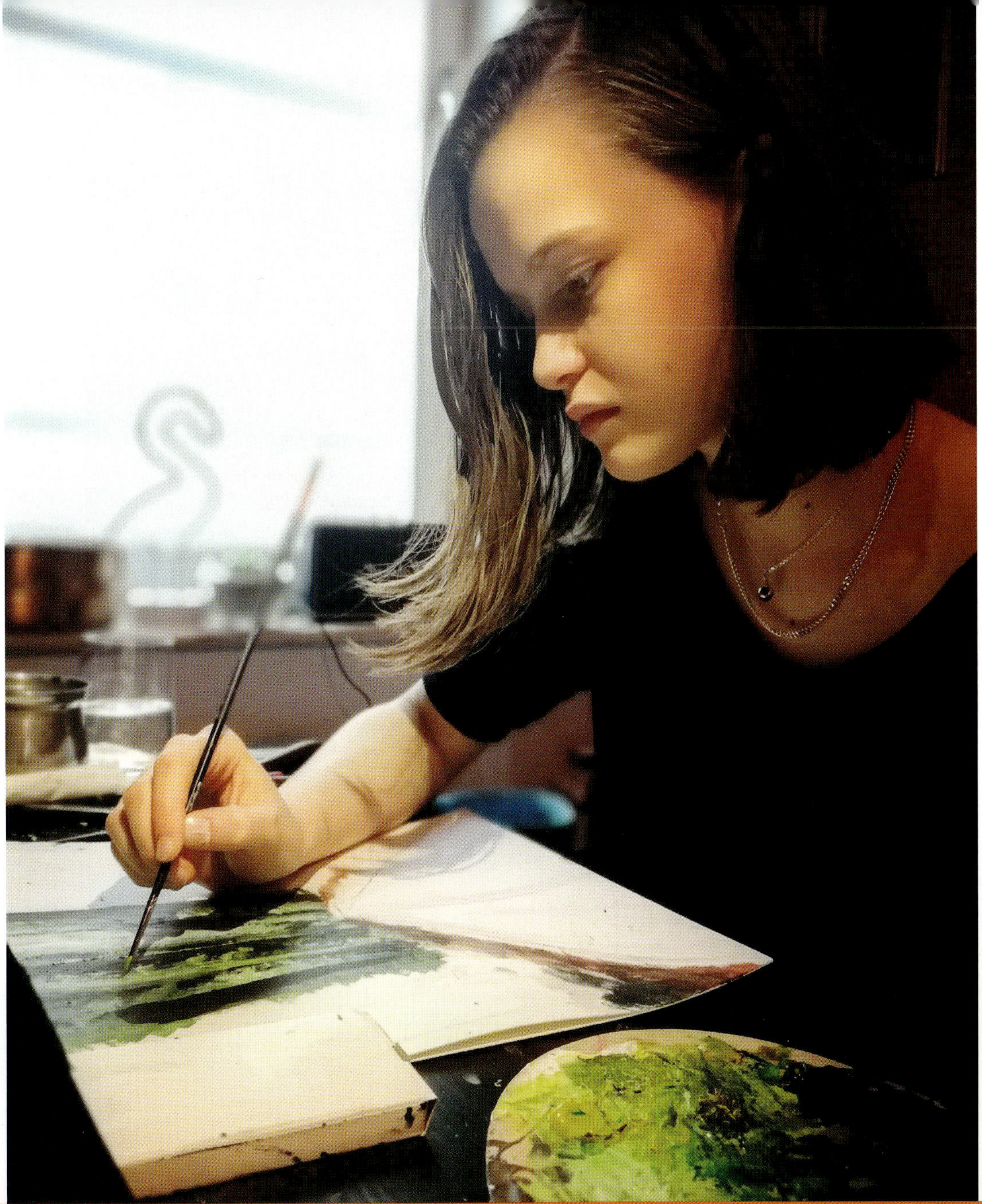

## ONLINE RESOURCES

Visit HK*Propel* to access audio supplements, worksheets, and vocabulary flash cards for this chapter.

## DISCUSSION QUESTIONS

1. What comes to mind when you hear the word *yoga*? How has this chapter changed your own ideas about yoga? If you had to engage in one form of yoga discussed in this chapter, which would you choose and why? How do you think it would improve your life?
2. Utilizing any form of breathing exercise has been shown to improve stress management, yet many people do not engage in breathing exercises. Create an argument to convince someone to incorporate breathing exercises as part of their daily routine.
3. How do meditation and mindfulness help with stress management? Describe how you would incorporate meditation or mindfulness into your life.
4. Paint or draw a picture of a place that helps you relax. What is it about this place that helps you relax?

11

# Proactive Approaches

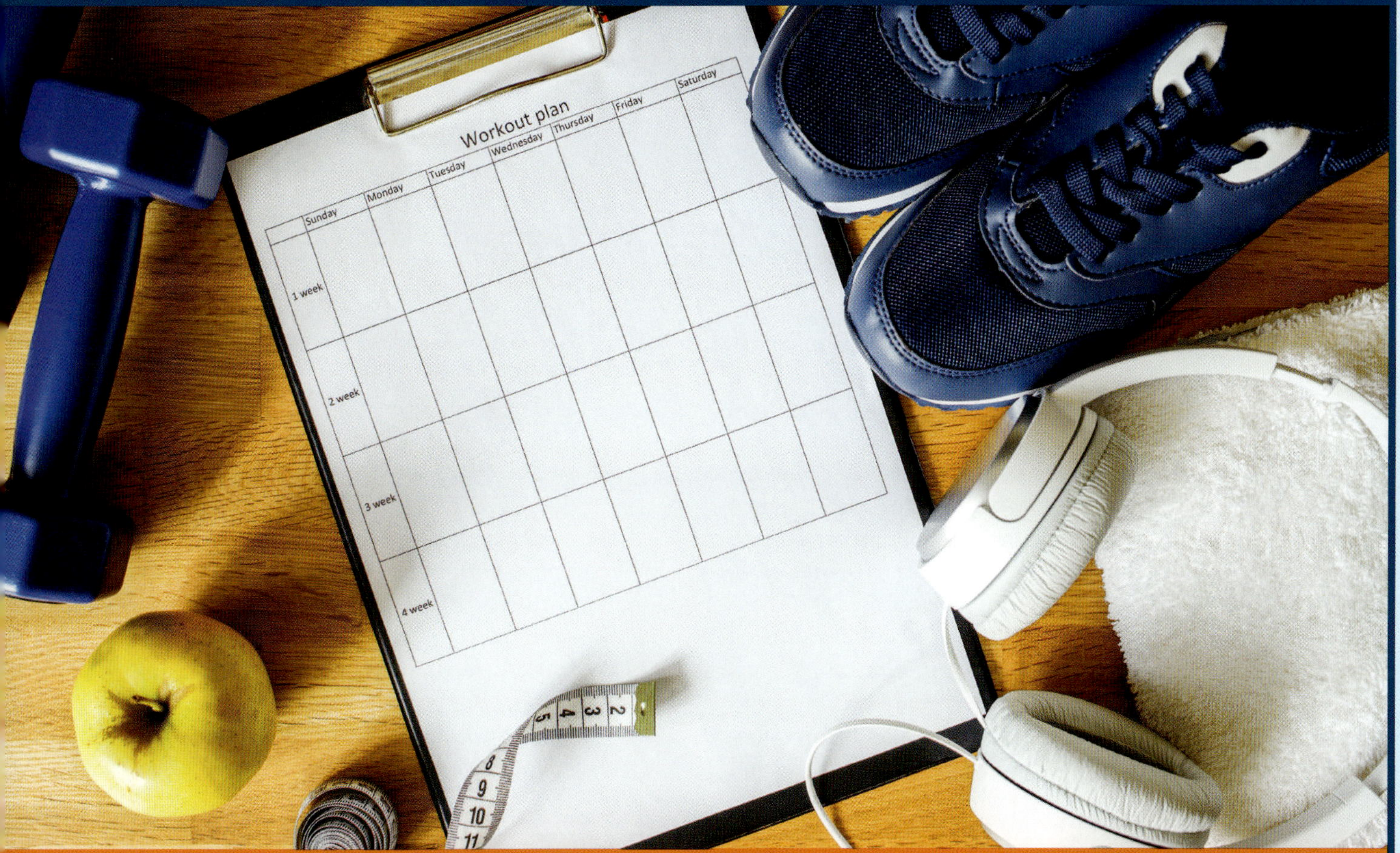


## LEARNING OBJECTIVES

After reading this chapter, you will be able to do the following:

- Justify the use of a strengths-based approach to manage stress
- Evaluate your own stress triggers and how to better manage them
- Explain the importance of self-care
- Identify at least four approaches to time management
- Describe ways to manage your own resources to avoid stress
- Examine ways to reduce the likelihood of getting burnout
- Identify sources of support that can help you proactively manage stress

# KEY TERMS

burnout
Eisenhower matrix
Most Important Task (MIT) strategy
Parkinson's law
Pomodoro technique
strengths-based approach
time blocking
trigger
work–life balance

Have you ever found that when you adequately plan for something, it tends to be easier and less stressful? In the previous chapter, you learned about ways to manage existing stress. This chapter will present proactive strategies for self-care, planning, time management, and other ways to help prevent or reduce the severity of stress.

## Strengths-Based Approach to Stress Management

Chapter 1 presented the historical views on wellness, which viewed health from a deficit approach. For instance, a person who has low levels of wellness was thought of as lacking health. This has a negative connotation and can end up feeling like patient blaming (Osborne et al., 2022). On the other hand, a **strengths-based approach** asks you to identify current strengths and build on them to maximize your likelihood of success (Bryant et al., 2020). To highlight the difference between these two concepts, imagine you are cooking dinner. In a deficit approach, you would locate a recipe, create a list of ingredients you are missing, and go out and get them before you can begin cooking. In a strengths-based approach, you would search for recipes that utilize the ingredients you already have. Which do you feel would be an easier approach to making dinner?

How would you go about starting a strengths-based approach? The following are the six hallmarks of the strengths-based approach (Rapp, Saleebey, & Sullivan, 2005):

1. *Identify your goals.* This approach invites you to determine what areas you would like to improve. This is central to the strengths-based approach—no one likes being told what to do. Identifying what is important to you makes the goal more meaningful.
2. *Identify your strengths.* This step has you identify the strengths you already possess, including past accomplishments, current progress, or a positive attitude. What do you see yourself as doing really well? What are activities you already enjoy doing? Identifying what you currently excel at and enjoy provides you with a solid groundwork to build on.
3. *Identify your resources.* This step identifies the strengths of your environment and how to utilize those resources to promote healthy change. For example, if you are looking to improve your fitness levels, what resources are available in your community to help you reach your goal? Are there fitness centers that offer classes? Are there running or walking trails?
4. *Use your strengths and resources to plan for goal attainment.* In this step, you can go about planning for healthy behavior change using the strengths and assets identified in previous steps. What do you plan on doing to reach your goal? What specific activities will help you move forward? What actions will you take?
5. *Create a goal that inspires hope.* When utilizing a strengths-based approach, it is very important to create a goal that is hopeful and looks to the future. Consider setting smaller goals that can be achieved along the way. For example, some gyms display photos marking workout milestones (100 workouts, birthday workouts, etc.); these serve to reward and celebrate gymgoers and motivate them to return.

**Success helps you stay motivated to continue working toward your goal.**

6. *Keep meaningful choices central to your goal.* You are responsible for making your own choices. The entire process is person first.

## Identifying Your Triggers

Another way to help prevent stress is to identify the things that cause it. A **trigger** is anything that gives rise to an emotional reaction. It can be an approaching deadline, an upcoming first date, a fear of spiders, or taking an exam. Triggers can also result in happy emotions (e.g., a photograph that reminds you of a happy time), but in the context of stress, it is referring to those that result in the activation of your fight-or-flight response.

The ultimate goal of stress management is not to eliminate all stress from your life but to effectively manage that stress so it motivates you and does not negatively impact your health. Because a stress-related trigger response tends to be overreactive and not helpful, avoiding triggers is one way to manage stress before it becomes worse. There are steps you can take to better manage your triggers.

1. *Name your trigger.* You cannot begin to manage the trigger causing your stress until you have identified it. There may be times when you are not sure what the trigger is. If that is the case, try keeping a journal. At the end of each day, write down how you felt during the day, noting any ups or downs and the events that led to them. This may allow you to identify your triggers to help you avoid them in the future.
2. *Know your backstory.* What about the trigger made it a trigger? Was it a previous experience with the situation? What is your personal history with the trigger?
3. *Consider positive reframing.* Start thinking about your trigger differently. What would it feel like to have a different reaction? How can you use positive self-talk to help you better manage the trigger?
4. *Use interruption.* When you encounter your trigger, use those positive reframing thoughts to interrupt your negative thought pattern. Utilize one of the stress management techniques mentioned in chapter 10. Get yourself relaxed and back to a mindset that allows you to remain neutral when managing the trigger.

Everyone has triggers. For example, consider Elijah, who has had a fear of small planes since he was a child. He once flew on a small plane that had terrible turbulence, which scared him badly, and he has avoided small planes since. Now in his early 20s, Elijah had a flight to catch back home. After getting a coffee and checking in, Elijah realized he was scheduled to fly on a small plane. He could feel his heart beating quickly and his palms getting sweaty—a reaction exacerbated by the coffee. He looked into changing flights, but unfortunately, nothing else was available. Elijah knew if he wanted to get back home today, he would have to fly on the small plane. He found a quiet spot to sit down and started mentally preparing himself for the flight. He used visualization to imagine himself confidently getting on the plane and relaxing during the flight. He also used positive self-talk to encourage himself to get on the plane. Although Elijah wasn't completely relaxed on the plane, he didn't feel nearly as nervous about it. After an uneventful flight, he feels better about flying on small planes—although he has vowed never to drink coffee before a flight again!

Triggers can also occur in relationships. There are times when a friend or partner may be your trigger. For example, Maya and Sophia have been friends for many years. Although Sophia is engaged, she would occasionally see someone outside of her relationship and ask Maya to cover for her. Initially Maya didn't mind, but as time wore on, it became a burden. Maya didn't like having to lie to Sophia's partner and would get nervous every time she was around him, worrying that she would forget what she was supposed to say. It soon progressed so that every time Sophia called her, Maya would dread answering the phone. For Maya, just seeing Sophia's name on the screen was becoming a trigger for stress. Although Maya didn't like confrontation, she finally told herself that confronting Sophia was better than dealing with the stress she was feeling. After practicing her part of the conversation in her head and taking a few deep breaths, she decided to tell her friend that she wasn't judging her behavior, but she couldn't be a part of it anymore. Sophia was upset that she was losing her cover story but also felt the friendship was important. She agreed to stop putting Maya in the middle of it, and their friendship got back on track.

These two examples highlight ways to manage your triggers. In both situations, the first thing to do is to label the stressor. Then, in both examples, they needed to step away from the trigger to gain a better understanding of what caused it. For Elijah, it was the negative experience of flying in a small plane as a child. For Maya, it was the fear of getting caught in a lie. The next step is to reframe your thoughts on the trigger—again, both Elijah and Maya had to spend some time thinking about what needed to be done to eliminate them. In both cases, they used positive thinking and reframing to move forward and address the trigger.

## Practicing Self-Care

One way to proactively manage stress is to take good care of yourself. In chapter 1 you learned about the dimensions of wellness and their relationship to stress. Practicing self-care helps keep your dimensions of wellness at high levels. When you feel good (physically, emotionally, intellectually, socially, spiritually, and environmentally) you are more likely to feel good about yourself, which helps reduce the effects of stress.

When we get busy, we tend to ignore self-care. Too often, when time is tight, we engage in so-called fast care—eating fast food, "forgetting" or "running out of time" to exercise, and perhaps using alcohol and other substances as a way to reduce the physical symptoms of stress. Although these provide short-term relief, they can often intensify your stressor because they do not deal with the stress.

When you are healthy and engage in behaviors to support your physical health, you give yourself the energy to deal with life's stressors. This includes eating nutritious foods, engaging in exercise a few times a week, and getting enough sleep at night (see chapter 4). When your body feels good, you feel good. You are strong and mentally fit. When your body is worn down, you feel worn down, which makes it more difficult to manage daily stressors.

Another aspect of self-care is making time in your schedule to practice active relaxation. Our lives are hectic, and we often fail to plan adequate time to rest. Take a few minutes every day to practice one of the exercises discussed in chapter 10.

**It is important to make time for yourself.**

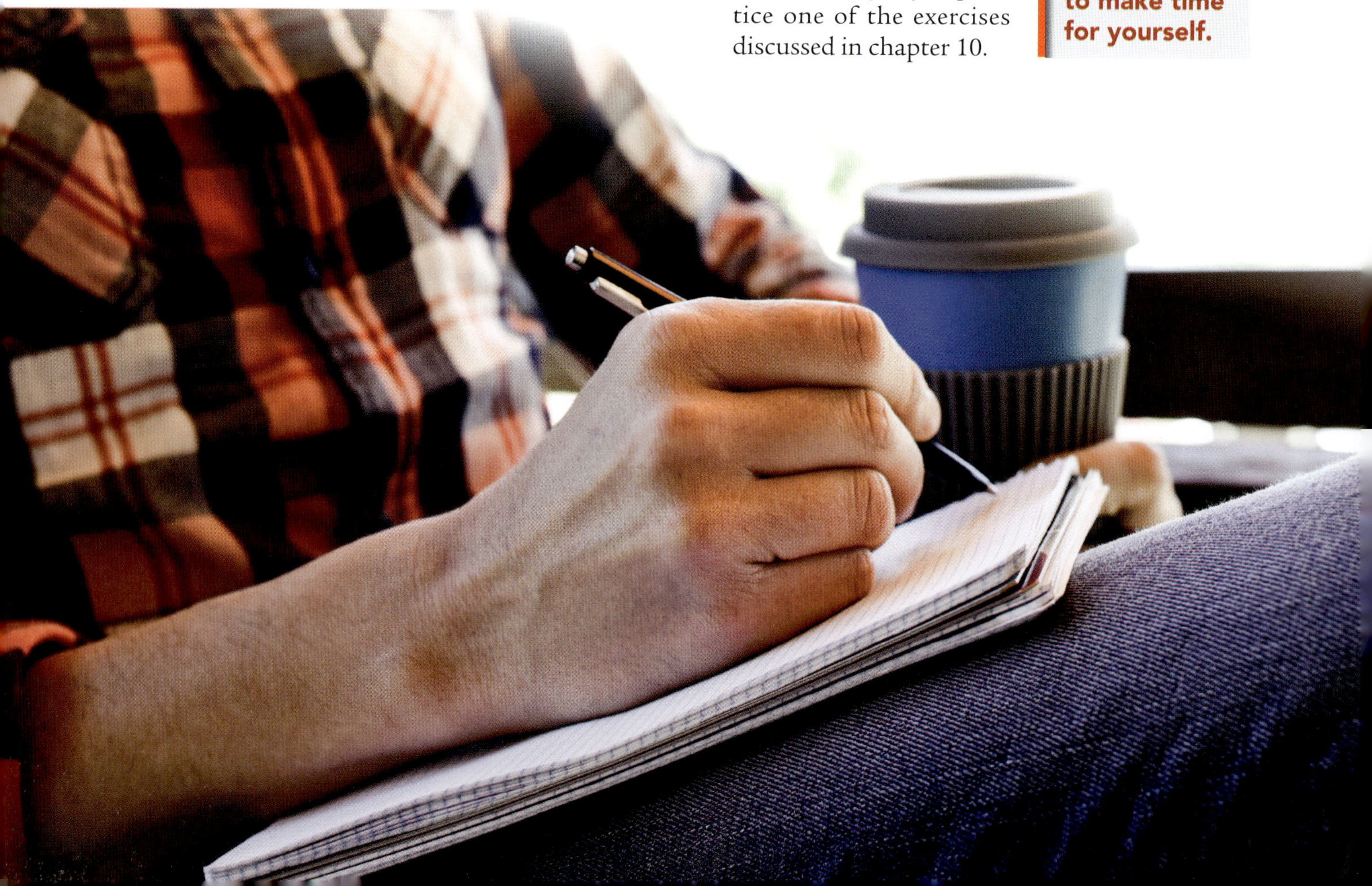

Case Study

## Put Yourself First

If you have ever flown on a plane, you have likely heard the following announcement: *"In case of emergency, oxygen masks will drop from the ceiling. If you are traveling with a child or someone who requires assistance, secure your own mask before assisting others."* For many people, the idea of helping yourself first is hard to grasp. It is our instinct to want to immediately help our children or someone who is unable to care for themselves. However, if you follow this instinct, there is a chance you would both pass out from lack of oxygen, which places both of your lives at risk.

This is a great analogy that you can take with you in life. In life, perhaps oxygen represents your energy level, time, or resources. If you care for yourself first, then you can care for others around you. On the other hand, if you care for others first, eventually your energy, time, or resources will run out, and you will no longer be able to help anyone.

Many people schedule their lives around the needs of others while ignoring their own needs. What if you created a schedule that prioritized your own needs so that you could not only survive but thrive? When you schedule time to practice self-care—practicing breathing exercises, making a nutritious meal, or just reading a book—you will find you feel more energized to tackle the day. Studies show a relationship among self-care and perceived stress levels: Those who prioritize and practice self-care generally show lower levels of stress than those who do not (Luis et al., 2021).

### Discussion Questions

1. How do you think it would feel to focus on your needs first? Does it make you nervous to put yourself ahead of others, or do you feel a sense of relief?
2. Why do you think people have a hard time putting their needs in front of others?
3. What is one thing you can do right now to put yourself first? How do you see it impacting your stress levels?

## Setting Limits Ahead of Time

Ella is overwhelmed with her coursework. She feels very stressed and is getting tension headaches. When her roommates invite her to a party, Ella has a few drinks to unwind. She ends up staying up pretty late and sleeps later than she was intending to. Ella wakes up with another headache and finds it hard to focus. As a result, she doesn't get a lot accomplished and falls further behind, and she now feels more stressed than before.

Ella engaged in behaviors that temporarily suppressed her stress. However, the next morning, the stressors resurfaced and were stronger than before. Practicing self-care can help you better plan to manage stress before it becomes overwhelming. If Ella had recognized that she really wanted to go out with her friends but also how much she needed to do the next day, she could have planned to go out but avoided drinking alcohol. She could have had a good time and woken up the next day feeling ready to focus and complete her tasks.

## Set Realistic Goals

Do you ever get stressed because you failed to achieve something you had set out to do? Sometimes the goals we set for ourselves are unrealistic, which sets us up for failure and stress. Some might think that avoiding setting goals would help reduce stress, but this is not true. Goals, like stress, help motivate you to achieve something. Without goals, it would be difficult to set an action plan and maintain focus and energy levels (see chapter 6 for more about the goal-setting theory). Setting realistic goals can also be a proactive way to manage stress that may occur from not reaching an unattainable goal.

# Planning and Prioritizing

Planning and prioritizing your tasks so you can complete them on time can be helpful in preventing stress. Whether it is planning a party, studying for an exam, or writing a paper, creating a plan or schedule can be a useful tool. There are several strategies for prioritizing and planning; a few techniques will be highlighted in this section.

## Sticky Notes

An easy way to manage your workload is by putting sticky notes near your workstation or computer. Write tasks that you need to accomplish immediately or in a short amount of time on a single note. For those that require a longer amount of time to complete, write the steps on multiple sticky notes. This helps break up the larger projects into smaller, more manageable tasks. The beauty of sticky notes is that each time you finish a task, you get to physically throw the note out. It is a nice activity that allows you to see the progress you made.

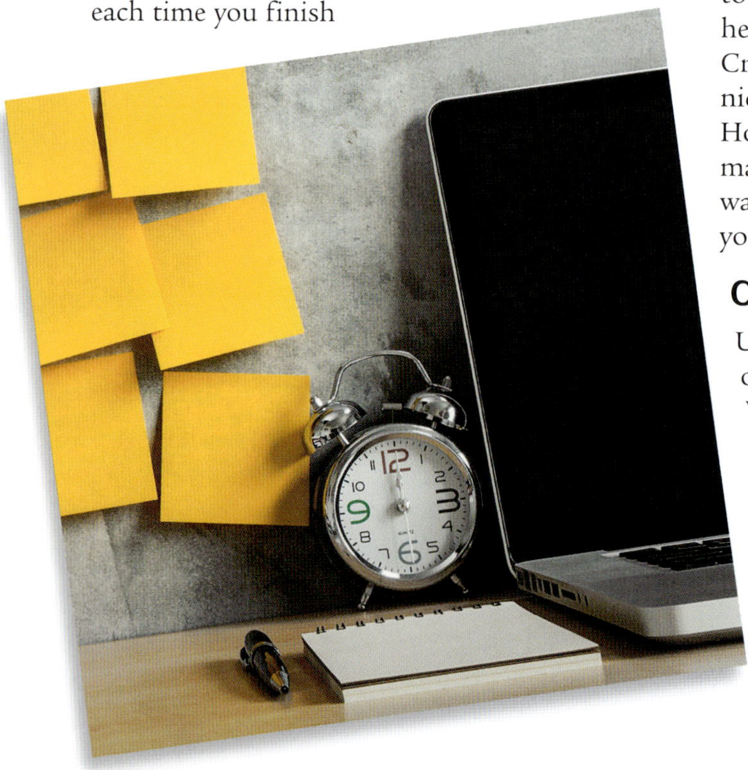

The drawback of sticky notes is they tend to be focused on short-term tasks. It may be harder to see the bigger picture. You also need to make sure you are paying attention to the notes. If you continually add sticky notes without completing tasks and throwing them out, the buildup can cause you to get overwhelmed, making it more difficult to get started on any type of task. You may also use note or reminder apps for this purpose, although you can "hide" notes from view, which may defeat the purpose.

## Lists

Another way to prioritize and plan is to create lists of all the tasks you need to complete. It may also be helpful to write down due dates next to your tasks to help you plan, as well as to create sublists to help you break up larger tasks into smaller items. Cross off items as you complete them to serve as a nice visual of all the work you have already done. However, as you continue to add to your list, it may become overwhelming to see it grow. You may want to rewrite your list daily, weekly, or whenever you feel it is getting too messy.

## Calendars

Utilizing a calendar—whether paper, online, or via app—can help you see the big picture. Write in the final due date for a project, and then identify the tasks that need to be done to complete it and place these on earlier dates to help keep you on track. This can also help you make plans while providing flexibility in that planning. For example, Karim has a large research paper due in two weeks and has set a deadline of having his outline done by Friday. This will give him enough time to present

## Waiting Until the Last Minute

Liam always waits until the last minute to write papers and finish assignments. When a deadline is close, Liam feels immense pressure to get things done and becomes very irritable and cranky with the people around him. This is a common scenario among college students. However, it doesn't have to be this way. Creating a schedule to better help with time management would greatly reduce the stress Liam feels when he is rushing to get his assignments completed.

the outline to his teacher on Monday to obtain feedback before starting on his draft. However, Karim was invited to his friend's house Thursday night to hang out and play games. Looking at his calendar, Karim is able to shift some work around to give him Thursday night free. Now Karim can go out and enjoy himself and still have his outline ready to present by Monday.

## Eisenhower Matrix

The **Eisenhower matrix** is a tool that helps you organize and prioritize tasks using a matrix. It was developed by President Dwight Eisenhower to help him prioritize the work he faced when he was a U.S. Army general (Monsalve et al., 2020). To create the matrix, draw a 2 × 2 table (see figure 11.1). Across the top (x-axis), write "urgent" on the left square and "not urgent" on the right. On the side (y-axis), write "important" on the top square and "not important" on the bottom.

The different quadrants are as follows:

1. *Urgent and important (upper left quadrant).* These items are the ones you need to take care of right away. This could be returning a phone call or finishing a project that is due later today. This is also called the "do it" quadrant.
2. *Important but not urgent (upper right quadrant).* These are important tasks, but they do not need to be done now. Examples include exercise or planning when to meet with your group to work on a project. This is also called the "plan it" quadrant.
3. *Not important but urgent (lower left quadrant).* These are items that need to be done immediately but don't require your specific skill set or personal attention to complete them. As such, they can be delegated to other people (if they are willing, of course). Examples of items that may go in this category are mailing a package or putting gas in the car. This quadrant is also called "delegate it."
4. *Neither important nor urgent (lower right quadrant).* This is also known as the "delete it" quadrant. These tend to be left over or unnecessary tasks that remain on your to-do list but serve no immediate purpose (Bratterud et al., 2020). They are leftover items that do not contribute to your work or academic success but may hold personal value—for example, watching your favorite television show. These items can be done during your personal or free time but not during the time you designate for work.

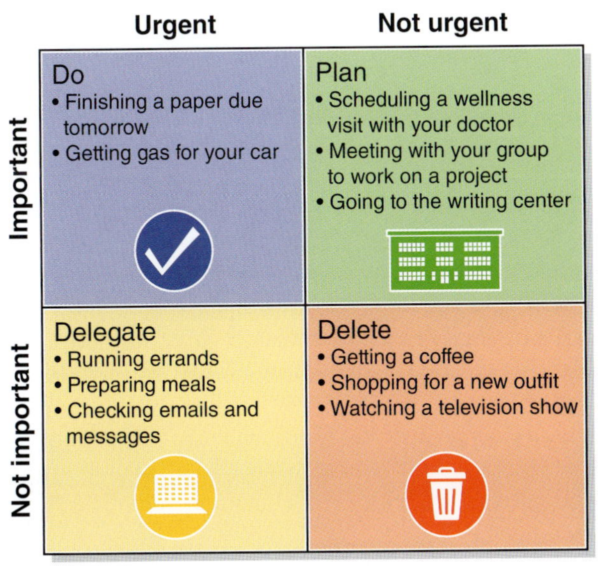


**Figure 11.1** Eisenhower matrix.

## Saying No

It is a common problem for college students to say yes to too many outside commitments (Somerville, Van Bavel, Lewis, Gruber, & Cunningham, 2021). At some point, however, your schedule will not be able to accommodate any additional requests and you may begin to feel the burden of being agreeable to everyone's requests.

**It may feel weird at first to say no to certain requests, but give yourself permission to have boundaries.**

Before you are quick to agree to a request, think about your own commitments. What does your schedule look like over the next few weeks? Do you have the time to take on another task? How will taking on another task impact your life? Will you have to sacrifice seeing family and friends? Will you have to sacrifice sleep? Do you have enough time and energy to take on more work?

If you feel like you can't handle another task, you need to say no. Some strategies for saying no include:

- *Be a broken record.* Say no. If asked again, repeat your no. You do not need to justify your response.
- *Suggest alternatives.* If you are interested in the request but do not have the time at this moment, you can say, "I would love to, but my schedule is busy for the next two weeks. If you can wait two weeks, then I will help out."
- *Offer less.* If you are somewhat interested in the task, but can't take the whole thing on, offer partial help: "I would love to work on this, but I don't have the time to complete all of it. What if I contributed [X]?"
- *Get more information.* Sometimes the size of the commitment is unclear. If so, ask: "I may be interested in working on that, but I need a bit more information. What all is involved? What is the time commitment?"

## Managing Your Time

This thing all things devours:
Birds, beasts, trees, flowers;
Gnaws iron, bites steel;
Grinds hard stones to meal;
Slays king, ruins town,
And beats high mountain down.

**J.R.R. Tolkien**

Time can sometimes elude us. It moves slowly during dreaded events and quickly during enjoyable ones. It is impossible to catch and hold, but it can be managed. Learning how to manage your time can help you achieve your goals while managing your stress levels. Those with good time management skills have greater productivity, improved efficiency, and a greater opportunity to achieve career and life goals (Nayak, 2018). There are many different methods you can use to help you better manage your time. A few will be highlighted next.

### Most Important Task (MIT) Strategy

Mark Twain said, "If it is your job to eat a frog, do it first thing in the morning. And if it's your job to eat two frogs, eat the biggest one first." In other words, get the hard jobs done first. The **Most Important Task (MIT) strategy** asks you to focus on the critical tasks first. It also suggests that you only focus on one or two tasks per day, but this can be subjective based on the size of the task. In this strategy, you will first set your goal and then decide on what tasks you need to complete to reach your goal.

For example, Kurt is a full-time college student who works part-time and is a student athlete. To help organize his day, he writes a to-do list every morning. He first works on the tasks that must be completed that day. With any extra time, he works on the tasks that are due later. His list Monday morning includes reading a chapter for class tomorrow, forming a study group for the exam next week, studying for a quiz on Friday, getting a haircut, and researching a paper due in four weeks. Some of his tasks are quite large and need more than one day to be completed. For example, forming a study group may take a few days, so he breaks the task into smaller ones. First, he emails his classmates to see if anyone is interested in creating a study group. Then he plans to schedule a meeting and later meet with the study group. For the research paper due in four weeks, he also creates smaller tasks, such as picking a topic, researching the topic, creating an outline, writing the rough draft, and finally writing the final paper. Now his list, including the smaller tasks, is in order from most important to least: read chapter, email classmates about a study group, study for quiz, pick a topic for the research paper, and get a haircut. Using the MIT strategy, Kurt is able to complete the more difficult and most important tasks first.

## Time Blocking

**Time blocking** is a great strategy if you feel you do not have enough time in the day. Often, we do have more than enough time to get everything done, but we waste a lot of time with distractions. (More about avoiding distractions will be discussed later.) Time blocking allows you to intentionally set your schedule every day and track how you spend each unit of time. For this strategy, use a daily planner—most will have 30- to 60-minute intervals. Write in your schedule for the day, including your classes, work schedule, and meetings or appointments. Now, decide what tasks you want to complete that day, such as read a chapter or start your term paper. Think about how much time each task will require and write it in the schedule. Don't forget to add in time for self-care (eating, exercise, relaxation exercises, sleep). You may also want to add in buffer time to transition from one activity to the next.

## Pomodoro Technique

Large projects can feel overwhelming—you may start to think about the time and energy required and just give up. In this case, the **Pomodoro technique** may be perfect for you. It was created by Francesco Cirillo, who used a kitchen timer in the shape of a tomato—*pomodoro* meaning *tomato* in Italian (Ismail, Putri, & Noviyanti, 2022). Here is how to use this technique:

1. Set your timer for 25 minutes.
2. When the timer goes off, stop working and take a 5- to 10-minute break.
3. After the break, set the timer again for 25 minutes and repeat.
4. After four repetitions, take a longer break (20 to 30 minutes).

This technique is great if you are worried about a task taking too long or you are working on something you do not particularly enjoy. It is easier to tackle something when you know you will only spend a short time on it.

## Parkinson's Law

**Parkinson's law** states that a task will take as long as the time you set aside for it. For example, if you give yourself two hours to write an email, it will take you two hours to complete it. This doesn't mean that you can complete a two-hour task in 30 minutes—you still need to be realistic—but if you give yourself too much time to complete a task, you will use up all of the allotted time to complete it. Similarly, if you tell yourself you will answer an email before you leave work, you will be rushed at the end of your workday to answer that email. On the other hand, if you tell yourself you will answer it before lunch, you will get to it before lunch. Be realistic about how much time you need to complete a task to avoid wasting time or waiting until the last minute.

## Avoid Distractions

One of the keys to having good time management is the ability to avoid distractions and focus on one task at a time. Many people believe they are good at multitasking, but studies show this is not true. Studies show that multitasking impairs your cognitive ability and mimics work overload (Howard, Evans, Innes, Brown, & Eidels, 2020). When you multitask, you are spreading your cognitive energy across several tasks, meaning that

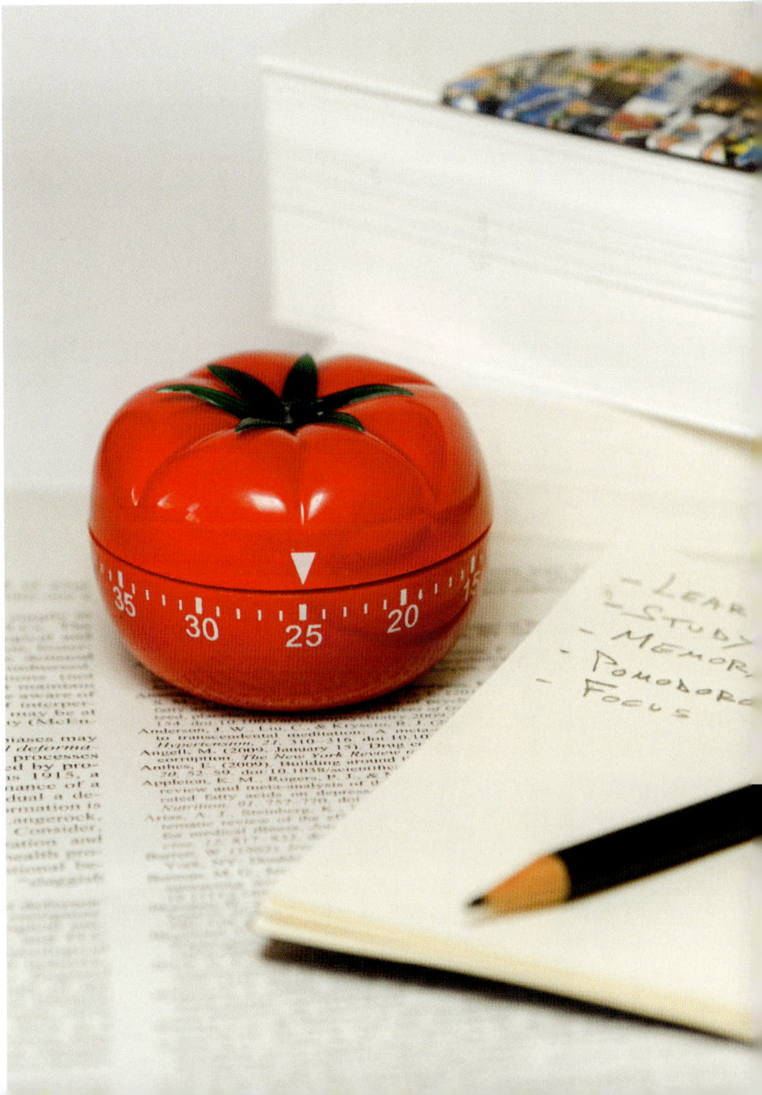

none get your full attention. Instead, you work on one task, then stop and work on another, then go back and work on the first task. This is distracting and ineffective, making it difficult to complete tasks (Biedermann, Schneider, & Drachsler, 2021).

Although personal electronic devices are great to have (it is hard to imagine life before), they are another major distraction in our lives. Having instant access to the Internet makes it easy to stop what we are doing and play around for a bit. However, it is just as easy to lose time as you scroll through social media—and before you know it, your day is almost over, and you didn't get your work completed. One way to manage this distraction is to put your phone away. Turn it facedown, or better yet, put it in a drawer. Turn off notifications or put it on silent. Give yourself breaks to check your phone, but if you easily lose track of time, it may be helpful to set a timer. Give yourself 10 to 15 minutes and then put the phone away again. This will also help with distracting personal communications, such as phone calls, texts, and direct messages that are not work related. It is nice to keep in touch with people, but there is a time and place to do it.

Whether you are working in an office, at the library, or in your bedroom, interruptions from others can also make it difficult to stay focused. One way to manage interruptions is to put a sign on your door. You can write "studying in progress," "on a conference call," or "quiet time"—anything that lets others know not to distract you. If needed, you can set time aside in your day to visit with people and then politely tell them you need to get back to work. Sometimes just standing and walking to another area (kitchen, bathroom, etc.) can serve as a hint that the visit is nearing its end.

**Schedule time each day to engage in personal communication.**

## Managing Your Resources

What are some resources you possess that can help you be proactive in managing your stress levels? Learning how to leverage your resources can help prevent stress by allowing you to stay on top of things.

### Money

Being in college is expensive. The majority of college students use loans to pay for college (The Ohio State University, 2016), and almost 40 percent of students rate their current financial situation as "often" or "always" stressful (Cadaret & Bennett, 2019). Furthermore, just under half of all college dropouts cite money stressors as the driving force for leaving school (Britt, Ammerman, Barrett, & Jones, 2017). However, dropping out of school to reduce financial obligation may have potential negative consequences down the

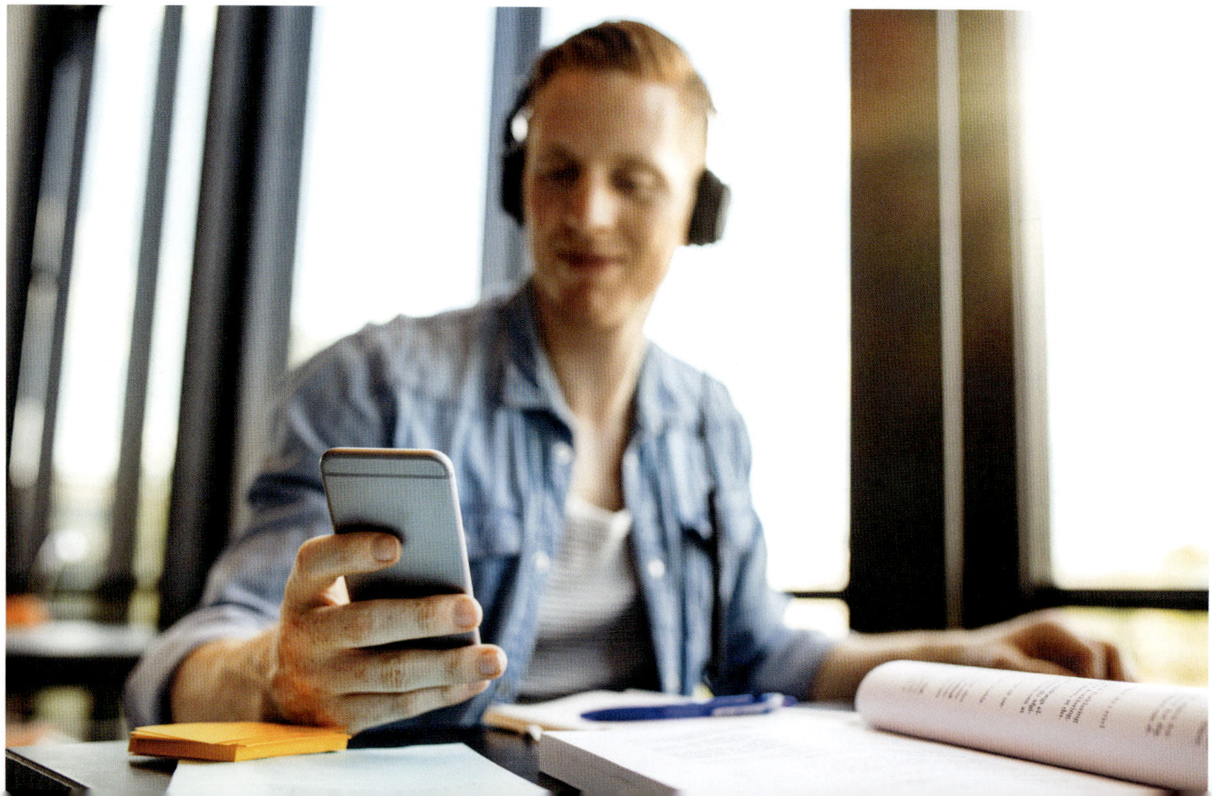

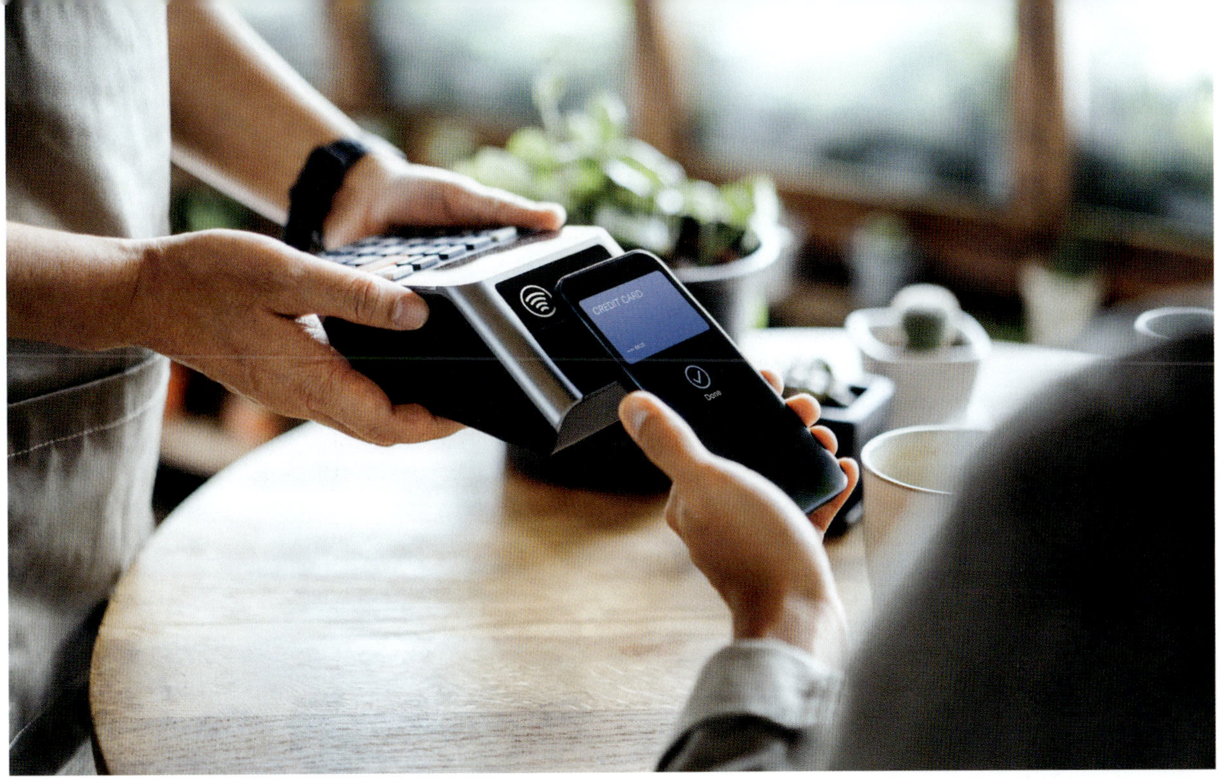


**Learning to manage your money helps set you up for financial success.**

line. Getting a college degree has been shown to improve your marketability (even during economic downfalls), increase your chances of being employed for a lifetime, increase your economic stability, increase your earning potential, increase your job satisfaction, and improve happiness and health after college (Nikolaev, 2016). Learning how to manage your money now can help you avoid financial hardships later on.

To start creating a budget, you first need to understand where your money goes. Use a spreadsheet, a notebook, or an app to keep track of your spending for one month. Place your spending into categories, which may include food, car, gasoline, rent, utility bills, and entertainment. After one month, look over your spending and compare it to your monthly income. Do they match up? Is there leftover money at the end of the month? Next, you will create your budget. Use the same categories and set your limits. See how your budget works and make adjustments as necessary.

Another important skill in money management is building a savings account to serve as a safety net in case of an emergency. Many people live paycheck to paycheck, which can place them in a difficult situation when they encounter a financial emergency (e.g., car breaks down, injury). Rather than put aside money at the end of the month only when there is extra money left, consider Warren Buffett's advice: "Do not save what is left over after spending, but spend what is left over after saving." When thinking of your monthly budget, first pay your bills, then contribute to your savings, and then spend what is left. This mindset will help you make saving a priority.

Learning how to create and live within a budget will help relieve your financial stress. Start slowly and remember there is a learning curve to money management. It takes time and practice, but don't give up. Financial management is a skill that will help you for the rest of your life, no matter how little or how much money you make.

> The bad news is time flies. The good news is you're the pilot.
>
> **Michael Altshuler**

## Work–Life Balance

**Work–life balance** describes the relationship between the demands of work and the demands of personal life. Work is anything that is not related to your personal life and health, including your job, schoolwork, childcare, and housework. Personal life demands include spending time with family and friends and practicing self-care. Think of work–life balance as a scale. When you spend too much time on one side, the other side dips. Figuring out how to balance work and life demands is a challenge that will look different for each person.

College students are usually working while going to college and trying to manage their personal lives, and it can become a lot to bear. Additionally, many students do not realize how much time they are expected to spend on schoolwork outside of the classroom. The general consensus is that for every hour spent in class, students should spend two hours studying, possibly more for certain classes. However, many college students are not aware of this commitment and overschedule themselves, and then they must pull all-nighters to finish their work. As discussed, this technique is not very effective for your academic performance or stress levels. It also greatly tips the scale on work–life balance.

Most people tend to push aside their personal lives to meet the demands of work and school. When you spend more time on work and less time and energy practicing self-care, it can increase stress and negatively impact your health. Studies show that work–life conflict is related to poorer physical and mental health, increased psychological distress, and greater life dissatisfaction (Mensah & Adjei, 2020). You become more likely to feel overburdened at work and are at risk of burnout (Pattnaik, Samanta, & Mohanty, 2022). **Burnout** is a type of workplace stress that results in emotional and physical exhaustion along with a general sense of reduced pleasure at the workplace. Burnout is bad for both you and your organization.

Burnout among college students has also been on the rise. It is associated with increased levels of psychological distress, anxiety, and depression, as well as decreased levels of motivation, decreased academic performance, and negative attitudes

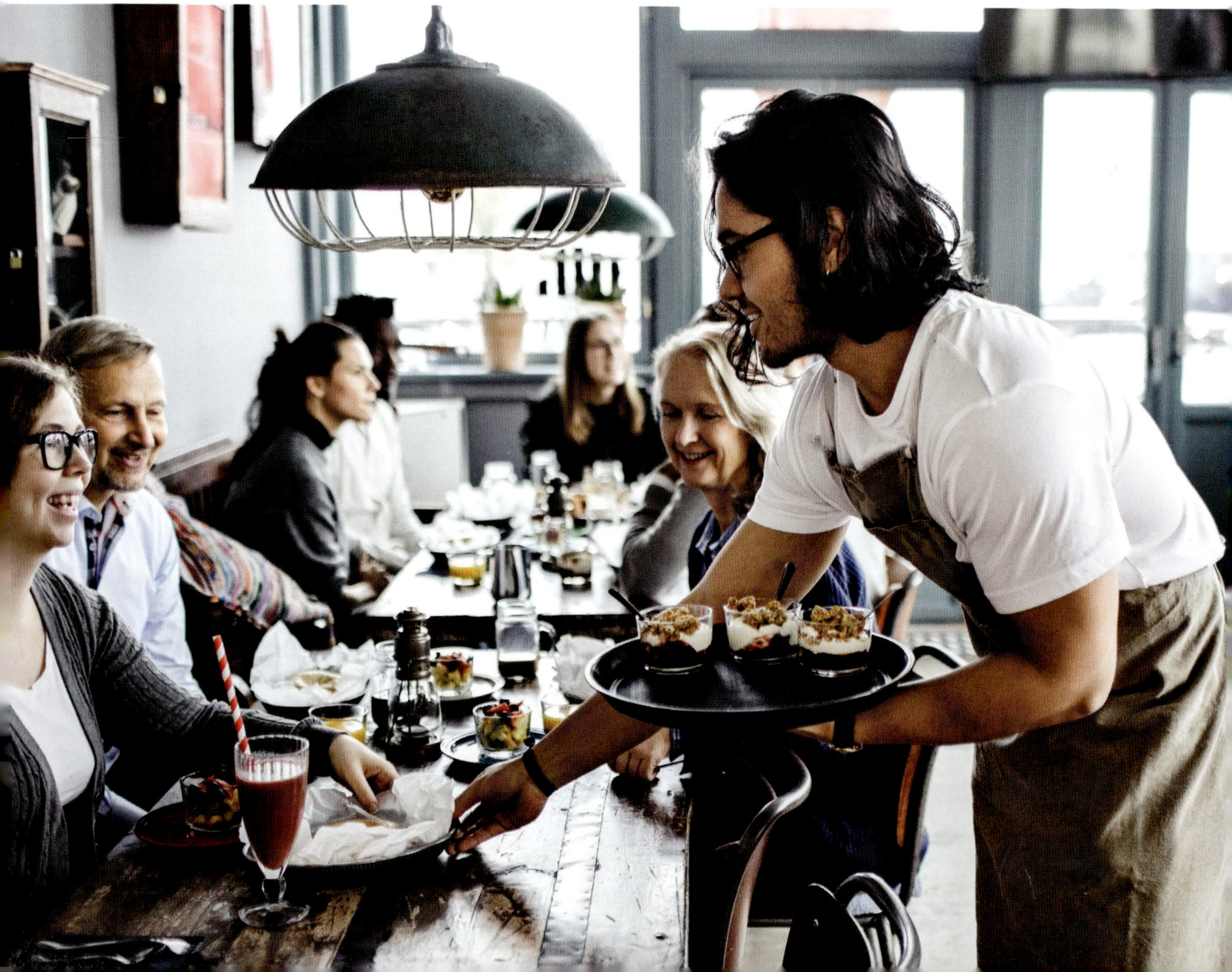

toward oneself and others (Saville, Bureau, Eckenrode, & Maley, 2018). The following signs indicate you might be suffering from burnout:

- Fatigue
- Lack of motivation
- Difficulty completing works that require creativity
- Increased susceptibility to illness
- Increased anxiety and depression
- Difficulty focusing
- Irritability
- Lack of interest in work

## Study Better

Adam is a full-time college student who works 15 to 20 hours a week. He studies only when there is an upcoming test or quiz and tends to feel underprepared. Adam stresses about his grades because he gets tuition assistance based on his academic performance, and if his grades drop too much, he will lose the scholarship. He knows there has to be a better way to schedule his time to study. After doing some research on time management and studying strategies, Adam reworks his schedule. Initially, his schedule looked like this (blue represents classes, green represents work, and orange represents his intramural basketball league):

| | Monday | Tuesday | Wednesday | Thursday | Friday | Saturday | Sunday |
|---|---|---|---|---|---|---|---|
| 8:00 | SOC 100 | | SOC 100 | | SOC 100 | | |
| 9:00 | | BIO 200 | | BIO 200 | | | |
| 10:00 | | | | | | Work | |
| 11:00 | ENG 101 | | ENG 101 | | ENG 101 | | |
| 12:00 | | | | | | | |
| 1:00 | MTH 115 | BIO 200- | MTH 115 | BIO 200- | MTH 115 | | |
| 2:00 | | Lab | | Lab | | | |
| 3:00 | | | | | | | |
| 4:00 | PHL 105 | | PHL 105 | | PHL 105 | | |
| 5:00 | | Work | | Work | | | |
| 6:00 | | | | | | | |
| 7:00 | Intramural | | | | | | |
| 8:00 | basketball | | | | | | |
| 9:00 | league | | | | | | |

Adam could see he had plenty of time to study—he just wasn't making it a priority. He comes up with the following schedule (yellow is study time):

| | Monday | Tuesday | Wednesday | Thursday | Friday | Saturday | Sunday |
|---|---|---|---|---|---|---|---|
| 8:00 | SOC 100 | | SOC 100 | | SOC 100 | | |
| 9:00 | | BIO 200 | | BIO 200 | | | Study |
| 10:00 | Study | | Study | | Study | Work | |
| 11:00 | ENG 101 | Study/break | ENG 101 | Study/break | ENG 101 | | |
| 12:00 | | | | | | | Study |
| 1:00 | MTH 115 | BIO 200- | MTH 115 | BIO 200- | MTH 115 | | |
| 2:00 | | Lab | | Lab | | | |
| 3:00 | Study | | Study | | Study | | |
| 4:00 | PHL 105 | | PHL 105 | | PHL 105 | | |
| 5:00 | | Work | | Work | | | |
| 6:00 | | | | | | | |
| 7:00 | Intramural | | | | | | |
| 8:00 | basketball | | Study | | Study | | |
| 9:00 | league | | | | | | |

Adam tries out the new schedule and finds that it works really well. He feels that because he scheduled in his study time, it is easier to commit to getting it done, and he still has free time to spend as he chooses. (Some people even like to schedule their free time as a reminder to perform self-care!) Adam also feels that spending shorter chunks of time studying works better for him. After a few weeks of following this schedule, he feels better about his performance and is more confident in class.

Research Spotlight

### Online Success

Online classes provide flexibility and convenience compared to traditional classes—however, they also generally have lower rates of success (Bettinger, Fox, Loeb, & Taylor, 2017). To be successful, online students must be independent and self-regulated learners. Students who do not possess these qualities report falling behind and feeling isolated from the instructor and other students, leading to higher rates of burnout (Barratt & Duran, 2021). The following strategies can help you be successful in online classes while reducing the risk of burnout.

1. *Time management.* Create a study schedule or set specific times each week to work on your online class, then stick to it.
2. *Put in the same effort as a face-to-face class.* Online courses, though flexible, still require the same amount of time as a traditional course (Broadbent & Poon, 2015). However, many students do not put in the time, which leaves them behind.
3. *Sign on a few times a week.* Studies suggest that signing on a few times a week and being actively engaged in the class leads to high levels of course success (Cho & Yoo, 2017). Set your learning management system page as your homepage to remind you to complete your work.
4. *Eliminate distractions.* Working with a television show or music on can distract you from learning. Create a space that is free from distractions and find ways to maintain your attention during your online class.
5. *Actively participate.* Participate in discussion boards and get to know your instructor. Ask questions and get additional help when needed.

Burnout can occur in any area of your life. To avoid this risk, it is important to have a healthy work–life balance. When you start to feel burnout, take a step back and identify the cause. Are you behind in schoolwork? Do you feel unprepared for a big exam? Once you identify the source of your burnout, you can decide how to deal with it. You might need to start eating more nutritious foods and engaging in physical activity, you might benefit from relaxation exercises, or perhaps you just need to spend some time with your friends. Realize that you may need to develop a new routine if your current routine doesn't provide enough time for you to engage in self-care. Sometimes you may have to give up something or even lower your expectations (perhaps utilizing humor–remember that "Cs get degrees!"). It may be helpful to give yourself permission to perform less well in one area in order to care for yourself and still accomplish your core goals. The goal is to create balance in your life so that you can remain healthy while still being productive.

## Leveraging Support

There are times when you may need additional strategies to proactively manage stress. The following section will help you learn how and where to seek out additional support.

Colleges often have a plethora of support options for students. Most colleges have a student success center or similar department that offers a variety of resources from studying tips to time management tools to managing test anxiety. Become familiar with these options at the beginning of the semester to lay out a foundation for how you will tackle your classes. Many will host open houses to introduce you to their services. Services may include the following:

- *Advisors.* They are trained to help you achieve your goals and will help you choose the courses that will fulfill the requirements for your major. If you are struggling, whether from stress, a family crisis, or coursework, they can provide you with resources to help you.

- *Writing center*. Because most courses you take will have a writing component, the writing center is a great resource. They recommend visiting early in the writing process to help you plan out your paper.
- *Tutoring*. If you are struggling in a particular course, visit the tutoring center. They can help you with study techniques and time management skills. Many colleges also offer a separate math tutoring lab.
- *Career services*. This is a valuable resource to help you find a job after you graduate. They can help with the job search process, writing a resume and cover letter, and polishing your interview skills.
- *Financial aid*. They can help you find financial resources to help pay for college.
- *Library*. Librarians can help you with your research. Many college libraries have different areas for quiet study and collaborative group work. Libraries are becoming the social hub of colleges.
- *Recreational services*. It is important not to forget to focus on you. Recreational services offer programs geared toward enhancing your physical and social health. Many also have fitness centers that are either free to use or offered at a greatly discounted rate.
- *Health services*. Many colleges have a health service center to help you when you are sick.

## Knowing When to Seek Professional Help

Whether you are mentally distressed or in a crisis, seeking out professional help is often the hardest step to take. Even though it has become more socially accepted, there are some who feel there is a negative stigma attached to seeking out mental health help. They may fear being judged or feel they do not really need help. However, knowing when and how to seek out professional help can benefit you in the long run. Seeing a mental health professional may not be a quick solution, but it can help you deal with mental anguish or distress. Unfortunately, many people do not seek out a mental health professional until their anguish is so severe, they cannot take anymore, and then end up wishing they had not waited so long.

**There may be times in your life when you need extra help.**

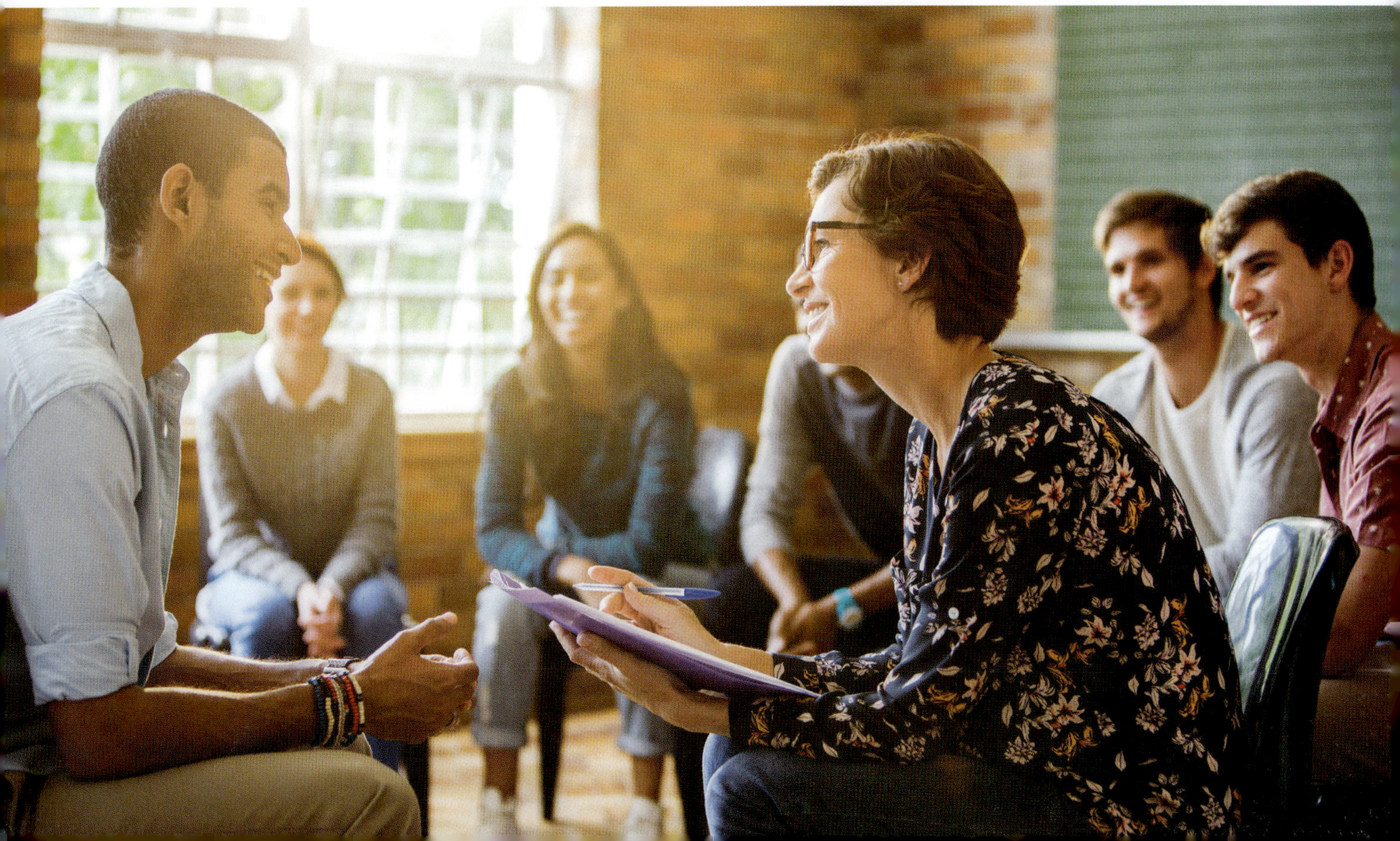

Many people are unsure when they should seek out mental health help. Generally, questioning whether you need mental health help is a sign that you may need it. Other signs that may indicate it is time to seek mental health help include the following:

- Prolonged depression or sadness
- Self-harm
- Thoughts of suicide
- Excessive fears
- Increased use of alcohol
- Increased use of drugs
- Change in sleep patterns
- Change in eating patterns

One of the best places to start your search for a mental health professional is at your college. Most colleges offer mental health services for free or included with your tuition and student fees. Campus health professionals understand the unique challenges of being a college student and can direct you to additional resources on campus. Another option is to speak with your primary care physician. They can provide you with referrals and resources on where to get help. If you do not have a primary care physician or are not comfortable talking to yours, there are other options. If you have health insurance, you can call the number on the back of your card and ask for referrals. If you belong to a religious organization, you can ask your clergy or other trusted official; they have often undergone training and can point you in the right direction. If you work for a company that offers an employee assistance program (EAP), you can contact them for resources, and some will even help you make your first appointment. Finally, if you are comfortable, you can ask friends and family members for recommendations. Many people visit mental health professionals, with 45 to 65 percent of adults with a mental disorder utilizing a mental health service in the past year (Substance Abuse and Mental Health Services Administration, 2021).

The majority of people who see a mental health professional are happy with their experience. A professional can help you better understand and manage your emotions and stressors, and they will work with you to help you set and achieve your goals.

## Types of Mental Health Professionals

There are a variety of different mental health professionals, each with their own qualifications and areas of expertise. This section will help describe their different titles, qualifications, and treatment options so you can figure out which is right for your needs.

- *Psychologist.* They hold a doctoral degree in clinical psychology or similar. They are trained to evaluate, diagnose, and provide treatment in the form of individual and group therapy.
- *Counselor, clinician, or therapist.* They hold a master's degree in their field. They are trained to evaluate a person's mental health and use therapeutic techniques to help clients discover better and more positive ways of thinking, feeling, and living.
- *Clinical social worker.* They hold a master's degree in social work. They are trained to evaluate a person's mental health and use therapeutic techniques. They are also trained in case management and advocacy efforts.
- *Psychiatrist.* The main difference between a psychiatrist and the other types of mental health professionals is that a psychiatrist holds a medical degree. They are trained to prescribe and monitor medication, diagnose mental health conditions, and provide therapy.
- *Psychiatric or mental health nurse practitioner.* These are specially trained nurses who hold at least a master's degree. They can provide assessment, diagnosis, and therapy for mental health conditions. In some states, they can also prescribe and monitor medications.

## Summary

Stress is inevitable, but too much stress places a strain on your health. This chapter focused on ways you can proactively manage and reduce stress. From time management skills to self-care, when you proactively plan your life, you will find you are better equipped to manage your day-to-day activities and more able to handle stress. The ultimate goal is not stress avoidance but stress management.

## ONLINE RESOURCES

Visit HK*Propel* to access audio supplements, worksheets, and vocabulary flash cards for this chapter.

## DISCUSSION QUESTIONS

1. What are two or three triggers you have that result in stress? What are some ways you can plan to avoid those triggers? Do you feel your plan would ultimately help you better manage your stress? Why or why not?
2. How can having effective time management skills help reduce stress? How would you describe your time management skills?
3. Write down your schedule for one week. How much time do you spend on schoolwork? How much time do you spend on work and chores? How would you describe your work–life balance? What can you change to make it more balanced?
4. How would you convince a friend to seek out professional help?

# GLOSSARY

**4-7-8 breathing**—technique in which you breathe in for four seconds, hold for seven seconds, and breathe out for eight seconds

**acute stress**—stress that occurs over the short term

**adrenaline**—a hormone and neurotransmitter secreted by the adrenal gland in response to stress that stimulates the fight-or-flight response; also known as epinephrine

**adverse childhood experiences (ACEs)**—traumatic childhood events, such as physical and emotional abuse, neglect, or household violence

**affirmations**—self-talk used to promote self-confidence and self-efficacy

**air quality**—the degree to which the ambient air is free of pollution

**alarm stage**—the body's initial reaction to stress

**altruism**—a devotion to the welfare of others

**anchor breathing**—a breathing technique that focused your mind on a point

**anxiety**— a state of nervousness in anticipation of a future threat

**art therapy**—the use of creative expression to enhance mental health

**asana**—the physical practice of postures or poses in yoga

**autonomic nervous system**—the system responsible for managing the automatic functions in the body, including respiration, heart rate, digestion, and blood pressure

**avoidance**—ignoring, denying, or minimizing the problem or stressor

**bhramari**—a breathing exercise that uses humming along with breathing to promote calmness

**biophilia**—innate tendency to love and connect with nature

**biopsychosocial (BPS) model of challenge and threat**—a framework that describes how a person's response to stress is based on their perception of the stressor

**blue light**—short, high-energy wavelength used in LED technology that can block melatonin and interrupt sleep

**box breathing**—a breathing technique that uses equal counts of four (breathe in, hold, breathe out, hold)

**breath awareness**—a technique that involves being conscious of your breath

**breath work**—the foundation for stress relief that includes a variety of breathing exercises designed to enhance physical, spiritual, and mental health

**built environment**—the physical and manmade parts of where you live and work

**burnout**—a type of workplace stress that results in emotional and physical exhaustion along with a general sense of reduced pleasure at the workplace

**cardiovascular system**—closed system consisting of the heart and blood vessels; supplies oxygen and nutrients to the body's cells

**central nervous system**—the body system consisting of the brain and spinal cord

**chromotherapy**—use of visible light and colors to aid in healing

**chronic stress**—stress that lasts for weeks, months, or years

**compassion**—understanding another person's suffering and wanting to do something to relieve it

**connotative meaning**—the meaning you assign to words based on your own experiences and beliefs

**cortisol awakening response (CAR)**—a rise in cortisol that occurs when waking from sleep

**cortisol**—a steroid hormone secreted by the adrenal gland in response to stress

**creative thinking**—the ability to gain new insight on an issue and to generate original and useful ideas

**denotative meaning**—the standardized definition of a word

**diaphragmatic breathing**—a slow and deep breathing exercise that focuses on controlling the diaphragm

**dietary patterns**—combination of food and beverages that constitute a person's diet

**dispositional gratitude**—your general orientation to perceiving and appreciating the positives in life

**distorted thinking**—negative and overexaggerated thought patterns

**distress**—stress that places strain on the body and mind

**divergent thinking**—the ability to view a problem from different perspectives

**Eisenhower matrix**—a task management tool that utilizes a matrix to help you organize and prioritize tasks

**emotional competency**—the ability to recognize, interpret, and respond to your emotions

**emotional hunger**—hunger that occurs as a response to emotion, not physical need

**emotional wellness**—an awareness and understanding of one's emotions and the ability to effectively manage those emotions

**emotion-focused coping**—how a person manages and regulates emotions under stress

**emotions**—neurological response to stimuli based on your environment, relationship, circumstance, or mood

**empathy**—understanding the thoughts and feelings of another person

**endocrine system**—responsible for making and releasing hormones

**enteric nervous system**—part of the autonomic nervous system responsible for controlling digestion

**environmental noise**—the sounds made from external sources such as traffic, airports, and construction

**environmental wellness**—your sense of safety, comfort, and connection with your physical environment

**euphemism**—a word used to substitute for ones that are socially awkward or negative

**eustress**—stress that is positive and can result in growth

**exercise**—a planned and structured activity with the goal of improving or maintaining physical fitness

**exhaustion stage**—the final stage of general adaptation syndrome, when the body's energy levels become depleted from stress

**external self-awareness**—the ability to accurately understand how others see you

**fight-or-flight response**—the physical reaction to stress that occurs during the alarm stage and provides the body with a burst of energy

**flow**—a state of mind when you are fully engrossed in an activity

**food desert**—an area where access to fresh, high-quality food is lacking

**food insecurity**—not having access to sufficient food or food quality

**forest bathing**—the act of walking in the forest to combat stress

**freeze response**—an adaptive stress response that causes physical immobility

**general adaptation syndrome**—the body's three-stage response to stress (alarm, resistance, exhaustion)

**generalized anxiety disorder**—persistent anxiety experienced for a period of six months

**genetics**—traits that are passed down from a parent to a child

**glucocorticoids**—steroid hormones secreted by the adrenal glands in response to stress

**goal disengagement**—the process of reducing your efforts at obtaining a goal that is not attainable

**goal reengagement**—the process of finding a new and attainable goal

**goal-setting theory**—theory stating that challenging, specific, and realistic goals lead to better task performance than goals that are too easy, too difficult, or not specific enough

**gratitude**—a appreciation for what you have and an acknowledgement of the goodness in your life

**growth mindset**—the idea that intelligence can be developed with practice and effort

**health**—a state of complete physical, mental, and social well-being

**homeostasis**—the body's process of self-regulating the internal environment while adjusting to a changing external environment

**hyperpalatable foods**—foods that have a high fat and sugar content and low nutrition value; may have addictive properties

**hypertension**—high blood pressure (higher than 120/80)

**hyperventilation**—rapid breathing caused by stress

**hypothalamus-pituitary-adrenal axis (HPA axis)**—stress response system that connects the central nervous system and endocrine system

**immersion**—total engagement in work

**immune system**—the body system responsible for identifying illnesses, infections, diseases, and injury and combatting them

**incubation**—a period of rest and recovery away from an activity

**insight**—a period of reflection and an emergence of new ideas

**integumentary system**—the outermost layer of the body, consisting of skin, hair, and nails

**intellectual wellness**—the ability and desire to continue learning throughout a lifetime

**internal self-awareness**—how you understand your thoughts, feelings, and emotions and how they impact others

**internalized racism**—when negative stereotypes of minority populations are internalized within those populations

**interpersonal**—relations with other people and groups

**interpersonal communication**—the way you exchange information with other people; includes both verbal and nonverbal communication

**intrapersonal**—the thoughts, feelings, and processes occurring within a person

**leisure physical activity**—any physical activity that is not part of essential daily activities

**light pollution**—the excessive use of artificial lighting

**locus of control**—where you place feelings of control (internal or external)

**loneliness**—the state of distress when you perceive a gap between your desired social connection with others and actual social connection with others

**mantra**—a word or sound used in repetition to aid in concentration

**meditation**—the practice of spending time in contemplation to achieve a mentally clear state of mind

**melatonin**—a hormone produced by the body in response to darkness to help you fall asleep

**mental imagery**—the ability to produce an image in the mind's eye without sensory input

**mentalization**—the ability to understand your own and other's mental states and intentions

**metacognition**—ability to understand how you think and learn

**microbiota**—bacteria in the intestine that protect against harmful pathogens

**mindful breathing**—an exercise that links diaphragmatic breathing and mindfulness

**mindful breathing meditation**—the act of focusing your attention on your breathing

**mindfulness**—the act of fully paying attention to something to appreciate it with all senses

**morbidity**—the state of having an illness; usually chronic

**mortality**—the number of deaths from a specific illness

**Most Important Task (MIT) strategy**—complete the critical tasks first

**movement therapy**—any type of mindfulness-based movement practices used to treat the mind, body, and spirit

**musculoskeletal system**— the body system responsible for movement and stability

**nadi shodhana**—a breathing exercise that uses alternative nostril breathing

**neuroplasticity**—the brain's ability to form and modify neural connections to adapt to its environment

**nomophobia**—a psychological condition describing the intense fear of being separated from one's mobile device

**nonverbal communication**—the use of nonlanguage components (facial expressions, gestures, and posture) to convey a message

**nutrient-dense foods**—foods that provide vitamins, minerals, and other health-promoting components while remaining low in sugar and fat

**obesity**—abnormal or excessive fat accumulation in the body that may impair health

**obesogenic diet**—a diet high in fat and sugar

**optimism**—an inclination to have a positive outlook on the future

**parasympathetic nervous system (PNS)**—part of the autonomic nervous system that works to relax the body, performs necessary body functions when the body is at rest (e.g., digestion), and helps return the body back to homeostasis after being exposed to stress

**Parkinson's law**—a law stating that your tasks will take as long as the time you set aside for them

**perceived social support**—the social support you feel is available if needed

**perception**—an interpretation of sensation

**peripheral nervous system**—the nerves that branch out from the brain and spinal cord to the rest of the body

**physical fitness**—a set of health- and skill-related attributes that enable you to be active and carry out daily tasks with vigor and alertness

**physical wellness**—caring for your body to maximize your quality of life

**plant parenting**—having and caring for houseplants

**Pomodoro technique**—a time management technique that breaks tasks into timed chunks

**positive self-talk**—using inner dialogue in a manner that promotes self-esteem, uses optimism to support your efforts, and encourages you to try new things

**posttraumatic stress disorder (PTSD)**—a psychiatric disorder that develops in people who have experienced or witnessed a traumatic event

**pranayama**—ancient Indian practice that focuses on breathing

**prebiotic**—fiber-rich foods that feed healthy gut bacteria

**probiotic**—live bacteria that improve and maintain the health of the digestive system

**problem-focused coping**—focuses on the problem that causes stress

**psychobiotic diet**—foods that contain prebiotics and probiotics to improve gut health

**received social support**—quality and quantity of support received

**reframing**—a technique used to identify and replace distorted thinking

**relaxation response**—physiologic state of quietude induced by a repetitive activity

**religiosity**—the extent to which one is committed to a formal religion and its practices

**reflective listening**—a technique used to help confirm the understanding of a speaker's message and ideas

**renal system**—the body system responsible for creating urine and consists of the kidney, ureters, and the urethra

**reproductive system**— the body system responsible for procreation

**resilience**—the ability to adapt to difficult situations

**resistance stage**—the second stage of general adaptation syndrome, when the parasympathetic nervous system tries to counteract the stress and resume a normal state

**respiratory system**— the body system responsible for delivering oxygen and nutrients to the body's cells

**rest**—the pausing of an activity (mental and physical) necessary to maintain health and recover from illness and stress

**reticular activating system (RAS)**—a bundle of nerves in the brain stem responsible for processing and filtering information; helps regulate arousal and attention

**rumination**—a unhealthy thinking pattern that revolves around thoughts and feelings about a negative experience

**sarcopenia**—gradual loss of muscle mass

**self-awareness**—being objectively aware of your thoughts, feelings, behaviors, and emotions

**self-care**—anything you do to keep yourself healthy

**self-compassion**—the practice of being kind and understanding to yourself when you are confronted with what you deem as personal failings

**self-esteem**—a person's level of confidence and sense of their own worth

**self-regulation**—the ability to monitor and modify behavior to achieve a goal

**sleep**—an altered state of consciousness and a reduction in physical and mental activity

**sleep hygiene**—healthy practices that promote sleep

**social network**—your relationships with people around you

**social referencing**—process that helps you read the emotional cues of others in order to regulate your own behavior

**social support**—the extent to which people in your life support you and can provide a buffer against adverse life experiences

**social wellness**—the ability to form and maintain healthy relationships

**spiritual wellness**—having a purpose and meaning in life or feeling a sense of connectedness with a higher power or the universe

**spirituality**—a human desire for interconnectedness and personal quest for meaning in life

**strengths-based approach**—an approach to wellness that identifies a person's strengths and assets to improve wellness

**stress**—the body's response to events or thoughts that cause physical or emotional strain

**stress buffering hypothesis**—theory that a strong social support system can reduce or eliminate the negative impact of stress

**stress eating**—increasing food intake to manage stress

**stress modulation effect**—the ability to control and manage stress levels

**stressors**—anything that disrupts the body's homeostasis

**stress reactivity**—an individual's capacity to respond to stress, which varies based on individual characteristics

**stress recovery theory**—a theory used to describe the benefits people receive when immersed in nature

**sympathetic nervous system (SNS)**—part of the autonomic nervous system responsible for the initial response to stress

**technostress**—the inability to cope with new technologies in a healthy manner

**time blocking**—intentionally setting your schedule including classes, work, meetings, tasks, homework, and projects

**trauma**—an emotional response to a disturbing event

**trigger**—anything that brings about an emotional reaction

**ujjayi**—a breathing exercise using only the nostrils to create a rushing sound

**verbal communication**—the use of language (written or spoken) to convey a message

**visualization**—using mental imagery to imagine a scene or outcome of an upcoming event

**wellness**—an active process an individual undergoes to achieve an optimal state of well-being

**work–life balance**—the relationship between the demands of work and the demands of personal life

**yoga**—a practice that focuses on bridging the mind–body connection

# REFERENCES


## Preface

Epstein, R. (2011, September/October). *Fight the frazzled mind: Proactive steps manage stress*. Retrieved November 23, 2021, from www.scientificamerican.com/article/fight-the-frazzled-mind

## Chapter 1

Abdullah, T., Brown, T.L., & Corrigan, P.W. (2020). Diagnostic labeling and mental illness stigma among Black Americans: An experimental vignette study. *Stigma and Health, 5*(1), 11-21.

Akbari, M., & Hossaini, S.M. (2018). The relationship of spiritual health with quality of life, mental health, and burnout: The mediating role of emotional regulation. *Iranian Journal of Psychiatry*, 22-31.

Ali, M.M., West, K., Teich, J.L., Lynch, S., Mutter, R., & Dubenitz, J. (2019). Utilization of mental health services in educational settings by adolescents in the United States. *Journal of School Health, 89*(5), 393-401.

Anyeyer, D., Leach, M.J., Klose, P., Dobos, G., & Cramer, H. (2019). Mindfulness-based stress reduction for treating chronic headache: A systematic review and meta-analysis. *Cephalalgia, 39*(4), 544-555.

Arsian, G., Yildirim, M., Tanhan, A., Bulus, M., & Allen, K.-A. (2022). Coronavirus stress, optimism-pessimism, psychological inflexibility, and psychological health: Psychometric properties of the coronavirus stress measure. *International Journal of Mental Health and Addiction, 19*, 2423-2439.

Bae, Y.J., Reinelt, J., Netto, J., Uhlig, M., Willenberg, A., Ceglarek, U., . . . Kratzsch, J. (2019). Salivary cortisone, as a biomarker for psychosocial stress, is associated with state anxiety and heart rate. *Psychoneuroendocrinology, 101*, 35-41.

Bandura, A. (1995). *Self-efficacy in changing societies*. Cambridge University Press.

Bandura, A. (1997). *Self efficacy: The exercise of control*. Worth Publishing.

Baumeister, R.F., & Vohs, K.D. (2007). Self-regulation, ego depletion, and motivation. *Social and Personality Compass*, 115-128.

Ben-Ami, N. (2020). Associations between backache and stress among undergraduate students. *Journal of American College Health, 68*(1), 61-67.

Bernecker, K., & Jon, V. (2020). Too exhausted to go to bed: Implicit theories about willpower and stress predict bedtime procrastination. *The British Journal of Psychology, 111*(1), 126-147.

Bub, K.L., Robinson, L.E., Curtis, D.S., & Kazak, A.E. (2016). Longitudinal associations between self-regulation and health across childhood and adolescence. *Health Psychology, 35*(11), 1235-1245.

Budhwani, H., Hearld, K.R., & Chavez-Yenter, D. (2015). Depression in racial and ethnic minorities: The impact of nativity and discrimination. *Journal of Racial and Ethnic Health Disparities*, 34-42.

Centers for Disease Control. (2011, June). *Impact of the built environment on health*. Retrieved June 22, 2021, from www.cdc.gov/nceh/publications/factsheets/impactofthebuiltenvironmentonhealth.pdf

Centers for Disease Control. (2020, May 13). *About physical activity: Why it matters*. Retrieved June 28, 2021, from www.cdc.gov/physicalactivity/about-physical-activity/why-it-matters.html

Cervone, D., & Pervin, L.A. (2018). *Personality: Theory and research*. Wiley.

Clement, S., Schauman, O., Graham, T., Maggioni, F., Evans-Lacko, S., Bexborodovs, N., . . . Thornicroft, G. (2014). What is the impact of mental health-related stigma on help-seeking? A systematic review of quantitative and qualitative studies. *Psychological Medicine, 45*(1), 11-27.

Cobb, C.L., Xie, D., Meca, A., & Schwartz, S.J. (2017). Acculturation, discrimination, and depression among unauthorized Latinos/as in the United States. *Cultural Diversity and Ethnic Minority Psychology, 23*(2), 258-268.

Cornah, D. (2006). *The impact of spirituality on mental health*. Mental Health Foundation.

De Oliveira, G., Cianelli, R., Gattamorta, K., Kowalski, N., & Peragallo, N. (2016). Social determinants of depression among Hispanic Women. *Journal of the American Psychiatric Nurse Association, 23*(1), 28-36.

Dossett, M.L., Fricchione, G.L., & Benson, H. (2020). A new era for mind-body medicine. *The New England Journal of Medicine, 382*(15), 1390-1391.

Garfin, D.R., Poulin, M.J., Blum, S., & Silver, R.C. (2018). Aftermath of terror: A nationwide longitudinal study of posttraumatic stress and worry across the decade following the September 11, 2001 terrorist attack. *Journal of Traumatic Stress, 31*, 146-156.

Grad, F.P. (2002). The Preamble of the Constitution of the World Health Organization. *Bulletin of the World Health Organization, 80*(12), 981-984.

Iannotti, R.J., Janssen, I., Haug, E., Kololo, H., Annaheim, B., & Borraccino, A. (2009). Interrelationship of adolescent physical activity, screen-based sedentary behaviour, and social and psychological health. *International Journal of Public Health, 54*, 191-198.

Ilyas, M., Naseem, S., & Bibi, A. (2019). Role of stress prone type A personality and anxiety among heart patients. *Journal of Psychiatry and Behavioral Sciences, 2*(1), 1020.

Ivey-Stephenson, A.Z., Demissie, Z., Crosby, A.E., Stone, D.M., Gaylor, E., Wilkins, N., . . . Brown, M. (2020). Suicidal ideation and behaviors among high school students—Youth Risk Behavior Survey, United States, 2019. *MMWR, 69*(Suppl. 1), 47-55.

Jahre, H., Grotle, M., Smedbraten, K., Dunn, K.M., & Oiestad, B.E. (2020). Risk factors for non-specific neck pain in young adults. *BMC Musculoskeletal Disorders, 21*.

Janis, I.L., & Mann, L. (1979). *Decision making: A psychological analysis of conflict, choice, and commitment.* Free Press.

King, A. (2016). Rise of resilience: Stress can have a negative influence on the human brain, but increasingly it is the ability to withstand severe stress that is the focus of research. *Nature, 531*, S18.

Kitko, C.T. (2001). Dimensions of wellness and the Health Matters program at Penn State. *Home Health Care Management & Practice, 13*(4), 308-311.

Knowles, J.W., & Ashley, E.A. (2018). Cardiovascular disease: The rise of the genetic risk score. *PLoS Medicine*. Retrieved from https://journals.plos.org/plosmedicine/article?id=10.1371/journal.pmed.1002546

Lee, C., Oliffe, J.L., & Kelly, M.T. (2017). Depression and suicidality in gay men: Implications for health care providers. *American Journal of Men's Health, 11*(4), 910-919.

Lenthe, F.V., Borrell, L.N., Costa, G., Roux, A.R., Kauppinen, T.M., Marinacci, C., . . . Valkonen, T. (2005). Neighbourhood unemployment and all cause mortality: A comparison of six countries. *Journal of Epidemiology & Community Health, 59*(3), 231-237.

Levine, G.N. (2019). The mind-heart-body connection. *Circulation, 140*(17), 1363-1365.

Marshal, M.P., Dietz, L.J., Friedman, M.S., Stall, R., Smith, H.A., McGinley, J., . . . Brent, D.A. (2011). Suicidality and depression disparities between sexual minority and heterosexual youth: A meta-analytic review. *Journal of Adolescent Health, 49*(2), 115-123.

Mayo Clinic. (2020, August 29). *Social support: Tap this tool to beat stress.* Retrieved November 10, 2021, from www.mayoclinic.org/healthy-lifestyle/stress-management/in-depth/social-support/art-20044445

Mayo Clinic. (2021, July 28). *Healthy lifestyle stress management.* Retrieved November 5, 2021, from www.mayoclinic.org/healthy-lifestyle/stress-management/in-depth/stress-relief/art-20044464

Moritz, S., Kother, U., Hartmann, M., & Lincoln, T.M. (2015). Stress is a bad advisor. Stress primes poor decision making in deluded psychotic patients. *European Archives of Psychiatry and Clinical Neuroscience, 265*(6), 461-469.

Papanagnou, D., Linder, K., Shah, A., London, K.S., Chandra, S., & Naples, R. (2017). An assessment of emotional intelligence in emergency medicine resident physicians. *International Journal of Medical Education, 8*, 439-445.

Pawar, S.Y. (2020). Mind-body connection of illness. *MIMER Medical Journal, 4*(2), 22-25.

Planey, A.M., Smith, S.M., Moore, S., & Walker, T. (2019). Barriers and facilitators to mental health help-seeking among African American youth and their families: A systematic review. *Children and Youth Services Review, 101*, 190-200.

Potochnick, S.R., & Perreira, K.M. (2010). Depression and anxiety among first-generation immigrant Latino youth: Key correlates and implications for future research. *Journal of Nervous and Mental Disease, 198*(7), 470-477.

Redondo-Florez, L., Tornero-Aguilera, J.F., Ramos-Campo, D.J., & Clemente-Suarez, V.J. (2020). Gender differences in stress- and burnout- related factors of university professors. *BioMed Research International.*

Reinert, M., Fritze, D., & Nguyen, T. (2021). *The state of mental health in America 2022.* Mental Health America.

Safran, M.A., Mays, R.A., Huang, L.N., McCuan, R., Pham, P.K., Fisher, S.K., . . . Tractenberg, A. (2009). Mental health disparities. *American Journal of Public Health, 99*(11), 1962-1966.

Shaygannejad, V., Dahnavi, S.R., & Ashtari, F. (2013). Study of type A and B behavior patterns in patients with multiple sclerosis in an Iranian population. *International Journal of Preventive Medicine, 4*, 279-283.

Slavich, G.M., & Auerbach, R.P. (2018). Stress and its sequelae: Depression, suicide, inflammation, and physical illness. In J.N. Butcher & J.M. Hooley (Eds.), *APA handbook of psychopathology: Psychopathology: Understanding, assessing, and treating adult mental disorders* (pp. 375-402). American Psychological Association.

Specht, J., Egloff, B., & Schmukle, S.C. (2011). Stability and change of personality across the life course: The impact of age and major life events on mean-level and rank-order stability of the Big Five. *Journal of Personality and Social Psychology, 101*(4), 862-882.

Substance Abuse and Mental Health Services Administration. (2016). *Creating a healthier life: A step-by-step guide to wellness.* Retrieved from https://store.samhsa.gov/sites/default/files/d7/priv/sma16-4958.pdf

Substance Abuse and Mental Health Services Administration. (2021). *Key substance use and mental health indicators in the United States: Results from the 2020 National Survey on Drug Use and Health.* Rockville, MD: Center for Behavioral Health Statistics and Quality.

Tavares, I.M., Schlagintweit, H.E., Nobre, P.J., & Rosen, N.O. (2019). Sexual well-being and perceived stress in couples transitioning to parenthood: A dyadic analysis. *International Journal of Clinical and Health Psychology, 19*(3), 198-208.

Taylor, S., Jaques, N., Nosakhare, E., Sano, A., Klerman, E.B., & Picard, R.W. (2017). Importance of sleep data in predicting the next-day stress, happiness, and health in college students. *Sleep, 40*, 294-295.

United States Dietary Association. (2019, July 17). *What is a healthy diet?* Retrieved June 25, 2021, from https://ask.usda.gov/s/article/What-is-a-healthy-diet

Uzan, P. (2021). Mind-body connection and causation: Conceptual and experimental approaches. *Foundations of Science, 26*(4), 901-915.

Uzum, B., Ozdemir, Y., Kose, S., Ozkan, O.S., & Seneldir, O. (2022). Crab barrel syndrome: Looking through the lens of type A and type B personality theory and social comparison process. *Frontiers in Psychology, 13*.

Vlagutu, D., Popescu, S.M., Mercut, R., Ionescu, M., Scrieciu, M., Glodeanu, A.D., . . . Mercut, V. (2022). Associations between bruxism, stress, and manifestations of temporomandibular disorders in young students. *International Journal of Environmental Research and Public Health, 19*(9).

Welnitzova, K. (2021). Stress in students' speeches. *INTED 2021 Proceedings*, 9490-9498.

Wiggins, G.A., Walker, L.C., & Pearson, J.F. (2020). Genome-wide gene expression analyses of BRCA1- and BRCA2-associated breast and ovarian tumors. *Cancers, 12*(10), 3015.

Williams, D.R. (2018). Stress and the mental health of populations of color: Advancing our understanding of race-related stressors. *Journal of Health and Social Behavior, 59*(4), 466-485.

Witzel, D., Turner, S., & Hooker, K. (2021). Daily perceived stress and physical health symptoms: Moderation by self-perceptions of aging. *Innovations in Aging, 5*, 602.

Yu, C.C., Tou, N.X., & Low, J.A. (2022). A comparative study on mental health and adaptability between older and younger adults during the COVID-19 circuit breaker in Singapore. *BMC Public Health, 22*(1), 507-507.

Zvonarev, V. (2019). Takotsubo cardiomyopathy: Medical and psychiatric aspects. Role of psychotropic medications in the treatment of adults with 'Broken Heart' syndrome. *Cureus, 11*(7), 5177-5177.

## Chapter 2

AMCHA Initiative. (2018). *Zionists off our campus! Campus Antisemitism in 2017*. Retrieved from https://amchainitiative.org/wp-content/uploads/2018/09/Campus-Antisemitism-2017.pdf

American Psychiatric Association. (2020, August). *What is posttraumatic stress disorder*. Retrieved November 15, 2021, from www.psychiatry.org/patients-families/ptsd/what-is-ptsd

American Psychological Association. (2020). Stress in America™ 2020: A national mental health crisis.

Anthenelli, R.M. (2012). Overview: Stress and alcohol use disorders revisited. *Alcohol Research, 34*(4), 386-390.

Bendall, S., Eastwood, O., & Scanlan, F. (2020). A systematic review and synthesis of trauma-informed care within outpatient and counseling health settings for young people. *Child Maltreatment, 26*(3).

Bhattacharya, S., Basher, A., Srivastava, A., & Singh, A. (2019). NOMOPHOBIA: NO MObile PHone PhoBIA. *Journal of Family Medicine and Primary Care, 8*(4), 1297-1300.

Billman, G.E. (2020). Homeostasis: The underappreciated and far too often ignored central organizing principles of physiology. *Frontiers in Physiology*.

Bondanini, G., Giorgi, G., Ariza-Montes, A., & Vega-Munoz, A. (2020). Technostress dark side of technology in the workplace: A scientometric analysis. *International Journal of Environmental Research and Public Health, 17*(21).

Bracha, H.S., Ralston, T.C., Matsukawa, J.M., Williams, A.E., & Bracha, A.S. (2004). Does "fight or flight" need updating? *Psychosomatics: Journal of Consultation and Liaison Psychiatry, 45*(5), 448-449.

Breslau, N. (2002). Gender differences in trauma and posttraumatic stress disorder. *The Journal of Gender-Specific Medicine, 5*(1), 34-40.

Brod, C. (1984). *Technostress: The human cost of the computer revolution*. Addison-Wesley.

Buchanan, T.W., & Lovallo, W.R. (2019). The role of genetics in stress effects on health and addiction. *Current Opinion in Psychology, 27*, 72-76.

Burgess, L. (2017, November 28). *What to know about general adaptation syndrome*. Retrieved March 25, 2021, from www.medicalnewstoday.com/articles/320172

Cannon, W.B. (1915). *Bodily changes in pain, hunger, fear, and rage: An account of recent research into the function of emotional excitement*. D. Appleton & Company.

Chaby, L.E., Sheriff, M.J., Hirrlinger, A.M., & Braithwaite, V.A. (2015). Can we understand how developmental stress enhances performance under future threat with the Yerkes-Dodson law? *Communicative & Integrative Biology, 8*(3).

Chiu, S. (2014). The relationship between life stress and smartphone addiction on Taiwanese university student: A mediation model of learning self-efficacy and social self-efficacy. *Computers in Human Behavior, 34*, 49-57.

Cianconi, P., Betrò, S., & Janiri, L. (2020). The impact of climate change on mental health: A systematic descriptive review. *Frontiers in Psychiatry, 11*(74). https://doi.org/10.3389/fpsyt.2020.00074

Ciria, L.F., Suarez-Pinilla, M., Williams, A.G., Jahannathan, S.R., Sanabria, D., & Bekinschtein, T.A. (2021). Different underlying mechanisms for high and low arousal in probabilistic learning in humans. *bioRxiv*.

Cooke, J.E., Eirich, R., Racine, N., & Madigan, S. (2020). Prevalence of posttraumatic and general psychological stress during COVID-19: A rapid review and meta-analysis. *Psychiatry Research, 292*.

Fuse, T., Forsyth, J.P., Marx, B., Gallup, G.G., & Weaver, S. (2007). Factor structure of the Tonic Immobility Scale in female sexual assault survivors: An exploratory and confirmatory factor analysis. *Journal of Anxiety Disorders, 21*(3), 265-284.

Garcia, G.L., Porto, L.G., Gomes da Cruz, C.J., & Molina, G.E. (2022). Can resting heart rate explain the heart rate and parasympathetic response during rest, exercise, and recovery? *PLoS ONE, 17*(12).

Gu, Y., Ocampo, J.M., Algoe, S.B., & Oveis, C. (2022). Gratitude expressions improve teammates' cardiovascular stress responses. *Journal of Experimental Psychology: General*.

Guinosso, S.A., Johnson, S.B., & Riley, A.W. (2016). Multiple adverse experiences and child cognitive development. *Pediatric Research, 79*, 220-226.

Hackett, R.A., & Steptoe, A. (2017). Type 2 diabetes mellitus and psychological stress—a modifiable risk factor. *Nature Reviews Endocrinology, 13*(9).

Hefner, D., Knop, K., Schmitt, S., & Vorderer, P. (2019). Rules? Role model? Relationship? The impact of parents on their children's problematic mobile phone involvement. *Media Psychology, 22*(1).

Holman, E.A., Thompson, R.R., Garfin, D R., & Silver, R.C. (2020). The unfolding COVID-19 pandemic: A probability-based, nationally representative study of mental health in the United States. *Science Advances*, 1-7. https://doi.org/10.1126/sciadv.abd5390

Ising, M., & Holsboer, F. (2006). Genetics of stress response and stress-related disorders. *Dialogues of Clinical Neuroscience, 8*(4), 433-444.

Kok, R., Luijk, M.P., Lucassen, N., Prinzie, P., Jongerling, J., van IJzendoorn, M.H., . . . Bakermans-Kranenburg, M.J. (2022). The role of supporting parenting and stress reactivity in the development of self-regulation in early childhood. *Journal of Child and Family Studies, 31*, 2424-2435.

Konok, V., Pogány, Á., & Miklosi, A. (2017). Mobile attachment: Separation from the mobile induces physiological and behavioural stress and attentional bias to separation-related stimuli. *Computers in Human Behavior, 71*, 228-239. https://doi.org/10.1016/j.chb.2017.02.002

Levy, K.N., Hlay, J.K., Johnson, B.N., & Witmer, C.P. (2019). An attachment theoretical perspective on tend-and-befriend. *Evolutionary Psychological Science, 5*, 426-439.

Macdonald, G., Livingstone, N., Hanratty, J., McCartan, C., Cotmore, R., Cary, M., . . . Churchill, R. (2016). The effectiveness, acceptability and cost-effectiveness of psychosocial interventions for maltreated children and adolescents: In evidence synthesis. *Health Technology Assessment, 20*.

Mahapatra, S. (2019). Smartphone addiction and associated consequences: Role of loneliness and self-regulation. *Behaviour and Information Technology*, 1-12.

Mayo Clinic. (2019, March 19). *Healthy lifestyle stress management*. Retrieved March 26, 2021, from www.mayoclinic.org/healthy-lifestyle/stress-management/in-depth/stress/art-20046037

Mayo Clinic. (n.d.). *Post-traumatic stress disorder (PTSD)*. Retrieved March 29, 2021, from www.mayoclinic.org/diseases-conditions/post-traumatic-stress-disorder/symptoms-causes/syc-20355967

Merrick, M.T., Ford, D.C., Ports, K.A., & Guinn, A.S. (2018). Prevalence of adverse childhood experiences from the 2011-2014 Behavioral Risk Factor Surveillance System in 23 states. *JAMA Pediatrics, 172*(11), 1038-1044.

Moller, A., Sondergaard, H.P., & Helstrom, L. (2017). Tonic immobility during sexual assault—a common reaction predicting post-traumatic stress disorder and severe depression. *Acta Obstetricia et Gyncologica Scandinavica, 96*(8), 932-938.

Montenegro, R.E. (2016). My name is not "Interpreter." *JAMA, 315*(19), 2071-2071.

Moss, H.B., Ge, S., Trager, E., Saavedra, M., Yau, M., Ijeaku, I., & Deas, D. (2020). Risk for substance use disorders in young adulthood: Associations with developmental experiences of homelessness, foster care, and adverse childhood experiences. *Comprehensive Psychiatry, 100*.

Mouzon, D.M., & McLean, J.S. (2017). Internalized racism and mental health among African-Americans, US-born Caribbean Blacks, and foreign-born Caribbean Blacks. *Ethnicity & Health, 22*(1), 36-48.

National Health Service. (2018, September 27). *Causes—Post-traumatic stress disorder*. Retrieved November 15, 2021, from www.nhs.uk/mental-health/conditions/post-traumatic-stress-disorder-ptsd/causes

Norris, G., & Norris, H. (2021). Building resilience through sport in young people with adverse childhood experiences. *Frontiers in Sports and Active Living, 3*, 663587.

Pew Research Center. (2019, August 15). *Sharp rise in the share of Americans saying Jews face discrimination*. Retrieved from www.pewresearch.org/politics/2019/04/15/sharp-rise-in-the-share-of-americans-saying-jews-face-discrimination

Pletcher, B.A., O'Connor, M., Swift-Taylor, M.E., & DallaPiazza, M. (2019). Adverse childhood experiences: A case-based workshop introducing medical students to trauma-informed care. *MedEdPORTAL, 15*.

Porges, S.W. (2022). Polyvagal theory: A science of safety. *Frontiers in Integrative Neuroscience, 16*.

Potapchuk, M., Leiderman, S., Bivens, D., & Major, B. (2005). *Flipping the script: White privilege and community building*. MP Associates.

Ren, Y., Zou, S., Wang, H., Ying, J., Wang, X., & Wu, X. (2022). Fathers and mothers' parenting stress and adolescent depressive symptoms: the mediating roles of overt and covert coparenting conflict behaviors. *Child and Adolescent Psychiatry and Mental Health, 16*(1), 102.

Repp, R.A. (2020). The great action Jackson coachwhip capers. *Bulletin of the Chicago Herpetological Society, 55*(5), 106-110.

Royce, J.B. (2021). The effects of poverty on childhood development. *Journal of Mental Health and Social Behaviour, 132*.

Russell, A.L., Tasker, J.G., Lucion, A.B., Fiedler, J., Munhoz, C.D., Wu, T.-Y.J., & Deak, T. (2018). Factors promoting vulnerability to dysregulated stress reactivity and stress-related disease. *Journal of Neuroendocrinology, 30*(10), e12641.

Russell, G., & Lightman, S. (2019). The human stress response. *Nature Reviews Endocrinology, 15*, 525-534.

Sattizahn, J.R., Moser, J.S., & Beilock, S.L. (2016). A closer look at who "chokes under pressure." *Journal of Applied Research in Memory and Cognition, 5*, 470-477.

Saw, A., Yellow Horse, A.J., & Russell, J. (2021, May 27). *Stop the AAPE Hate Mental Health Report*. Retrieved from https://stopaapihate.org/mental-health-report

Schmidt, N.B., Richey, J.A., Zvolensky, M.J., & Maner, J.K. (2008). Exploring human freeze responses to a threat stressor. *Journal of Behavior Therapy and Experimental Psychiatry, 39*(3), 292-304.

Shevlin, M., McBride, O., Murphy, J., Miller, J.G., Hartman, T.K., Levita, L., . . . Bentall, R.P. (2020). Anxiety, depression, traumatic stress and COVID-19-related anxiety in the UK general population during the COVID-19 pandemic. *BJPsych Open, 6*(6).

Solomon, Z., Ginzburg, K., Ohry, A., & Mikulincer, M. (2021). Overwhelmed by the news: A longitudinal study of prior trauma, posttraumatic stress disorder trajectories, and news watching during the COVID-19 pandemic. *Social Science & Medicine, 278.*

Sosoo, E.E., Bernard, D.L., & Neblett Jr., E.W. (2020). The influence of internalized racism on the relationship between discrimination and anxiety. *Cultural Diversity and Ethnic Minority Psychology, 26*(4), 570-580.

Sripada, R.K., Swain, J.E., Evans, G.W., Welsh, R.C., & Liberzon, I. (2014). Childhood poverty and stress reactivity are associated with aberrant functional connectivity in default mode network. *Neuropsychopharmacology, 39,* 2244-2251.

Steckler, T., Kalin, N.H., & Reul, J.H. (2005). *Handbook of stress and the brain part 2: Stress: Integrative and clinical aspects* (Vol. 15). Elsevier.

Stop the Hate & AARP. (2022). *Anti-Asian hate, social isolation, and mental health among Asian American elders during COVID-19.* Retrieved from https://stopaapihate.org/elder-report-2022

Stroud, L.R., Salovey, P., & Epel, E.S. (2002). Sex differences in stress responses: social rejection versus achievement stress. *Biological Psychiatry, 52*(4), 318-327.

Tan, S.Y., & Yip, A. (2018). Hans Seyle (1907-1982): Founder of the stress theory. *Singapore Medical Journal, 59*(4), 170-171.

Tandon, A., Dhir, A., Almugren, I., AlNemer, G.N., & Mantymaki, M. (2021). Fear of missing out (FoMO) among social media users: A systematic literature review, synthesis and framework for future research. *Internet Research, 31*(3), 782-821.

Taylor, S.E., Klein, L.C., Lewis, B.P., Gruenewald, T.L., Gurung, R.A., & Updegraff, J.A. (2000). Biobehavioral responses to stress in females: Tend-and-befriend, not fight-or-flight. *Psychological Review, 107*(3), 411-429.

Turecki, G., & Meaney, M.J. (2017). Effects of the social environment and stress on glucocorticoid receptor gene methylation: A systemic review. *Biological Psychiatry, 79,* 87-96.

United States Department of Veterans Affairs. (n.d.). *PTSD: National Center for PTSD.* Retrieved March 29, 2021, from www.ptsd.va.gov/understand_tx/tx_basics.asp

Uphill, M.A., Rossato, C.J., Swain, J., & O'Driscoll, J. (2019). Challenge and threat: A critical review of the literature and an alternative conceptualization. *Frontiers in Psychology.*

Viner, R. (1999). Putting stress in life: Hans Selye and the making of stress theory. *Social Studies of Science*, 391-410.

Wang, H., Xia, Q., Xiong, Z., Li, Z., Xiang, W., Yuan, Y., & Li, Z. (2020). The psychological distress and coping styles in the early stages of the 2019 coronavirus disease (COVID-19) epidemic in the general mainland Chinese population: A web-based survey. *PLoS ONE, 15*(5).

Weir, K. (2016). Climate change in threatening mental health. *American Psychological Association, 47*(7).

Williams, D.R. (2018). Stress and the mental health of populations of color: Advancing our understanding of race-related stressors. *Journal of Health and Social Behavior, 59*(4), 466-485. https://doi.org/10.1177/0022146518814251

Wright, G., Volodarsky, S., Hecht, S., & Saxe, L. (2021). Trends in Jewish young adult experiences and perceptions of antisemitism in America from 2017-2019. *Contemporary Jewry, 41,* 461-481.

Yan, L., Gan, Y., Ding, X., Wu, J., & Duan, H. (2021). The relationship between perceived stress and emotional distress during the COVID-19 outbreak: Effects of boredom proneness and coping style. *Journal of Anxiety Disorders, 77.*

Yau, M.Y., Ge, S., Moss, H.B., Cooper, T., Osei, O., Ijeaku, I., & Deas, D. (2022). Regional prevalence of adverse childhood experiences in the United States using a nationally represented school-based sample. *SSM Population Health, 19,* 101145.

Yerkes, R.M., & Dodson, J.D. (1908). The relation of strength of stimulus to rapidity of habit-formation. *Journal of Comparative Neurology and Psychology, 18*(5), 459-482.

Ziviani, J., Feeney, R., Cuckelly, M., Meredith, P., & Hunt, K. (2012). Effectiveness of support services for children and young people with challenging behaviours related to or secondary to disability, who are in out-of-home care: A systematic review. *Children and Youth Services Review, 34*(4), 758-770.

## Chapter 3

Abdel-Haq, R., Schlachetzki, J.C., Glass, C.K., & Mazmanian, S.K. (2019). Microbiome-microglia connections via the gut-brain axis. *The Journal of Experimental Medicine, 216*(1), 41-59.

American Psychological Association. (2018, November 1). *Stress effects on the body.* Retrieved December 15, 2021, from American Psychological Association: https://www.apa.org/topics/stress/body.

Assaf, A.M. (2013). Stress-induced immune-related diseases and health outcomes of pharmacy students: A pilot study. *Saudi Pharmacy Journal, 21*(1), 35-44.

Bahrami-Nejad, Z., Zhao, M.L., Tholen, S., Hunderdosse, D., Tkach, K.E., van Schie, S., . . . Teruel, M.N. (2018). A transcriptional circuit filters oscillating circadian hormonal inputs to regulate fat cell differentiation. *Cell Metabolism, 27*(4), 854-868.

Camilleri, M. (2019). Leaky gut mechanisms, measurement and clinical implications in humans. *Gut, 68,* 1516-1526.

Chan, Y., Ho-Wai, S.S., Mak, A.D., Siah, K.T., Wai Chan, J., & Wu, C.Y. (2019). The temporal relationship of daily stress, emotions, and bowel symptoms in irritable bowel syndrome-diarrhea subtype: A smartphone-based experience sampling study. *Neurogastroenterology & Motility, 31*(3).

Chen, H., Zhang, T., Xu, X., Wan, S., & Wang, Y. (2022). Review of skin problems caused by stress. *Journal of Clinical Medicine Research, 3*(3), 116-122.

Chrousos, G.P. (2009). Stress and disorders of the stress system. *Nature Reviews Endocrinology, 5*(7), 374-381.

Dar, T., Radfar, A., Abohashem, S., Pitman, R.K., Tawakol, A., & Osborne, M.T. (2019). Psychosocial stress and cardiovascular disease. *Prevention, 21.*

De Couck, M., Caers, R., Musch, L., Fliegauf, J., Giangreco, A., & Gidron, Y. (2019). How breathing can help you make better decisions: Two studies on the effects of breathing patterns on the heart rate variability and decision making in business cases. *International Journal of Psychophysiology, 139*, 1-9.

Eckerling, A., Ricon-Becker, I., Sorski, L., Sandbank, E., & Ben-Eliyahu, S. (2021). Stress and cancer: mechanisms, significance, and future directions. *Nature reviews. Cancer,* 21(12), 767-785.

Gao, Y., & Rodriquez, L.V. (2022). The effect of chronic psychological stress on lower urinary tract function: An animal model perspective. *Frontiers in Physiology, 13.*

Henley, D.E., Kaye, J.M., & Lightman, S.L. (2011). The endocrine response to stress. In J.A. Wass, P.M. Stewart, S.A. Amiel, & M.J. Davies (Eds.), *Oxford textbook of endocrinology and diabetes.* Oxford University Press.

Iliades, C. (2018, October 16). *How stress affects digestion.* Retrieved December 15, 2021, from www.everydayhealth.com/wellness/united-states-of-stress/how-stress-affects-digestion

Jaurez-Rojas, L., Vigueras-Villasenor, R.M., Casillas, F., & Retana-Marquez, S. (2017). Graduate decrease in spermatogenesis caused by chronic stress. *Acta Histochemica*, 284-291.

Joseph, D.N., & Whirledge, S. (2017). Stress and the HPA axis: Balancing homeostasis and fertility. *International Journal of Molecular Science, 18*(10), 2224.

Madison, A., & Kiecolt-Glaser, J.K. (2019). Stress, depression, diet, and the gut microbiota: Human-bacteria interactions at the core of psychoneuroimmunology and nutrition. *Current Opinions in Behavioral Science, 28*, 105-110.

Magarinos, A.M., & Pfaff, D. (2015). Sexual motivation in the female and its opposition by stress. *Behavioral Neuroscience of Motivation,* 35-49.

Newton, E., Schosheim, A., Patel, S., Chitkara, D.K., & Tilburg, M.L. (2018). The role of psychological factors in pediatric functional abdominal pain disorders. *Neurogastroenterology and Motility,* 31(6).

Rooney, K.L., & Domar, A.D. (2018). The relationship between stress and infertility. *Dialogues in Clinical Neuroscience, 20*(1), 41-47.

Rosen, R.D., & Winters, R. (2020). *Physiology, lower esophageal sphincter.* StatPearls.

Scott, A., & Newson, L. (2020). Should we be prescribing testosterone to perimenopausal women? A guide to prescribing testosterone for women in primary care. *British Journal of General Practice, 70*(693), 203-204.

Seo, W., Kim, N., Kim, S., Lee, C., & Park, S.-M. (2019). Deep ECG-Respiration Network (DeepER Net) for recognizing mental stress. *Sensors, 19*(13).

Sharma, S.T., Nieman, L.K., & Feelders, R.A. (2015). Cushing's syndrome: Epidemiology and developments in disease management. *Clinical Epidemiology, 7.*

Shen, Y., He, D., He, L., Bai, Y., Wang, B., Xue, Y., & Hou, G. (2020). Chronic psychological stress, but not chronic pain stress, influences sexual motivation and induces testicular autophagy in male rats. *Frontiers in Psychology, 11.*

Stefanaki, C., Pervanidou, P., Boschiero, D., & Chrousos, G.P. (2018). Chronic stress and body composition disorders: Implications for health and disease. *Hormones, 17*, 33-43.

Swaney, M.H., Nelsen, A., Sandstrom, S., & Kalan, L.R. (2023). Sweat and sebum preferences of the human skin microbiota. *Microbiology Spectrum, 11*(1).

Torrico, T.J., & Abdijadid, S. (2019). *Neuroanatomy, limbic system.* StatPearls Publishing.

Turner, L., Galante, J., Vainre, M., Stochl, J., Dufour, G., & Jones, P.B. (2020). Immune dysregulation among students exposed to exam stress and its mitigation by mindfulness training: Findings from an exploratory randomized trial. *Scientific Reports, 10.*

Vafaee, F., Shirzad, S., Shamsi, F., & Boskabady, M.H. (2022). Neuroscience and treatment of asthma, new therapeutic strategies and future aspects. *Life Sciences,* 292.

Valsamakis, G., Chrousos, G., & Mastorakos, G. (2019). Stress, female reproduction, and pregnancy. *Psychoneuroendocrinology*, 48-57.

van der Valk, E.S., Savas, M., & van Rossum, E.F. (2018). Stress and obesity: Are there more susceptible individuals? *Current Obesity Reports, 7*(2), 193-203.

Vita, R., Lapa, D., Trimarchi, F., Vita, G., Fallahi, P., Antonelli, A., & Benvenga, S. (2016). Certain HLA alleles are associated with stress-triggered Graves' disease and influence its course. *Endocrine Genetics/Epigenetics*, 93-100.

Vogel, S., & Schwabe, L. (2016). Learning and memory under stress: Implications for the classroom. *NPJ Science of Learning.*

Vogel, S., Kluen, L.M., Ferandez, G., & Schwabe, L. (2018). Stress affects the neural ensemble for integrating new information and prior knowledge. *NeuroImage*, 176-187.

Yaribeygi, H., Panahi, Y., Sahraei, H., Johnston, T.P., & Sahebkar, A. (2017). The impact of stress on body function: A review. *Experimental and Clinical Sciences Journal, 16*, 1057-1072.

Zari, S., & Alrahmani, D. (2017). The association between stress and acne among female medical students in Jeddah, Saudi Arabia. *Clinical, Cosmetic and Investigational Dermatology, 10*, 503-506.

Zhang, B., Ma, S., Rachmin, I., He, M., Baral, P., Choi, S., . . . Hsu, Y.C. (2020). Hyperactivation of sympathetic nerves drives depletion of melanocyte stem cells. *Nature,* 676-681.

## Chapter 4

Ahghadir, A.H., Gabr, S.A., & Iqbal, Z. (2020). Effect of gender, physical activity and stress-related hormones on adolescent's academic achievements. *International Journal of Environmental Research and Public Health, 17*(11).

Ajabshir, S., Stumbar, S., Lachica, I., Gates, K., Qureshi, Z., & Huffman, F. (2021). Diet-related chronic diseases among a multi-ethnic group of uninsured adults. *Current Developments in Nutrition, 5*, 95-95.

Akerstedt, T., Orsini, N., Petersen, H., Axelsson, J., & Lekander, M. (2012). Predicting sleep quality from stress and prior sleep—A study of day-to-day covariation across six weeks. *Sleep Medicine, 13*(6), 674-679.

Allison, S.E. (1970). The meaning of rest: An exploratory nursing study. In *ANA clinical sessions* (pp. 191-198). Appleton-Century-Crofts.

American College Health Association. (2020). *National college health assessment III: Fall 2019 reference group data report.* Author.

American Heart Association. (2020, January 9). *What is the Mediterranean diet?* Retrieved November 26, 2021, from www.heart.org/en/healthy-living/healthy-eating/eat-smart/nutrition-basics/mediterranean-diet

Amir, S., Brown, Z.W., & Amit, Z. (1980). The role of endorphins in stress: Evidence and speculations. *Neuroscience & Biobehavioral Reviews, 4*(1), 77-86.

Anderson, S.C., Cryan, J.F., & Dinan, T. (2017). *The psychobiotic revolution: Mood, food, and the new science.* National Geographic.

Arnsten, A.F. (2009). Stress signaling pathways that impair prefrontal cortex structure and function. *Nature Reviews Neuroscience, 10*, 410-422.

Asp, M. (2015). Rest: A health-related phenomenon and concept in caring science. *Global Qualitative Nursing Research.*

Beiter, R., Nash, R., McCrady, M., Rhoades, D., Linscomb, M., Clarahan, M., & Sammut, S. (2015). The prevalence and correlates of depression, anxiety, and stress in a sample of college students. *Journal of Affective Disorders, 173*(1), 90-96.

Ben-Ami, N., & Korn, L. (2020). Associations between backache and stress among undergraduate students. *Journal of American College Health, 68*(1), 61-67.

Benham, G. (2010). Sleep: An important factor in stress-health models. *Stress and Health, 26*, 204-214.

Benham, G. (2021). Stress and sleep in college students prior to and during the COVID-19 pandemic. *Stress and Health, 37*(3), 504-515.

Bennett, G.G., Wolin, K.Y., Avrunin, J.S., Stoddard, A.M., Sorensen, G., Barbeau, E., & Emmons, K.M. (2006). Does race/ethnicity moderate the association between job strain and leisure time physical activity? *Annals of Behavioral Medicine,* 32(1), 60-67.

Benson, H., & Klipper, M.Z. (2009). *The relaxation response.* HarperCollins.

Berczik, K., Szabo, A., Griffiths, M.D., Kurimay, T., Kun, B., Urban, R., & Demetrovics, Z. (2012). Exercise addiction: Symptoms, diagnosis, epidemiology, and etiology. *Substance Use & Misuse, 47*(4).

Berding, K., Ahmed, M., Bastiaanssen, T., Long-Smith, C., Stanton, C., Dinan, T., & Cryan, J. (2020). A psychobiotic diet decreases stress and depressive mood in healthy volunteers. *European Neuropsychopharmacology, 40*, S132.

Bosland, P.W. (2016). Hot stuff—do people living in hot climates like their food spicy hot or not? *Temperature, 3*(1), 41-42.

Brown, J.D., & Siegal, J.M. (1988). Exercise as a buffer of life stress. *Health Psychology, 7*(4), 341-353.

Chang, K.K., Wong, F.K., Chan, K.L., Wong, F., Ho, H.C., Wong, M.S., . . . Yang, L. (2020). The impact of the environment of the quality of life and the mediating effects of sleep and stress. *International Journal of Environmental Research and Public Health, 17*(22).

Chao, A.M., Jastreboff, A.M., White, M.A., Grilo, C.M., & Sinha, R. (2017). Stress, cortisol, and other appetite-related hormones: Prospective prediction of 6-month changes in food cravings and weight. *Obesity, 25*(4), 713-720.

Cheng, L.-H., Liu, Y.-W., Wu, C.-C., Wang, S., & Tsai, Y.-C. (2019). Psychobiotics in mental health, neurodegenerative and neurodevelopmental disorders. *Journal of Food and Drug Analysis, 27*(3), 632-648.

Cheng, Y., Kawachi, I., Coakley, E.H., Schwartz, J., & Colditz, G. (2000). Association between psychological work characteristics and health functioning in American women: Prospective study. *BMJ, 320*(7247), 1432-1436.

Chou, R., Deyo, R., Friedly, J., Skelly, A., Hashimoto, R., Weimer, M., . . . Brodt, E.D. (2017). A systematic review for an American College of Physicians clinical practice guideline. *Annals of Internal Medicine, 166*(7), 493-505.

Cleveland Clinic. (2021, June 15). *Eat these foods to reduce stress and anxiety.* Retrieved November 26, 2021, from https://health.clevelandclinic.org/eat-these-foods-to-reduce-stress-and-anxiety

Colledge, F., & Meyer, M. (2022). Exercise addiction—status, identification and treatment. *Praxis, 111*(6), 317-321.

Connell, C.M. (1994). Impact of spouse caregiving on health behaviors and physical and mental health status. *American Journal of Alzheimer's Disease & Other Dementias, 9*(1).

Cryan, J.F., O'Riordan, K.J., Cowan, C.S., Sandhu, K.V., Bastiaanssen, T.F., Boehme, M., . . . Dinan, T.G. (2018). The microbiota-gut-brain-axis. *Psychological Reviews, 99*(4), 1877-2013.

Dar, T., Radfar, A., Abohashem, S., Pitman, R.K., Tawakol, A., & Osborne, M.T. (2019). Psychosocial stress and cardiovascular disease. *Prevention, 21*(23).

Delgado, I., Dexpert, S., Sauvant, J., Cryan, J.F., & Capuron, L. (2021). Influences of pro-obesogenic dietary habits on stress-induced cognitive alterations in healthy adult volunteers. *Neurobiology of Stress, 15.*

Doyle, K.L., Toepfer, M., Bradfield, A.F., Noffke, A., Ausderau, K.K., Andreae, S., & Pickett, K.A. (2021). Systematic review of exercise for caregiver–care recipient dyads: What is best for spousal caregivers—exercising together or not at all? *The Gerontologist, 61*(6), e283-e301.

Elsayed, E.B., Radwan, E.H., Elashri, N.I., & El-Gilany, A.-H. (2019). The effect of Benson's relaxation technique on anxiety, depression and sleep quality of elderly patients undergoing hemodialysis. *International Journal of Nursing Didactics, 9*(2).

Fazeli, M.S., Pourrahmat, M.-M., Massah, G., Lee, K., Lavoie, P.M., Fazeli, M., . . . Collet, J.-P. (2020). The effect of massage on the cardiac autonomic nervous system and markers of inflammation in night shift workers: A pilot randomized crossover trial. *International Journal of Therapeutic Massage & Bodywork, 13*(3), 6-17.

Field, T. (2014). Massage therapy research review. *Complementary Therapies in Clinical Practice, 20*(4), 224-229.

Fleshner, F. (2005). Physical activity and stress resistance: Sympathetic nervous system adaptations prevent stress-induced immunosuppression. *Exercise and Sport Sciences Review, 33*(3), 120-126.

Gearhardt, A.N., Grilo, C.M., DiLeone, R.J., Brownell, K.D., & Potenza, M.N. (2011). Can food be addictive? Public health and policy implications. *Addiction, 106*(7), 1208-1212.

Gonzalez-Zacarias, A.A., Mavarez-Martinez, A., Arias-Morales, C.E., Stoicea, N., & Rogers, B. (2016). Impact on demographic, socioeconomic, and psychological factors on glycemic self-management in adults with type 2 diabetes. *Frontiers of Public Health, 4*.

Greenwood, B.N., Spence, K.G., Crevling, D.M., Clark, P.J., Craig, W.C., & Fleshner, M. (2013). Exercise-induced stress resistance is independent of exercise controllability and the medial prefrontal cortex. *The European Journal of Neuroscience, 37*(3), 469-478.

Hales, C.M., Carroll, M.D., Fryar, C.D., & Ogden, C.L. (2017). *Prevalence of obesity among adults and youth: United States, 2015-2016.* National Center for Health Statistics Data Brief.

Hasan, Y.M., Heyat, M.B., Siddiqui, M.M., Azad, S., & Askhtar, F. (2015). An overview of sleep and stages of sleep. *International Journal of Advanced Research in Computer and Communication Engineering, 4*(12).

Helvig, A., Wade, S., & Hunter-Eades, L. (2016). Rest and the associated benefits in restorative sleep: A concept analysis. *Journal of Advanced Nursing, 72*(1), 62-72.

Herbert, C., Meixner, F., Wiebking, C., & Gilg, V. (2020). Regular physical activity, short-term exercise, mental health, and well-being among university students: The results of an online laboratory study. *Frontiers in Psychology, 11*.

Hirshkowitz, M., Whiton, K., Albert, S.M., Alessi, C., Bruni, O., DonCarlos, L., . . . Rawding, R. (2015). National Sleep Foundation's sleep time duration recommendations: Methodology and results summary. *Sleep Health, 1*(1), 40-43.

Honda, Y., Tsuda, A., & Horiuchi, S. (2012). Effect of a four-week self-administered acupressure intervention on perceived stress over the past month. *Open Journal of Medical Psychology, 1*(3).

House, L.A., Neal, C., & Kolb, J. (2019). Supporting the mental health needs of first generation college students. *Journal of College Student Psychotherapy, 34*(2), 157-167.

Hu, Y., Visser, M., & Kaiser, S. (2019). Perceived stress and sleep quality in midlife and later: Controlling for genetic and environmental influences. *Behavioral Sleep Medicine*.

Irkham, M. (2022). Reduce pain scale in post-surgery percutaneous coronary intervention (PCI) patients with Benson relaxation in the cathlab room AI Adan Hospital. *South East Asia Nursing Research, 4*(2).

Jimoh, F., Lund, E., Harvey, L.J., Frost, C., Lay, W.J., Roe, M.A., . . . Finglas, P.M. (2018). Comparing diet and exercise monitoring using smartphone app and paper diary: A two-phase intervention study. *JMIR Mhealth Uhealth, 6*(1).

Kamada, N., Seo, S.-U., Chen, G.Y., & Nunez, G. (2013). Role of the gut microbiota in immunity and inflammatory disease. *Nature Reviews Immunology, 13*, 321-335.

Lee, S.-Y., Wuertz, C., Rogers, R., & Chen, Y.-P. (2013). Stress and sleep disturbances in female college students. *American Journal of Health Behavior, 37*(6), 851-858.

Leserman, J., Stuart, E.M., Mamish, M.E., & Benson, H. (1989). The efficacy of the relaxation response in preparing for cardiac surgery. *Behavioral Medicine, 15*(3), 111-117.

Liu, X., Ping, S., & Gao, W. (2019). Changes in undergraduate students' psychological well-being as they experience university life. *International Journal of Environmental Research and Public Health, 16*(16).

Liu, Z., Heffernan, C., & Tan, J. (2020). Caregiver burden: A concept analysis. *International Journal of Nursing Sciences, 7*(4), 438-445.

Magness, S., & Stulberg, B. (2017). *Peak performance.* Rodale.

Magrone, T., Russo, M.A., & Jirillo, E. (2017). Cocoa and dark chocolate polyphenols: From biology to clinical applications. *Frontiers in Immunology*.

Mani, S., & Mishra, M. (2021). Are your employees getting their daily dose of DOSE? A neuroscience perspective to enhance employee engagement. *Development and Learning in Organizations, 35*(5), 11-14.

Martinez, M.A., Lewis, K., & Marquez, J. (2019). College ready at a cost: Underrepresented students overwhelmed, scared, increasingly stressed, and coping. *Education and Urban Society, 52*(5).

Middlekauff, H.R., Hui, K., Yu, J.L., Hamilton, M.A., Fonarow, G.C., Moriguchi, J., . . . Hage, A. (2002). Acupuncture inhibits sympathetic activation during mental stress in advanced heart failure patients. *Journal of Cardiac Failure, 8*(6), 399-406.

Moore, A., Nguyen, A., Rivas, S., Bany-Mohammed, A., Majeika, J., & Martinez, L. (2021). A qualitative examination of the impacts of financial stress on college students' well-being: Insights from a large private institution. *Sage Open Medicine, 9*, 1-8.

Murray, D.W., & Hamoudi, A. (2016). *A brief on self-regulation and toxic stress: How do acute and chronic stress impact the development of self-regulation?* U.S. Department of Health and Human Services.

National Center for Chronic Disease Prevention and Health Promotion. (2020, April 15). *Sleep and sleep disorders.* Retrieved October 27, 2021, from www.cdc.gov/sleep/index.html

Office of Disease Prevention and Health Promotion. (2020). *Healthy People 2030.* U.S. Department of Health and Human Services. Retrieved from https://health.gov/healthypeople/objectives-and-data

Otte, J.L., Lalevich, S.T., Hollingsworth, P., Chernyak, Y., & Manchanda, S. (2017). 1200 Sleep Great! A wellness program to promote sleep in the workplace. *Sleep, 40*, A447-A448.

Padden, D.L., Connors, R.A., & Agazio, J.G. (2011). Determinants of health-promoting behaviors in military spouses during deployment separation. *Military Medicine, 176*(1), 26-34.

Pecoraro, N., Reyes, F., Gomez, F., Bhargava, A., & Dallman, M.F. (2004). Chronic stress promotes palatable feeding, which reduces signs of stress: Feedforward and feedback effects of chronic stress. *Endocrinology, 145*(8), 3754-3762.

Permana, B., Lindayani, L., Hendra, A., & Juniarni, L. (2020). The effect of yoga exercise on reducing blood pressure among elderly with hypertension: A systematic review. *Journal Pendidikan Keperawatan Indonesia, 6*(2), 163-170.

Perrault, A.A., Bayer, L., Peuvrier, M., Alfyouni, A., Ghisletta, P., Brockmann, C., . . . Sterpenich, V. (2019). Reducing the use of screen electronic devices in the evening is associated with improved sleep and daytime vigilance in adolescents. *Sleep, 42*(9).

Pilozzi, A., Carro, C., & Huang, X. (2020). Roles of B-Endorphin in stress, behavior, neuroinflammation, and brain energy metabolism. *International Journal of Molecular Sciences, 22*(1).

Romero-Ramos, N., Gonzalez Suarez, A.J., & Ramos, O.R. (2022). Effects of meditation on biochemical markers in healthy people: A systematic review of the last 5 years. *LASE Journal of Sport Science, 13*(1), 90-107.

Sawyer, S.M., Azzopardi, P.S., Wickremarathne, D., & Patton, G.C. (2018). The age of adolescence. *The Lancet Child & Adolescent Health, 2*(3), 223-228.

Schroeder, S., Burnis, J., Denton, A., Krasnow, A., Raghu, T.S., & Mathis, K. (2017). Effectiveness of acupuncture therapy on stress in a large urban college population. *Journal of Acupuncture and Meridian Studies, 10*(3), 165-170.

Schultchen, D., Reichenberger, J., Mittl, T., Weh, T.R., Smyth, J.M., Blechert, J., & Pollatos, O. (2019). Bidirectional relationship of stress and affect with physical activity and healthy eating. *British Journal of Health Psychology, 24*(2), 315-333.

Sharp, E., & Barney, D. (2016). Required and non-required college physical activity classes effect on college students' stress. *American Journal of Health Studies, 31*(2).

Shively, C.A., Appt, S.E., Chen, H., Day, S.M., Frye, B.M., Shaltout, H.A., . . . Register, T.C. (2020). Mediterranean diet, stress resilience, and aging in non-human primates. *Neurobiology of Stress, 13.*

Shuttleworth, S., & Foster, R.G. (2020). Sleep and stress. *Interface Focus, 10*(3).

Simao, S., Horing, A.C., Lima, B.D., Silva, N.C., & Alfieri, F.M. (2021). Immediate effect of quick massage on muscle tension and pressure pain threshold. *Brazilian Journal of Pain*, 221-224.

Smith, A.R., Fink, E.L., Anestis, M.D., Ribeiro, J.D., Gordon, K.H., Davis, H., . . . Wonderlich, S. (2013). Exercise caution: Over-exercise is associated with suicidality among individuals with disordered eating. *Psychiatry Research, 206*(2-3), 246-255.

Stults-Kolehmainen, M.A., & Sinha, R. (2014). The effects of stress on physical activity and exercise. *Sports Medicine, 44*(1), 81-121.

Sun, N., Tu, J.F., Lin, L.L., Li, Y.T., Yang, J.W., Shi, G.X., . . . Liu, C.Z. (2019). Correlation between acupuncture dose and effectiveness in the treatment of knee osteoarthritis: A systematic review. *Acupuncture in Medicine, 37*(5), 261-267.

Sung, K.M., Yu, M., Kang, Y.S., Gu, M.O., Jung, M.S., Eun, Y., & Meon, M.Y. (2019). The effects of a tripod approach for cancer patients on illness stress, health-promoting lifestyle, hope, and resilience. *Cancer Nursing, 44*(2), 125-135.

Trigueros, R., Padilla, A.M., Aguilar-Parra, J.M., Rocamora, P., Morales-Gazquez, M.J., & Lopez-Liria, R. (2020). The influence of emotional intelligence on resilience, test anxiety, academic stress, and the Mediterranean diet. A study with university students. *International Journal of Environmental Research and Public Health, 17*(6).

Tucker, S.J., Weymillerr, A.J., Cutshall, S.M., Rhudy, L.M., & Lohse, C.M. (2012). Stress ratings and health promotion practices among RNs: A case for action. *Journal of Nursing Administration, 42*(5), 282-292.

U.S. Department of Agriculture and U.S. Department of Health and Human Services. (2020). *Dietary guidelines for Americans 2020-2025.* Retrieved from dietaryguidelines.gov

U.S. Department of Health and Human Services. (2018). *Physical activity guidelines for Americans* (2nd ed.). Author.

Vargas, I., & Lopez-Duran, N. (2014). Dissecting the impact of sleep and stress on the cortisol awakening response in young adults. *Psychoneuroendocrinology, 40*, 10-16.

Vernon, M.M., Young-Hyman, D., & Looney, S.W. (2010). Maternal stress, physical activity, and body mass index during new mothers' first year postpartum. *Women Health, 50*(6), 544-562.

Volkow, N.D., Wang, G.J., Fowler, J.S., Tomasi, D., & Baler, R. (2012). Food and drug reward: Overlapping circuits in human obesity and addiction. *Current Topics in Behavioral Neurosciences, 11*, 1-24.

Weidner, G., Boughal, T., Connor, S.L., Pieper, C., & Mendell, N.R. (1997). Relationship of job strain to standard coronary risk factors and psychological characteristics in women and men of the Family Heart Study. *Health Psychology, 16*(3), 239-247.

Yoon, E.S., Park, S.J., & Park, S.H. (2019). Associations between psychological stress and exercise in Korean adults: Findings from the Korean genome and epidemiology study. *Exercise Science, 28*(4), 355-364.

Zhao, J., Yin, H., Zhang, G., Li, G., Shang, B., Wang, C., & Chen, L. (2019). A meta-analysis of randomized controlled trials of laughter and humour interventions on depression, anxiety and sleep quality in adults. *Journal of Advanced Nursing, 75*(11), 2435-2448.

## Chapter 5

Arens, E.A., & Stangier, U. (2020). Sad as a matter of evidence: The desire for self-verification motivates the pursuit of sadness in clinical depression. *Frontiers in Psychology, 11.*

Avvenuti, G., Baiardini, I., & Giardini, A. (2016, March 2). Optimism's explicative role for chronic disease. *Frontiers in Psychology, 7.*

Bastiaansen, M., Lub, X.D., Mitas, O., Jung, T.H., Ascencao, M.P., Han, D.-I., . . . Strijbosch, W. (2019). Emotions as core building blocks of an experience. *International Journal of Contemporary Hospitality Management, 21*(2), 651-668.

Baumgartner, J.N., Schneider, T.R., & Capiola, A. (2018). Investigating the relationship between optimism and stress response: A biopsychosocial perspective. *Personality and Individual Differences, 129*(15), 114-118.

Blakely, M.L., Aronson, B.D., Chen, A.M., Kiersma, M.E., Wicker, E., & Draime, J.A. (2022). Establishing validity evidence for parallel patient-provider empathy scales to drive self-reflection. *American Journal of Pharmaceutical Education, 86*(8), 971-978.

Bloch, L., Haase, C.M., & Levenson, R.W. (2014). Emotion regulation predicts marital satisfaction: More than a wives' tale. *Emotion, 14*, 130-144.

Burrage, E., Marshall, K., Santanam, N., & Chantler, P. (2018). Cerebrovascular dysfunction with stress and depression. *Brain Circulation, 4*(2).

Chow, S.K., & Choi, E.K. (2019). Assessing the mental health, physical activity levels, and resilience of today's junior college students in self-financing institutions. *International Journal of Environmental Research and Public Health, 16*(17).

Contreras, J.A., Edwards-Maddox, S., Hall, A., & Lee, M.A. (2020). Effects of reflective practice on Baccalaureate nursing students' stress, anxiety, and competency: An integrative review. *Worldviews on Evidence-Based Nursing, 17*(3), 239-245.

Cordaro, D.T., Brackett, M., Glass, L., & Anderson, C.L. (2016). Contentment: Perceived completeness across cultures and traditions. *Review of General Psychology, 20*(3).

Covey, S. (2004). *The 7 habits of highly effective people.* New York: Free Press.

Cristiano, S. (2019). Suppressed anger and response to facial expressions of emotion. *Dissertation*. ALL.1069.

Du, J., Huang, J., An, Y., & Xu, W. (2018). The relationship between stress and negative emotion: The mediating role of rumination. *Clinical Research and Trials.*

Duval, S., & Wicklund, R.A. (1972). *The theory of objective self awareness.* The University of Michigan Press.

Dworkin, J.D., Waldinger, R.J., Zimmerman, V., & Schulz, M.S. (2019). Capturing naturally occurring emotional suppression as it unfolds in couple interactions. *Emotion, 19*(7), 1224-1235.

Ekman, P. (1999). Basic emotion. In R. Dalgleish, & M.J. Power, *Handbook of cognition and emotion* (pp.45-60). New York: John Wiley & Sons Ltd.

Ekman, P., & Cordaro, D. (2011). What is meant by calling emotions basic. *Emotion Review,* 3(4), 364-370.

Ehli, S., Wolf, J., Newen, A., Schneider, S., & Voigt, B. (2020). Determining the function of social referencing: The role of familiarity and situational threat. *Frontiers in Psychology, 11.*

Eurich, T. (2018, January 4). *What self-awareness really is (and how to cultivate it)*. Retrieved January 21, 2022, from https://hbr.org/2018/01/what-self-awareness-really-is-and-how-to-cultivate-it

Fujiwara, Y., & Okamura, H. (2018). Hearing laughter improves the recovery process of the autonomic nervous system after a stress-loading task: A randomized controlled trial. *BioPsychoSocial Medicine.*

Ghai, S., Ghai, I., & Effenberg, A.O. (2018). "Low road" to rehabilitation: A perspective on subliminal sensory neuroprosthetics. *Neuropsychiatric Disease and Treatment, 14*, 301-307.

Green, Z.A., Noor, U., & Ahmed, F. (2020). The body-mind-spirit dimensions of wellness mediate dispositional gratitude and life satisfaction. *Journal of Happiness Studies, 21*, 3095-3119.

Haase, C.M., Holley, S.R., Bloch, L., Verstaen, A., & Levenson, R.W. (2016). Interpersonal emotional behaviors and physical health: A 20-year longitudinal study of long-term married couples. *Emotion, 16*(7), 965-977.

Huang, K. (2022). The review of anxiety and working memory. *Proceedings of the 2022 International Conference on Sport Science, Education and Social Development.*

Hwang, H., & Matsumoto, D. (2022). Functions of emotions. In R. Biswas-Diener & E. Diener (Eds.), *Noba textbook series: Psychology.* DEF Publishers.

Kaplanova, A. (2018). Self-esteem, anxiety and coping strategies to manage stress in ice hockey. *Acta Gymnica, 49*(1), 19-15.

Kerahrodi, J.G., & Michal, M. (2020). The fear-defense system, emotions, and oxidative stress. *Redox Biology, 37.*

Klinnert, M.D., & Sorce, J.F. (1983). Emotions as behavior regulators: Social referencing in infancy. In R. Plutchik & H. Kellerman (Eds.), *Emotion: Theory, research, and experience* (pp. 57-86). Academic Press.

Kowalczyk, M., Aydin, S., Gulcz, K., Mela, T., & Roszak, J. (2022). Creation of a sense of belonging questionnaire and its links to self-esteem and meaning in life in collectivistic and individualistic cultures. *Research Gate.*

La, I.S., & Yun, E.K. (2019). Effects of trait anger and anger expression on job satisfaction and burnout in preceptor nurses and newly graduated nurses: A dyadic analysis. *Asian Nursing Research, 13*(4), 242-248.

Lakhani, R. (2021, September). *Bouncing back: From stress to joy.* Retrieved February 7, 2022, from www.stress.org/bouncing-back-from-stress-to-joy

Levy, S., Heruti, I., & Avitsur, R. (2019). Physical injury, stress, and health: Protective role of dispositional optimism. *Stress & Health: Journal of the International Society for the Investigation of Stress, 35*(3), 267-276.

London, M., Sessa, V.I., & Shelley, L.A. (2023). Developing self-awareness: Learning process for self-and interpersonal growth. *Annual Review of Organizational Psychology and Organizational Behavior, 10*, 261-288.

Lyubomirsky, S., Sheldon, K.M., & Schkade, D. (2005). Pursing happiness: The architecture of sustainable change. *Review of General Psychology, 9*(2), 111-131.

Manee, F.M., Khoiee, S.A., & Eghbal, M.K. (2015). Comparison of the efficiency of self-awareness, stress management, effective communication life skill trainings on the social and academic adjustment of first-year students. *Research in Psychology and Behavioral Sciences, 3*(2), 18-24.

Masood, A., Kamran, F., Qaisar, S., & Ashraf, F. (2018). Anger, impulsivity, academic stress and suicidal risk in suicide ideators and normal cohorts. *Journal of Behavioral Sciences, 28*(2).

Mayo Clinic. (2018, May 14). *Anxiety disorders*. Retrieved February 1, 2022, from www.mayoclinic.org/diseases-conditions/anxiety/symptoms-causes/syc-20350961

Mayo Clinic. (2020, July 14). *Self-esteem: Take steps to feel better about yourself*. Retrieved February 1, 2022, from www.mayoclinic.org/healthy-lifestyle/adult-health/in-depth/self-esteem/art-20045374

Nes, R.B., & Roysamb, E. (2017). Happiness in behaviour genetics: An update on heritability and changeability. *Journal of Happiness Studies, 18*, 1533-1552.

Olyaiekhachic, R., Bozorgnejad, M., Haghani, S.H., Khayeri, F., & Seyedfatemi, N. (2020). Evaluating the effect of positive self-talk on job stress among nurses working in the emergency ward. *Iran Journal of Nursing, 33*(127), 89-102.

Pekrun, R., Lichtenfeld, S., Marsh, H.W., Murayama, K., & Goetz, T. (2017). Achievement emotions and academic performance: Longitudinal models of reciprocal effects. *Child Development, 88*(5), 1653-1670.

Piryaei, S., Mohebbi, M., Khademi Ashkzari, M., & Khademi Ashkzari, E. (2017). Academic stress and emotion regulation in the Iranian female students with high and low academic performance. *European Psychiatry, 41*(S1), S787-S788.

Puig-Perez, S., Hackett, R.A., Salvador, A., & Steptoe, A. (2017). Optimism moderates psychophysiological responses to stress in older people with type 2 diabetes. *Psychophysiology, 54*(4), 536-543.

Rector, N.A., & Roger, D. (1997). The stress buffering effects of self-esteem. *Personality and Individual Differences, 23*(5), 799-808.

Rozin, P., & Haidt, J. (2013). The domains of disgust and their origins: contrasting biological and cultural evolutionary accounts. *Trends in Cognitive Sciences,* 17(8), 367-368.

Salari, N., Hosseinian-Far, A., Jalali, R., Vaisi-Raygani, A., Rasoulpoor, S., Mohammadi, M., . . . Khaledi-Paveh, B. (2020). Prevalence of stress, anxiety, depression among the general population during the COVID-19 pandemic: A systematic review and meta-analysis. *Globalization and Health, 16*.

Shepherd, G., & Cant, M. (2020). Difficult to change? The difference between successful and not-so-successful participation in anger management groups. *Counselling and Psychotherapy Research, 20*(2), 214-223.

Sherman, A., Shavit, T., & Barokas, G. (2020). A dynamic model on happiness and exogenous wealth shock: The case of lottery winners. *Journal of Happiness Studies, 21*, 117-137.

Shirai, M., Soshi, T., & Suzuki, N. (2021). Knowledge of sadness: Emotion-related behavioral words differently encode loss and failure sadness. *Current Psychology, 40*(2), 895-909.

Soma, C.S., Baucom, B.R., Xiao, B., Butner, J.E., Hilpert, P., Narayanan, S., . . . Imel, Z.E. (2020). Coregulation of therapist and client emotion during psychotherapy. *Psychotherapy Research, 30*(5), 591-603.

Sorid, S.D., Wedell, E., Herchenroeder, L., & Bravo, A.J. (2021). Anxiety symptoms and alcohol-related problems among college students: A moderated-mediation model of rumination and emotion dysregulation. *Substance Use & Misuse, 56*(4), 471-478.

Sparks, N. (1999). *A walk to remember.* Warner Books.

Stangor, C., & Walinga, J. (2017). Positive emotions: The power of happiness. In J.A. Cummings & L. Sanders (Eds.), *Introduction to psychology*. Pressbooks. Retrieved from https://openpress.usask.ca/introductiontopsychology/chapter/positive-emotions-the-power-of-happiness

Tarmizi, R., Sugiharto, D.Y., & Sutoyo, A. (2020). The effectiveness of group counseling with self-management and cognitive restructuring techniques to reduce student aggression. *Jurnal Bimbingan Konseling, 9*(1).

Terrill, A.L., Ruiz, J.M., & Garofalo, J.P. (2010). Look on the bright side: Do the benefits of optimism depend on the social nature of the stressor? *Journal of Behavioral Medicine, 33*, 399-414.

Tolksdorf, N.F., Crawshaw, C.E., & Rohlfing, K.J. (2021). Comparing the effects of a different social partner (social robot vs human) on children's social referencing in interaction. *Frontiers in Education, 5*.

van der Wal, N., & Kok, R.N. (2019). Laughter-inducing therapies: Systematic review and meta-analysis. *Social Science & Medicine, 232*, 473-488.

Vo, T.N., Chiu, H.-Y., Chuang, Y.-H., & Huang, H.-C. (2022). Prevalence of stress and anxiety among nursing students: A systematic review and meta-analysis. *Nurse Educator*.

Watkins, E.R., & Roberts, H. (2020). Reflecting on rumination: Consequences, causes, mechanisms and treatment of rumination. *Behaviour Research and Therapy, 127*.

Willcox, G. (1982). The feeling wheel. *Transactional Analysis Journal, 12*(4), 274-276.

Wolff, J.M., Rospenda, K.M., & Colaneri, A.S. (2017). Sexual harassment, psychological distress, and problematic drinking behavior among college students: An examination of reciprocal causal relations. *The Journal of Sex Research, 54*(3), 362-373.

Yilmaz, H.A. (2022). Self-awareness and self-consciousness: A review from a social psychology perspective. *Current Approaches in Psychiatry, 14*(4), 437-445.

Yim, J. (2016). Therapeutic benefits of laughter in mental health: A theoretical review. *The Tohoku Journal of Experimental Medicine*, 243-249.

Yogeswaran, V., & El Morr, C. (2021). Effectiveness of online mindfulness interventions on medical students' mental health: a systematic review. *BMC Public Health, 21*(1).

Zarrin, S.A., Gracia, E., & Paixao, M.P. (2020). Prediction of academic procrastination by fear of failure and self-regulation. *Educational Sciences: Theory and Practice, 20*(3).

Zein, M.E., Wyart, V., & Grezes, J. (2015, December 29). *Anxiety dissociates the adaptive function of sensory and motor response enhancements to social threats*. Retrieved February 1, 2022, from https://elifesciences.org/articles/10274

Zsido, A.N., Arato, N., Ihasz, V., Basler, J., Matuz-Budai, T., Inhof, O., . . . Coelho, C.M. (2021). 'Finding an emotional face' revisited: Differences in own-age bias and the happiness superiority effect in children and young adults. *Frontiers in Psychology*.

## Chapter 6

Aarts, H. (2019). Goal setting theory and the mystery of setting goals. *Motivation Science, 106*.

Abdi, M., & Sharyati, A. (2019). Comparing the training effects of problem solving and coping skills with stress. *Global Journal of Psychology Research: New Trends and Current Issues, 9*(1).

Amabile, T.M. (1988). A model of creativity and innovation in organizations. *Research in Organizational Behavior, 10*(1), 123-167.

Belenky, D., & Nokes-Malach, T. (2012). Motivation and transfer: The role of mastery approach in goals in preparation for future learning. *Journal of the Learning Sciences, 21*(3), 399-432.

Bell, H., Limberg, D., Jacobson, L., & Super, J.T. (2014). Enhancing self-awareness through creative experiential-learning play-based activities. *Journal in Creativity in Mental Health, 9*(3), 399-414.

Bennett, D.A., Schneider, J.A., Buchman, A.S., Barnes, L.L., Boyle, P.A., & Wilson, R.S. (2013). Overview and findings from the Rush Memory and Aging Project. *Current Alzheimer Research, 9*(6), 646-663.

Buenaventura, M.D., Fajatin, J.M., Samaniego, A.M., Villagracia, C.J., & Reyes, R.C. (2022). Elements of realistic goal-setting model. *The Philippine Journal of Allied Health Sciences, 5*(2).

Campbell, A., Craig, T., & Collier-Reed, B. (2020). A framework for using learning theories to inform "growth mindset" activities. *International Journal of Mathematical Education in Science and Technology, 51*.

Crane, M.F., Searle, B.J., Kangas, M., & Nwiran, Y. (2019). How resilience is strengthened by exposure to stressors: The systematic self-reflection model of resilience strengthening. *Anxiety, Stress & Coping, 32*(1).

Creed, P.A., Sawitri, D.R., Hood, M., & Hu, S. (2020). Career goal setting and goal pursuit in young adults: The role of financial distress. *Journal of Career Development*.

Dweck, C.S. (2006). *Mindset: The new psychology of success*. Random House.

Ekechukwu, E.N., Nzeakuba, I.C., Dada, O.O., Nwankwo, K.O., Olowoyo, P., Utti, V.A., & Owolabi, M.O. (2021). Virtual reality, a neuroergonomic and neurorehabilitation tool for promoting neuroplasticity in stroke survivors: A systematic review with meta-analysis. *Proceedings of the 21st Congress of the International Ergonomics Association*, 495-508.

Feldman, R. (2020). What is resilience: An affiliative neuroscience approach. *World Psychiatry, 19*(2), 132-150.

Garcia-Leon, M.A., Perez-Marmol, J.M., Gonzalez-Perez, R., Garcia-Rios, M.C., & Peralta-Ramirez, M.I. (2019). Relationship between resilience and stress: Perceived stress, stressful life events, HPA axis response during a stressful task and hair cortisol. *Physiology & Behavior, 202*, 87-93.

Gilbert, P. (1998). The evolved basis and adaptive functions of cognitive distortions. *British Journal of Medicine, 71*, 447-463.

Harris, S. (2021, February 10). *Reframing our thoughts to have positive feelings*. Retrieved from www.allhealthnetwork.org/colorado-spirit/reframing-our-thoughts-to-have-positive-feelings/#:~:text=Reframing%20Negative%20Thoughts,them%20with%20more%20balanced%20thoughts

Jha, A., Bhoi, A.K., Saha, S.K., Singh, A., Mukherjee, S., Sharma, B., & Jayarani. (2021). Impact of select cognitive distortions on emotional stress. *Cognitive Computing for Risk Management*.

Joesl, M., Pu, Z., Wiegert, O., Oitzl, M.S., & Krugers, H.J. (2006). Learning under stress: How does it work? *Trends in Cognitive Sciences, 10*(4), 152-158.

Kartoshkina, Y. (2022). *Conversations on culture, brain, and cognitive shifts*. Routledge.

Lathan, G. (2011). *Organizational collaboration*. Routledge.

Legg, T.J. (2020, June 16). *6 ways to rewire your brain*. Retrieved June 19, 2022, from www.healthline.com/health/rewiring-your-brain

Limeri, L.B., Carter, N.T., Choe, J., Harper, H.G., Martin, H.R., Benton, A., & Dolan, E.L. (2020). Growing a growth mindset: Characterizing how and why undergraduate students' mindsets change. *International Journal of STEM, 7*(35).

Lin, T.-W., Tasai, S.-F., & Kuo, Y.-M. (2018). Physical exercise enhances neuroplasticity and delays Alzheimer's disease. *Brain Plasticity, 4*(1), 95-110.

Liu, J.J., Reed, M., & Vickers, K. (2019). Reframing the individual stress response: Balancing our knowledge of stress to improve responsivity to stress. *Stress & Health*.

Locke, E.A., & Lathan, G.P. (2019). The development of goal setting theory: A half century retrospective. *Motivation Science, 5*(2), 93-105.

Madu, V.N. (2019). Rewiring the brain for adaptive teaching and learning. *International Journal of Education and Research, 7*(9), 117-124.

McCarroll, C.J. (2017). Looking the past in the eye: Distortion in memory and the costs and benefits of recalling from an observer perspective. *Consciousness and Cognition, 49*, 322-332.

Melnyk, B.M. (2018). Intellectual wellbeing: Learn how to keep your mind nimble for lifelong health benefits. *American Nurse Today, 13*(5).

Morris, L. (2020). Relationship between the effects of positivity and high school students perceived levels of stress. *South Carolina Junior Academy of Sciences*.

Mosanta, M. (2019). Exploring cultural intelligence relationships with growth mindset, grit, coping and academic stress in the United Arab Emirates. *Positive Psychology, 5*.

Muller, F., & Greif, S. (2022). Insights through coaching. In S. Greif, H. Moller, W. Scholl, J. Passmore, & F. Muller (Eds.), *International handbook of evidence-based coaching* (pp. 471-485). Springer, Cham.

Murphy, F., & Gash, H. (2020). I can't yet and growth mindset. *Constructivist Foundations, 15*(2), 83-94.

Olszewska, A.M., Gaca, M., Herman, A.M., Jednorog, K., & Marchewka, A. (2021). How musical training shapes the adult brain: Predispositions and neuroplasticity. *Frontiers in Neuroscience, 15.*

Parvar, S.Y., Ghamari, N., Pezeshkian, F., & Shahriarirad, R. (2022). Prevalence of anxiety, depression, stress, and perceived stress and their relation with resilience during the COVID-19 pandemic, a cross-sectional study. *Health Science Reports, 5*(1).

Puderbaugh, M., & Emmady, P.D. (2022). *Neuroplasticity.* StatPearls.

Ramos, M.A., Figueiredo, P.S., & Pereira-Guizzo, C. (2018). Antecedents of innovation in industry: The impact of work environment factors on creative performance. *Innovation & Management Review, 15*(3), 269-285.

Rastogi, R., Arora, N., Tawar, P.S., Satya, S., Chaturvedi, D., & Vyas, P. (2018). Statistical analysis for effect of positive thinking on stress management and creative problem solving for adolescents. *5th International Conference on Computing for Sustainable Global Development.* Bharati Vidyapeeth's Institute on Computer Applications and Management.

Ren, F., & Zhang, J. (2015). Job stressors, organizational innovation climate, and employees' innovative behavior. *Creativity Research Journal, 27*(1), 16-23.

Renner, F., Murphy, F.C., Ji, J.L., Manly, T., & Holmes, E.A. (2019). Mental imagery as a 'motivational amplifier' to promote activities. *Behavior Research and Therapy, 114*, 51-59.

Ritter, S.M., Gu, X., Crijns, M., & Biekens, P. (2020). Fostering students' creative thinking skills by means of a one-year creativity training program. *PLoS ONE, 15*(3).

Ronkainen, R., Kuusisto, E., & Tirri, K. (2019). Growth mindset in teaching: A case study of a Finnish elementary school teacher. *International Journal of Learning, Teaching and Educational Research.*

Rossi, E., Cheng, H., Kroll, J.F., Diaz, M.T., & Newman, S.D. (2017). Changes in white-matter connectivity in late second language learners: Evidence from diffusion tensor imaging. *Frontiers in Psychology.*

Setiawati, Y., Wahyuhadi, J., Joestandari, F., Maramis, M.M., & Atika, A. (2021). Anxiety and resilience of healthcare workers during COVID-19 pandemic in Indonesia. *Journal of Multidisciplinary Healthcare, 14.*

Sharouni, T.-J., McClymont, R.G., Alcorn, C., Rebar, A.L., Law, K.H., Jackson, B., . . . Dimmock, J.A. (2022). Within- and between-person relationships between spontaneous self-affirmations, coping style, and wellbeing. *Stress & Health.*

Skalski, S.B., Konaszewski, K., Bussing, A., & Surzykiewics, J. (2022). Resilience and mental well-being during the COVID-19 pandemic: Serial mediation by persistent thinking and anxiety about coronavirus. *Frontiers in Psychiatry, 12.*

Smiley, P.A., Buttitta, K.V., Chung, S.Y., Dubon, V.X., & Chang, L.K. (2016). Mediation models of implicit theories and achievement goals predict planning and withdrawal after failure. *Motivation and Emotion, 40*(6), 878-894.

Surmai, M., & Duff, E. (2022). Cognitive behavioural therapy: A strategy to address pandemic-induced anxiety. *The Journal for Nurse Practitioners, 18*(1), 36-39.

Vaisvaser, S. (2021). Creative therapies, complex childhood trauma, and neurological improvement: How the arts can enhance neuroplasticity: A literature review. *Frontiers in Psychology.*

Walsh, P., Owen, P.A., Mustafa, N., & Beech, R. (2020). Learning and teaching approaches promoting resilience in student nurses: An integrated review of the literature. *Nurse Education in Practice, 45.*

Wang, X., Duan, H., Kan, Y., Wang, B., Qi, S., & Hu, W. (2019). The creative thinking process influenced by acute stress in humans: An electroencephalography study. *The International Journal on the Biology of Stress, 22*(4).

Weintraub, J., Cassell, D., & DePatie, T.P. (2021). Nudging flow through 'SMART' goal setting to decrease stress, increase engagement, and increase performance at work. *Journal of Occupational and Organizational Psychology, 94*, 230-258.

Wickramarathne, P.C., Phuoc, J.C., & Albattat, A.R. (2020). A review of wellness dimension models: For the advancement of the society. *European Journal of Social Sciences Studies, 5*(1).

Wignall, N. (2018, December 5). *Divergent thinking: The mental muscle behind consistent creativity.* Retrieved from nickwignall.com/divergent-thinking/

Yadolahzadeh, A. (2020). The role of mental imagery and stress management training in the performance of female swimmers. *Atena Journal of Sport Sciences.*

Yu, W., & Wang, Z. (2022). Dual influencing paths of time pressure on employee creativity. *International Journal of Stress Management.*

Zechner, M.R., Pratt, C.W., Barrett, N.M., Dreker, M.R., & Santos, S. (2019). Multi-dimensional wellness interventions for older adults with serious mental illness: A systematic literature review. *Psychiatric Rehabilitation Journal, 42*(4), 382-393.

Zhang, X.X., Tian, Y., Wang, Z.T., Ma, Y.H., Tan, L., & Yu, J.T. (2021). The epidemiology of Alzheimer's disease modifiable risk factors and prevention. *The Journal of Prevention of Alzheimer's Disease, 8*, 313-321.

## Chapter 7

Agbaria, Q., & Mokh, A.A. (2022). Coping with stress during the coronavirus outbreak: The contribution of the big five personality traits and social support. *International Journal of Mental Health and Addiction, 20*, 1854-1872.

Baroona, P. (2019). The impact of non-verbal communication in the learning process. *Journal of Education, Linguistics, Literature and Language Teaching,* (2), 2.

Berretz, G., Cebula, C., Wortelmann, B.M., Papadopoulou, P., Wolf, O.R., Ocklenburg, S., & Packheiser, J. (2022). Romantic partner embraces reduce cortisol release after acute stress induction in women but not in men. *PLoS ONE.*

Bibi, A., & Khalid, M.A. (2020). Death, anxiety, perceived social support, and demographic correlates of patients with breast cancer in Pakistan. *Death Studies, 44*(12), 787-792.

Bourassa, K.J., Ruiz, J.M., & Sbarra, D.A. (2019). The impact of physical proximity and attachment working models on cardiovascular reactivity: Comparing mental activation and romantic partner presence. *Psychophysiology, 56*(5).

Brauer, K., Proyer, R.T., & Chick, G. (2021). Adult playfulness: An update to an understudied individual differences variable and its role in romantic life. *Social and Personality Psychology Compass, 15*(4).

Brenner, R.E., Heath, P.J., Vogel, D.L., & Crede, M. (2017). Two is more valid than one: Examining the factor structure of the self-compassion scale. *Journal of Counseling Psychology, 64*, 696-707.

Brinkley-Rubinstein, L., Sivaraman, J., Rosen, D.L., Cloud, D.H., Junker, G., Proescholdbell, S., . . . Ranapurwala, S. (2019). Association of restrictive housing during incarceration with mortality after release. *JAMA Network Open, 2*(10).

Brkjacic, T., Sucic, I., Lucic, L., Tkalic, R.G., & Lipovcan, L.K. (2020). The beginning, the end, and all the happiness in between: Pet owners' wellbeing from pet acquisition to death. *Anthrozoos, 33*.

Buchholz, K. (2022, April 29). *Which countries spend the most time on social media?* Retrieved July 7, 2022, from www.weforum.org/agenda/2022/04/social-media-internet-connectivity/#:~:text=Global%20internet%20users%20spend%20an,by%20country%2C%20a%20study%20finds

Chadick, C., Batastini, A., Levulis, S., & Morgan, R. (2018). The psychological impact of solitary: A longitudinal comparison of general population and long-term administratively segregated male inmates. *Legal and Criminological Psychology, 23*(2), 101-116.

Chang, C.-M., Chou, Y.-H., Hsieh, H.-H., & Huange, C.-K. (2020). The effect of participation motivations on interpersonal relationships and learning achievement of female college students in sports club: Moderating the role of club involvement. *International Journal of Environmental Research and Public Health, 17*(18).

Chickering, A.W., & Reisser, L. (1993). *Education and identity.* San Francisco: Jossey-Bass.

Counts, C.J., & John-Henderson, N.A. (2020). Risk in childhood family environments and loneliness in college students: Implications for health. *Journal of American College Health, 68*(4), 381-386.

Department of Communication, Indiana State University. (2016). *Introduction to public communication.* Indiana State University.

Doron, J., Trouillet, R., Gana, K., Boiche, J., Neveu, D., & Ninot, G. (2014). Examination of the hierarchical structure of the BRIEF COPE in a French sample: Empirical and theoretical convergences. *Journal of Personality Assessment, 96*(5), 567-575.

Dreisoerner, A., Junker, N.M., Schlotz, W., Heimrich, J., Bloemeke, S., Ditzen, B., & Dick, R.V. (2021). Self-soothing touch and being hugged reduce cortisol response to stress: A randomized controlled trial on stress, physical touch, and social identity. *Comprehensive Psychoneuroendocrinology, 8*.

Ein, N., Li, L., & Vickers, K. (2018). The effect of pet therapy on the physiological and subjective stress response: A meta-analysis. *Stress Health, 34*(4), 477-489.

Every-Palmer, S., Jenkins, M., Gendall, P., Joek, J., Beaglehole, B., Bell, C., . . . Stanley, J. (2020). Psychological distress, anxiety, family violence, suicidality, and wellbeing in New Zealand during the COVID-19 lockdown: A cross-sectional study. *PLoS ONE, 15*(11).

Freedman, A., & Nicolle, J. (2020). Social isolation and loneliness: The new geriatric giants. *Canadian Family Physician, 66*(3), 176-182.

Friedman, A., Homma, D., Bloem, B., Gibb, L.G., Amemori, K.-I., Hu, D., . . . Arana, S.E. (2017). Chronic stress alters striosome-circuit dynamics, leading to aberrant decision-making. *Cell, 171*(5), 1191-1205.

Garcia-Leon, M.A., Perez-Marmol, J., Gonzalez-Perez, R., Garcia-Rios, M.D., & Peralta-Ramirez, M.I. (2019). Relationship between resilience and stress: Perceived stress, stressful life events, HPA axis response during a stress task and hair cortisol. *Physiology & Behavior, 202*, 87-93.

Gellert, P., Hausler, A., Suhr, R., Gholami, M., Rapp, M., Kuhlmey, A., & Nordheim, J. (2018). Testing the stress-buffering hypothesis of social support in couples coping with early-stage dementia. *PLoS ONE, 13*(1).

Gifford, A., Fouche, H., & Beadle, J. (2021). Effects of loneliness and stress management on perceived stress in older adults. *Innovation in Aging*, 924.

Gottman, J.M. (1994). *What predicts divorce? The relationship between marital processes and marital outcomes.* Lawrence Erlbaum.

Griffiths, M.D., Kuss, D.J., & Demetrovics, Z. (2014). Social networking addiction: An overview of preliminary findings. In K.P. Rosenberg & L.C. Feder (Eds.), *Behavioral addictions criteria, evidence, and treatment.* London, UK: Academic Press.

Heerde, J.A., & Hemphill, S.A. (2018). Examination of associations between informal help-seeking behavior, social support, and adolescent psychosocial outcomes: A meta-analysis. *Developmental Review, 47*, 44-62.

Herring, T. (2020, December 8). *The research is clear: Solitary confinement causes long-lasting harm.* Retrieved June 29, 2022, from www.prisonpolicy.org/blog/2020/12/08/solitary_symposium

House, J.S. (1981). *Work stress and social support.* Addison-Wesley.

Howard, L. (2018, February 22). *Here's why sharing passwords with your partner can be so risky.* Retrieved from www.bustle.com/p/should-partners-share-passwords-in-a-relationship-heres-why-its-not-always-a-good-idea-according-to-experts-8296206

Hu, T., Zheng, X., & Huang, M. (2020). Absence and presence of human interaction: The relationship between loneliness and empathy. *Frontiers in Psychology, 11*.

Hysi, G. (2015). Conflict resolution styles and health outcomes in married couples: A systematic literature review. *ICRAE Conference Paper Proceedings*.

Ionut, C. (2020). Dealing with conflicts in social work: A discussion on Thomas-Kilmann model of applicability in social work. *Revista de Asistenta Sociala, 19*(2), 33-44.

Jessen, M.A., Pallesen, A.V., Kriegbaum, M., & Kristiansen, M. (2018). The association between loneliness and health—a survey-based study among middle aged and older adults in Denmark. *Aging & Mental Health, 22*(10), 1338-1343.

Kalenkoski, C.M., & Korankye, T. (2021). Enriching lives: How spending time with pets is related to the experiential well-being of older Americans. *Applied Research in Quality of Life, 17*, 489-510.

Kapoor, R. (2020). Psychiatrists and solitary confinement in US prisons. *The International Journal of Forensic Psychotherapy, 2*(2), 127-134.

Kline, J.A., VanRyzin, K., Davis, J.C., Parra, J.A., Todd, M.L., Shaw, L.L., . . . Beck, A.M. (2020). Randomized trial of therapy dogs versus deliberate coloring (art therapy) to reduce stress in emergency medicine providers. *Academic Emergency Medicine, 27*(4), 266-275.

Kothgassner, O.D., Goreis, A., Kafka, J.X., Kaufmann, M., Attender, K., Buetl, L., . . . Felnhofer, A. (2019). Virtual social support buffers stress response: An experimental comparison of real-life and virtual support prior to a social stressor. *Journal of Behavior Therapy and Experimental Psychiatry, 63*, 57-65.

Krhae, C., Paloyelis, Y., Condon, H., Jenkinson, P.M., Williams, S.C., & Fotopoulou, A. (2015). Attachment style moderates partner presence effects on pain: A laser-evoked potentials study. *Social Cognitive and Affective Neuroscience, 10*(8), 1030-1037.

Lau, K.K., Randall, A.K., Duran, N.D., & Tao, C. (2018). Examining the effects of couples' real-time stress and coping process on interaction quality: Language use as a mediator. *Frontiers in Psychology, 9*.

Lazarus, R.S., & Folkman, S. (1984). *Stress, appraisal, and coping.* Springer Publishing Company.

Lin, C.-Y., Namdar, P., Griffiths, M.D., & Pakpour, A.H. (2021). Mediated roles of generalized trust and perceived social support in the effects of problematic social media use on mental health: A cross sectional study. *Health Expectations, 24*(1), 165-173.

Madigan, D.J., Rumbold, J.L., Gerber, M., & Nicholls, A.R. (2020). Coping tendencies and changes in athlete burnout over time. *Psychology of Sport and Exercise, 48*.

Mathews, J., & Shajan, S. (2018). Interpersonal communication: A stress reducing remedy. *International Journal of New Technology and Research, 4*(11), 71-72.

Maymon, R., Hall, N.C., & Harley, J.M. (2019). Supporting first-year students during the transition to higher education: The importance of quality and source of received support for student well-being. *Student Success, 10*(3).

McLean, L., Gaul, D., & Penco, R. (2022). Perceived social support and stress: A study of 1st year students in Ireland. *International Journal of Mental Health and Addiction*, 1-21.

McNaughton-Cassill, M.E., Lopez, S., Knight, C., Perrotte, J., Mireles, N., Cassill, C.K., . . . Cassill, A. (2021). Social support, coping, life satisfaction, and academic success among college students. *Psi Chi Journal of Psychological Research, 26*(2), 150-156.

Mertika, A., Mitskidou, P., & Stalikas, A. (2020). "Positive relationships" and their impact on wellbeing: A review of current literature. *Psychology, 25*(1), 115-127.

Mosadeghrad, A.M., & Mojbafan, A. (2019). Conflict and conflict management in hospitals. *International Journal of Health Care Quality Assurance, 32*(3), 550-561.

Orellana, M. (2019). The anti-stress effects of therapy dogs on college students. *Psychoneuroendocrinology, 100*.

Ortiz, D.V., Horner, P.S., Sato, M., Nelson, A., & Lamas, D. (2023). Separate but not divided: Art-based inquiry on attachment and resiliency among displaced Puerto Rican families in Central Florida post Hurricane Maria. *International Journal of Disaster Risk Reduction, 85*.

Ozamiz-Etxebarria, N., Mondragon, N.I., Santamaria, M., & Gorrotxategi, M.P. (2020). Psychological symptoms during the two stages of lockdown in response to the COVID-19 outbreak: An investigation in a sample of citizens in Northern Spain. *Frontiers in Psychology, 11*, 1491.

Pendry, P., & Vandagriff, J.L. (2019). Animal visitation program (AVP) reduces cortisol levels of university students: A randomized controlled trial. *AERA Open, 5*(2).

Pietrabissa, G., & Simpson, S.G. (2020). Psychological consequences of social isolation during COVID-19 outbreak. *Frontiers in Psychology, 11*.

Pilcher, J.J., & Bryant, S.A. (2016). Implications of social support as a self-control resource. *Frontiers in Behavioral Neuroscience, 10*, 228.

Pretorius, T.B., & Padmanabhanunni, A. (2023). Toward a positive life beyond COVID-19: Problem-solving appraisal as a resistance resource in the relationship between stress and well-being in students. *Healthcare, 11*(3).

Reiter, K., Ventura, J., Lovell, D., Augustine, D., Barragan, M., Blair, T., . . . Strong, J. (2020). Psychological distress in solitary confinement: Symptoms, severity, and prevalence in the United States, 2017-2018. *American Journal of Public Health, 110*(S1), S56-S62.

Reynolds, E.K., Schreiber, W.M., Geisel, K., MacPherson, L., Ernst, M., & Lejuez, C.W. (2013). Influence of social stress on risk-taking behavior in adolescents. *Journal of Anxiety Disorders, 27*(3), 272-227.

Riu, J.R., & Guo, J. (2022). Differentiating the stress buffering functions of perceived versus received social support. *Current Psychology*, 1-11.

Rueda, H.A., Yndo, M., Williams, L.R., & Shorey, R.C. (2018). Does Gottman's marital communication conceptualization inform teen dating violence? Communication skill deficits analyzed across three samples of diverse adolescents. *Journal of Interpersonal Violence, 36*(11-12).

Selkie, E., Adkins, V., Masters, E., Bajpai, A., & Shumer, D. (2020). Transgender adolescents' uses of social media for social support. *Journal of Adolescent Health, 66*(3), 275-280.

Sirois, F.M. (2023). Procrastination and stress: A conceptual review of why context matters. *International Journal of Environmental Research and Public Health, 20*(6).

Skelton, K.R., Evans, R., LaChenaye, J., Amsbary, J., Wingate, M., & Talbott, L. (2018). Exploring social media group use among breastfeeding mothers: Qualitative analysis. *JMIR Pediatrics and Parenting, 1*(2).

Skelton, K., Evans, R., & LaChenaye, J. (2020). Hidden communities of practice in social media groups: Mixed methods study. *JMIR Pediatrics and Parenting, 3*(1).

Smithsonian Institution. (2020, October 27). *Human characteristics: Social life.* Retrieved June 29, 2022, from https://humanorigins.si.edu/human-characteristics/social-life#:~:-text=Over%20time%2C%20early%20humans%20began,social%20lives%20of%20modern%20humans

Spohr, S.A., Suzuki, S., Marshall, B., Tasman, F.S., & Walters, S.T. (2016). Social support quality and availability affects risk behaviors in offenders. *Health & Justice, 4,* 2.

Stanislawski, K. (2019). The coping circumplex model: An integrative model of the structure of coping with stress. *Frontiers in Psychology, 10.*

Suciu, P. (2021, June 24). *Americans spent on average more than 1,300 hours on social media last year.* Retrieved July 7, 2022, from www.forbes.com/sites/petersuciu/2021/06/24/americans-spent-more-than-1300-hours-on-social-media/?sh=482641dc2547

Szkody, E., & McKinney, C. (2019). Stress-buffering effects of social support on depressive problems: Perceived vs. received social support and moderation by parental depression. *Journal of Child and Family Studies, 28,* 2209-2219.

Tamir, D.I., Templeton, E.M., Ward, A.F., & Zaki, J. (2018). Media usage diminished memory for experiences. *Journal of Experimental Social Psychology, 76,* 161-168.

Thomas, K.W., & Kilmann, R.H. (1976). Thomas-Kilmann conflict mode instrument. *Group & Organization Studies, 1*(2), 249-251.

Tiggemann, M., & Anderberg, I. (2019). Social media is not real: The effect of 'Instagram vs reality' images on women's social comparison and body image. *New Media & Society, 22*(12).

Twenge, J.M., & Martin, G.N. (2020). Gender differences in associations between digital media use and psychological well-being: Evidence from three large datasets. *Journal of Adolescence, 79,* 91-102.

Umberson, D., & Montez, J.K. (2010). Social relationships and health: A flashpoint for health policy. *Journal of Health and Social Behavior, 51*(Suppl. 1), S54-S66. https://doi.org/10.1177/0022146510383501

Vandenbosch, L., Fardouly, J., & Tiggemann, M. (2022). Social media and body image: Recent trends and future directions. *Current Opinion in Psychology, 45.*

Wang, X., Cai, L., Wian, J., & Peng, J. (2014). Social support moderates stress effects on depression. *International Journal of Mental Health Systems, 8*(1).

Ward, M., May, P., Normand, C., Kenny, R.A., & Nolan, A. (2021). Mortality risk associated with combinations of loneliness and social isolation. Findings from the Irish Longitudinal Study on Ageing (TILDA). *Age and Ageing, 50*(4), 1329-1335.

Wilksch, S.M., O'Shea, A., Ho, P., Byrne, S., & Wade, T.D. (2020). The relationship between social media use and disordered eating in young adolescents. *The International Journal of Eating Disorders, 53*(1), 96-106.

Wu, F., Ren, Z., Wang, Q., He, M., Xiong, W., Ma, G., . . . Zhang, X. (2021). The relationship between job stress and job burnout: The mediating effects of perceived social support and job satisfaction. *Psychology, Health & Medicine, 26*(2).

Young, J., Pritchard, R., Nottle, C., & Banwell, H. (2020). Pets, touch, and COVID-19: Health benefits from non-human touch through times of stress. *Journal of Behavioral Economics for Policy, 4*(2), 25-33.

Zemp, M., Nussbeck, F.W., Cummings, E.M., & Bodenmann, G. (2017). The spillover of child-related stress into parents' relationship mediated by couple communication. *Family Relations, 66*(2), 317-330.

## Chapter 8

Aknin, L.B., & Whillans, A.V. (2020). Helping and happiness: A review and guide for public policy. *Social Issues and Policy Review, 15*(1), 3-34.

Allen, S. (2018). *The science of gratitude.* Greater Good Science at Berkeley.

Anchour, M., Muhamad, A., Syihab, A.H., Nor, M.R., & Yusoff, M.Y. (2021). Prayer moderating job stress among Muslim nursing staff at the University of Malaya Medical Centre. *Journal of Religion and Health, 60,* 202-220.

Ashwini, U.R., & Indumathy, J. (2018). Altruism and general well-being among adults. *International Journal of Research in Social Sciences, 8*(4), 528-540.

Balboni, T.A., VanderWeele, T.J., Doan-Soares, S.D., Long, K.N., Ferrell, B.R., Fitchett, G., . . . Koh, H.K. (2022). Spirituality in serious illness and health. *Journal of the American Medical Association, 328*(2), 184-197.

Banks, R. (1980). Health and the spiritual dimension: Relationships and implications for professional preparation programs. *Journal of School Health, 50*(4), 195-202.

Bates, G.W., Elphinstone, B., & Whitehead, R. (2021). Self-compassion and emotional regulation as predictors of social anxiety. *Psychology & Psychotherapy: Theory, Research and Practice, 94*(3), 426-442.

Bennett, M.R., & Einolf, C.J. (2017). Religion, altruism, and helping strangers: A multilevel analysis on 126 countries. *Journal of the Scientific Study of Religion, 56*(2), 323-341.

Bonini, L., Rotunno, C., Arcuri, E., & Gallese, V. (2022). Mirror neurons 30 years later: Implications and applications. *Trends in Cognitive Sciences, 26*(9), 767-781.

Bravin, A.M., Dos Santos Trettene, A., Andrade, L.G., & Popim, R.C. (2019). Benefits of spirituality and/or religiosity in patients with chronic kidney disease: An integrative review. *Revista Brasileira de Enfermagem, 72*(2).

Carson, J.W., Keefe, F.J., Lynch, T.R., Carson, K.M., Goli, V., Fras, A.M., & Thorp, S.R. (2005). Loving-kindness meditation for chronic low back pain: Results from a pilot trial. *Journal of Holistic Nursing, 23*(3).

Chishima, Y., Mizuno, M., Sugawara, D., & Miyagawa, Y. (2018). The influence of self-compassion on cognitive appraisals and coping with stressful events. *Mindfulness, 9*, 1907-1915.

Chovanec, M.G. (2020). Transforming into men who matter: Increasing empathy in domestic abuse treatment. *Australian Social Work, 73*(3), 296-308.

Corso, L.D., Carlo, A.D., Carluccio, F., Colledani, D., & Falco, A. (2020). Employee burnout and positive dimensions of well-being: A latent workplace spirituality profile analysis. *PLoS ONE, 15*(11).

De Silva, P.N. (2022). Neurobiological and epigenetic perspectives on hedonism, altruism, and conscience. *BJPsych Advances, 29*(3).

Deb, S., Thomas, S., Bose, A., & Aswathi, T. (2020). Happiness, meaning, and satisfaction in life as perceived by Indian university students and their association with spirituality. *Journal of Religion and Health, 59*(5), 2469-2485.

Dillane, M., Murphy, M., O'Sullivan, D., & Di Blasi, Z. (2021). Pain is inevitable, but suffering is optional: A cross-sectional study of positive psychology variables in chronic back pain. *European Journal of Applied Positive Psychology, 5*(16).

Dong, S., Dong, Q., & Chen, H. (2022). Mothers' parenting stress, depression, marital conflict, and marital satisfaction: The moderating effect of fathers' empathy tendency. *Journal of Affective Disorders*, 682-690.

Ekman, P. (2010). Darwin's compassionate view of human nature. *JAMA Network, 303*(6), 557-558.

Esch, T., & Stefano, G.B. (2004). The neurobiology of pleasure, reward processes, addition and their health implication. *Neuroendocrinology, 25*(4), 235-251.

Fisher, J. (2011). The four domain model: Connecting spirituality, health, and wellbeing. *Religions, 2*, 17-28.

Ghiglieri, M., McAndrew, R., Baum, C.M., & Taff, S.D. (2021). Identity, civic engagement, and altruism: A phenomenological exploration of activity engagement in older adults. *Scandinavian Journal of Occupational Therapy, 28*(3), 225-238.

Gilbert, P. (2019). Explorations into the nature and function of compassion. *Current Opinion in Psychology, 28*, 108-114.

Gu, Y., Ocampo, J.M., Algoe, S.B., & Oveis, C. (2022). Gratitude expressions improve teammates' cardiovascular stress responses. *Journal of Experimental Psychology: General, 151*(12), 3281-3291.

Hagelquist, J.O. (2017). *The mentalization guidebook*. Routledge.

Han, K.H., Sun, C.K., Cheng, Y.S., Chung, W., & Kao, C.C. (2022). Impacts of extrinsic and intrinsic factors on psychiatric nurses' spiritual care attitudes. *Journal of Psychiatric and Mental Health Nursing, 30*(3), 481-491.

Hartanto, A., Lee, S.T., & Yong, J.C. (2018). Dispositional gratitude moderations the association between socioeconomic status and Interleukin-6. *Scientific Reports, 9*(1), 802.

Heyn, M. (2018). *What is spiritual health and why it matters*. Retrieved July 11, 2022, from https://www.spirituallyhealthyyou.com/definespiritualhealth/.

Hess, J.L., Strobel, J., & Pan, R. (2016). Voices from the workplace: Practitioners' perspectives on the role of empathy and care within engineering. *Engineering Studies, 8*(3), 212-242.

Heyes, C., & Catmur, C. (2022). What happened to mirror neurons? *Perspectives on Psychological Science, 17*(1), 153-168.

Huang, J., Shi, H., & Lui, W. (2018). Emotional intelligence and subjective well-being: Altruistic behavior as a mediator. *Social Behavior and Personality: An International Journal, 46*(5), 749-758.

Huang, N., Qui, S., Alizadeh, A., & Wu, H. (2020). How incivility and academic stress influence psychological health among college students: The moderating role of gratitude. *International Journal of Environmental Research and Public Health, 17*(9).

Hughes, P. (2021). Do religion and spirituality make a contribution to the public good? The association of religion and spirituality with volunteering. *Journal for the Academic Study of Religion, 34*(1), 96-121.

Hunt, P., Denieffe, S., & Gooney, M. (2019). Running on empathy: Relationship of empathy to compassion satisfaction and compassion fatigue in cancer healthcare professionals. *European Journal of Cancer Care, 28*(5).

Joseph, R. (2021). *Yahweh, my shepherd and my king*. Xlibris Corporation.

Karakilic, A., Kizildag, S., Kandis, S., Guvendi, G., Koc, B., Camsari, G.B., . . . Uysal, N. (2018). The effects of acute foot shock stress on empathy level in rats. *Behavioural Brain Research, 349*(3), 31-36.

Kilner, J.M., & Lemon, R.N. (2013). What we know currently about mirror neurons. *Current Biology, 23*(23), R1057-R1062.

Knabb, J.J., Vazquez, V.E., Wang, K.T., & Pate, R.A. (2021). The Christian Gratitude Scale: An emic approach to measuring thankfulness in every season of life. *Spirituality in Clinical Practice*.

Konrath, S.K., O'Brien, E.H., & Hsing, C. (2010). Changes in dispositional empathy in American college students over time: A meta-analysis. *Personality and Social Psychology Review*, 180-198.

Kulik, L. (2018). Through adversity comes strength: Volunteering and self-esteem among people with physical disabilities. *Voluntas, 29*, 174-189.

Kuswartanti, D.R. (2020). How positive thinking can affect stress in moms who worked during pandemic corona? *International Journal of Global Operations Research, 1*(4), 136-142.

LaBarbera, R., & Hetzel, J. (2016). Christian educators' use of prayer to cope with stress. *Journal of Religion and Health, 55*(4), 1433-1448.

Levin, J. (2016). Prevalence and religious predictors of healing prayer use in the USA: Findings from the Baylor Religion Survey. *Journal of Religion and Health, 55*, 1136-1158.

Li, Y., Deng, J., Lou, X., Wang, H., & Wang, Y. (2019). A daily diary study of the relationship among daily self-compassion, perceived stress and health promoting behaviours. *International Journal of Psychology, 55*(3), 364-372.

Luyten, P., Campbell, C., Allison, E., & Fonagy, P. (2020). The mentalizing approach to psychopathology. *Annual Review of Clinical Psychology, 16*, 297-325.

Mahurin-Smith, J., & Beck, A. (2021). Caregivers' experiences of infant feeding problems: The role of self-compassion and stress management. *American Journal of Speech-Language Pathology, 30*(4).

May, R.W., Cooper, A.N., & Fincham, F.D. (2020). Prayer in marriage to improve wellness: Relationship quality and cardiovascular functioning. *Journal of Religion and Health, 59*, 2990-3003.

McClintock, C.H., Worhunsky, P.D., Balodis, I.M., Sinha, R., Miller, L., & Potenza, M.N. (2019). How spirituality may mitigate against stress and related mental disorders: A review and preliminary neurobiological evidence. *Current Behavioral Neuroscience Reports*, 253-262.

Miller, L., Wickramaratne, P., Hao, X., McClintock, C.H., Pan, L., Svob, C., & Weissman, M.M. (2021). Altruism and 'love of neighbor' offer neuroanatomical protection against depression. *Psychiatry Research: Neuroimaging, 315*(30).

Murphy, J.L., & Rafie, S. (2021, December 7). *5 exercises to ease chronic pain with gratitude*. Retrieved July 13, 2022, from www.psychologytoday.com/us/blog/ease-pain/202112/5-exercises-ease-chronic-pain-gratitude

Nezlek, J.B., Krejtz, I., Rusanowka, M., & Holas, P. (2019). With-in person relationships among daily gratitude, well-being, stress and positive experiences. *Journal of Happiness Studies, 20*, 883-898.

Odrovakavula, L., & Mohammadnezhad, M. (2022). Psychological and spiritual dimensions of wellness among high school students: A descriptive study in Fiji. *International Journal of Child & Adolescent Health, 15*(1), 41-48.

Park, C.L. (2021). Intrinsic and extrinsic religious motivation: Retrospect and prospect. *The International Journal for the Psychology of Religion, 31*(3), 213-222.

Pong, H.-K. (2017). The relationship between the spiritual well-being of university students in Hong Kong and their academic performance. *International Journal of Children's Spirituality, 22*(3-4), 329-351.

Raghuveer, P., Bhatia, R., & Sachith, M. (2022). A cross-sectional study on assessment of spiritual health and its associated factors among undergraduate students in a medical college in Mangalore, Karnataka. *F1000 Research, 11*.

Raine, A., & Chen, F.R. (2018). The cognitive, affective, and somatic empathy scales (CASES) for children. *Journal of Clinical Child & Adolescent Psychology, 47*(1), 24-37.

Raine, L., & Page, D. (2015, August). *Americans' view on mobile etiquette*. Retrieved from www.pewinternet.org/2015/08/26/americans-views-on-mobile-etiquette

Ramsay, J.E., Tong, E.M., Chowdhury, A., & Ho, M.-H.R. (2019). Teleological explanation and positive emotion serially mediate the effect of religion on well-being. *Journal of Personality, 87*(3), 676-689.

Shoshani, A., Braverman, S., & Meirow, G. (2021). Video games and close relations: Attachment and empathy as predictors of children's and adolescents' video game social play and socio-emotional functioning. *Computers in Human Behavior, 114*.

Simpson, E.A., Murray, L., Paukner, A., & Ferrari, P.F. (2014). The mirror neuron system as revealed through neonatal imitation: Presence from birth, predictive power and evidence of plasticity. *Philosophical Transactions of the Royal Society B. Biological Sciences, 369*(1644).

Soguilon, W.K. (2022). A study on Catholic religious practices in the seminary as stress coping mechanisms and its effect on the well-being of grade 11 seminarians. *Academia Letters*.

Stewart, C., Whitworth, J., & Lawrence, S.A. (2022). The relationship between spirituality and empathy to attitudes towards addiction. *Journal of Social Work Practice in the Addictions, 22*.

Stockigy, B., Jeserich, F., Walach, H., Elies, M., Brinkhaus, B., & Teut, M. (2021). Experiences and perceived effects of Rosary praying: A qualitative study. *Journal of Religion and Health*, 3886-3906.

Thonhauser, G. (2022). Towards a taxonomy of collective emotions. *Emotion Review, 14*(1).

Villani, D., Sorgente, A., Iannello, P., & Antonietii, A. (2019). The role of spirituality and religiosity in subjective well-being of individuals with different religious studies. *Frontiers in Psychology*.

van Vliet, M., Jong, M., & Jong, M.C. (2017). Long-term benefits by a mind-body medicine skills course on perceived stress and empathy among medical and nursing students. *Medical Teacher, 39*(7), 710-719.

Zhang, Y., Xue, G., Chen, Y., An, K., & Chen, L. (2020). Factors related to spiritual health in Chinese haemodialysis patients: A multicentre cross-sectional study. *Nursing Open, 7*(5), 1536-1543.

## Chapter 9

Aidala, A.A., Wilson, M.G., Shubert, V., Gogolishvili, D., Globerman, J., Rueda, S., . . . Rourke, S.B. (2016). Housing status, medical care, and health outcomes among people living with HIV/AIDS: A systematic review. *American Journal of Public Health, 106*(1).

Al-Ayash, A., Kane, R.T., Smith, D., & Green-Armytage, P. (2016). The influence of color on student emotion, heart rate, and performance in learning environments. *Color Research and Application, 41*(2), 196-205.

American Academy of Ophthalmology. (2022, January 19). *Digital devices and your eyes*. Retrieved from www.aao.org/eye-health/tips-prevention/digital-devices-your-eyes

Arthur, K.N., Spencer-Hwang, R., Knutsen, S.F., Shavlik, D., Soret, S., & Montgomery, S. (2018). Are perceptions of community safety associated with respiratory illness among a low-income, minority adult population? *BMC Public Health*, 18(1).

Azeemi, S.T., Rafiq, H.M., Ismail, I., Kazmi, S.R., & Azeemi, A. (2019). The mechanistic basis of chromotherapy: Current knowledge and future perspectives. *Complementary Therapies in Medicine, 46*, 217-222.

Bedrosian, T.A., & Nelson, R.J. (2017). Timing of light exposure affects mood and brain circuits. *Translational Psychiatry, 7*(1).

Beukeboom, C.J., Langeveld, D., & Tanja-Dijkstra, K. (2012). Stress-reducing effects of real and artificial nature in a hospital waiting room. *Journal of Alternative and Complementary Medicine*, 329-333.

Bowers, S.J., Lambert, S., He, S., Lowry, C.A., Fleshner, M., Wright, K.P., . . . Vitaterna, M. (2021). Immunization with heat-killed bacterium, Mycobacterium vaccae NCTC 11659, prevents the development of cortisol hyperarousal and a PTSD-like sleep phenotype after sleep disruption and acute stress in mice. *Sleep, 44*(6).

Chalmin-Pui, L.S., Griffiths, A., Roe, J., Heaton, T., & Cameron, R. (2021). Why garden? Attitudes and the perceived health benefits of home gardening. *Cities, 112*.

Chameberlin, L.C., & Callmer, A. (2021). Spark joy and slow consumption: An empirical study of the impact of KonMari method on acquisition and wellbeing. *Journal of Sustainability Research, 3*(1).

Corazon, S.S., Sidenius, U., Poulsen, D.V., Gramkow, M.C., & Stigsdotter, U.K. (2019). Psycho-physiological stress recovery in outdoor nature-based interventions: A systematic review of the past eight years of research. *International Journal of Environmental Research and Public Health, 16*(10).

Crowe, J., Lacy, C., & Columbus, Y. (2018). Barriers to food security and community stress in an urban food desert. *Urban Science, 2*(2), 48.

Dao, T.N., & Ferrari, J.R. (2020). The negative side of office clutter: Impact on work-related well-being and job satisfaction. *North American Journal of Psychology, 22*(3), 397-410.

Davies, T.W., & Smyth, T. (2017). Why artificial light at night should be a focus for global change research in the 21st century. *Global Change Biology, 24*(3), 872-882.

Duyan, F., & Rengin, U. (2016). A research on the effect of classroom wall colours on student's attention. *A|Z ITU Journal of the Faculty of Architecture, 13*(2), 73-78.

Dzhambov, A.M., Lercher, P., Browning, M.H., Stoyanov, D., Petrova, N., Novakov, S., & Dimitrova, D.D. (2021). Does greenery experienced indoors and outdoors provide and escape and support mental health during the COVID-19 quarantine? *Environmental Research, 196*.

Environmental Protection Agency. (2022, July 6). *Improving indoor air quality*. Retrieved from www.epa.gov/indoor-air-quality-iaq/improving-indoor-air-quality

Ewert, A., & Chang, Y. (2018). Levels of nature and stress response. *Behavioral Science, 8*(5), 49.

Frone, M.R. (2016). Work stress and alcohol use: Developing and testing a biphasic self-medication model. *An International Journal of Work, Health & Organization, 30*(4).

Frumkin, H., Gratman, G.N., Breslow, S.J., Cochran, B., Kahn Jr., P.H., Lawler, J.J., . . . Wood, S.A. (2017). Nature contact and human health: A research agenda. *Environmental Health Perspectives, 125*(7).

Furuyashiki, A., Tabuchi, K., Norikoshi, K., Kobayashi, T., & Oriyama, S. (2019). A comparative study of the physiological and psychological effects of forest bathing (Shinrin-yoku) on working age people with and without depressive tendencies. *Environmental Health and Preventive Medicine, 24*(1), 46.

Fushimi, T., Inui, S., Nakajima, T., Ogasawara, M., Hosokawa, K., & Itami, S. (2012). Green light emitting diodes accelerate wound healing: Characterization of the effect and its molecular basis in vitro and in vivo. *Wound Repair and Regeneration, 20*, 226-235.

Grunt, M.L., Raap, T., Grunst, A. S., Pinxten, R., Parenteau, C., Angelier, F., & Eens, M. (2020). Early-life exposure to artificial light at night elevates physiological stress in free-living songbirds. *Environmental Pollution, 259*.

Gunes, E., & Olgunturk, N. (2020). Color-emotion associations in interiors. *COLOR Research & Application, 45*(1), 129-141.

Hahad, O., Prochaska, J.H., Daiber, A., & Munzel, T. (2019). Environmental noise-induced effects on stress hormones, oxidative stress, and vascular dysfunction: Key factors in the relationship between cerebrocadiovascular and psychological disorders. *Oxidative Medicine and Cellular Longevity*.

Haider, S., Smith, L., Markovic, L., Schuch, F.B., Sadarangani, K.P., Lopez Sanchez, G., . . . Grabovac, I. (2021). Associations between physical activity, sitting time, and time spent outdoors with mental health during the first COVID-19 lock down in Austria. *International Journal of Environmental Research and Public Health, 18*(17).

Hall, C., & Knuth, M. (2019). An update of the literature supporting the well-being benefits of plants: A review of the emotional and mental health benefits of plants. *Journal of Environmental Health, 37*(1), 30-38.

Hambly, B. (2022). *Pink flamingos and the Yellow Pages: The surprising stories behind the colors of our world.* Chronicle Books.

Han, K.-T., & Li-Wen, R. (2019). Effects of indoor plants on self-reported perceptions: A systematic review. *Sustainability, 11*(16).

Han, K.-T., Ruan, L.-W., & Liao, L.-S. (2022). Effects of indoor plants on human functions: A systematic review with meta-analysis. *International Journal of Environmental Research and Public Health, 19*(12).

Hartswick, K.J. (2004). *The gardens of Sallust: A changing landscape.* University of Texas Press.

Hunter, M.R., Gillespie, B.W., & Chen, S.Y. (2019). Urban nature experiences reduce stress in the context of daily life based on salivary biomarkers. *Frontiers in Psychology, 10*, 722.

Hwang, H.-J., Choi, Y.-J., & Hong, D. (2023). The association between self-rated health status, psychosocial stress, eating behaviors, and food intake according to the level of sunlight exposure in Korean adults. *International Journal of Environmental Research and Public Health, 20*(1).

International Dark Sky Association. (n.d.). *Light Pollution*. Retrieved July 20, 2022, from www.darksky.org/light-pollution

Jiang, B., He, J., Larsen, L., & Wang, H. (2020). Perceived green at speed: A simulated driving experiment raises new questions for attention restoration theory and stress reduction theory. *Environment and Behavior, 53*(3).

Khamis, S. (2019). The aestheticization of restraint: The popular appeal of de-cluttering after the global financial crisis. *Journal of Consumer Culture, 19*(4).

Killgore, W.G., Pace-Schott, E., Ozcan, M., Shepard, K.C., Burns, A.I., Grandner, M.A., . . . Alkozei, A. (2019). 0884 morning blue light exposure improves sleep and fear extinction recall in PTSD. *Sleep, 42*, A355-A356.

Kondo, M. (2014). *The life-changing magic of tidying up: The Japanese art of decluttering and organizing.* Random House.

Kraus, M., Senitkova, I., & Juhasova, C. (2021). Influence of houseplants on the indoor environment quality. *International Multidisciplinary Scientific Geoconference, 21*(6).

Lawrenson, J.G., Hull, C.C., & Downie, L.E. (2017). The effect of blue-light blocking spectacle lenses on visual performance, macular health, and the sleep-wake cycle: A systematic review of the literature. *Ophthalmic and Physiological Optics, 37*(6), 644-654.

Lee, M.J., Oh, W., Kim, J., & Jang, J.S. (2018). LED colors and worker stress response after a flower arrangement activity. *Horticulture Science and Technology*, 435-443.

Lee, M.S., Lee, J., Park, B.-J., & Miyazaki, Y. (2015). Interaction with indoor plants may reduce psychological and physiological stress by suppressing autonomic nervous system activity in young adults: A randomized crossover study. *Journal of Physiological Anthropology, 34*(1).

Li, M., Ferreira, S., & Smith, T.A. (2020). Temperature and self-reported mental health in the United States. *PLoS ONE, 15*(3).

Ma, J., Li, C., Kwan, M.-P., & Chai, Y. (2018). A multilevel analysis of perceived noise pollution, geographic contexts and mental health in Beijing. *International Journal of Environmental Research and Public Health, 15*(7).

Manav, B. (2007). Color-emotion associations and color preferences: A case study for residences. *COLOR Research and Application, 32*(2), 144-151.

Matsubara, E., & Kawai, S. (2018). Gender differences in the psychophysiological effects induced by VOCs emitted from Japanese cedar (Cryptomeria japonica). *Environmental Health and Preventive Medicine, 23*(10).

McArthur, L.H., Fasczewski, K.S., Farris, A.R., & Petrone, M. (2020). Use and perceptions of a campus food pantry among food insecure college students: An exploratory study from Appalachia. *Journal of Appalachian Health, 2*(2), 7-23.

Meza, A., Altman, E., Martinez, S., & Leung, C.W. (2018). "It's a feeling that one is not worth food": A qualitative study exploring the psychosocial experiences and academic consequences of food insecurity among college students. *Journal of the Academy of Nutrition and Dietetics, 119*(10), 1713-1721.

Morello-Frosch, R., Zuk, M., Jerrett, M., Shamasunder, B., & Kyle, A. (2011). Understanding the cumulative impacts of inequalities in environmental health: Implications for policy. *Health Affairs, 30*(5), 879-887.

Nollet, M., Wisden, W., & Franks, N.P. (2020). Sleep deprivation and stress: A reciprocal relationship. *Interface Focus, 103.*

Nunez-Gonzalez, S., Delgado-Ron, J.A., Gault, C., Lara-Vinueza, A., Calle-Celi, D., & Porreca, P. (2020). Overview of "systematic reviews" of the built environment's effects on mental health. *Journal of Environmental and Public Health.*

Nuyts, V., Nawrot, T.S., Scheers, H., Nemery, B., & Casas, L. (2019). Air pollution and self-perceived stress and mood: A one-year panel study on health in elderly persons. *Environmental Research, 177.*

O'Connor, Z. (2011). Colour psychology and colour therapy: Caveat emptor. *Color Research and Design, 36*(3), 229-234.

Oh, J., Lee, H., & Park, H. (2021). Effects on heart rate variability of stress level response to the properties of indoor environmental colors: A preliminary study. *International Journal of Environmental Research and Public Health, 18*(17).

Orru, K., Nordin, S., Harzia, H., & Orru, H. (2018). The role of perceived air pollution and health risk perception in health symptoms and disease: A population-based study combined with modelled levels of PM10. *International Archives of Occupational and Environmental Health*, 581-589.

Pagliccio, D., Herbstman, J.B., Perera, F., Tang, D., Goldsmith, J., Peterson, B.S., . . . Margolis, A.E. (2020). Prenatal exposure to polycyclic aromatic hydrocarbons modified the effects of early life stress on attention and thought problems in late childhood. *The Journal of Child Psychology and Psychiatry, 61*(11), 1253-1265.

Palar, K., Hufstedler, E.L., Hernandez, K., Chang, A., Ferguson, L., Lozano, L., . . . Weiser, S.D. (2019). Nutrition and health improvements after participation in an urban home garden program. *Journal of Nutrition Education and Behavior, 51*(9), 1037-1046.

Payne-Sturges, D.C., Tjaden, A., Caldeira, K.M., Vincent, K.B., & Arria, A.M. (2017). Student hunger on campus: Food insecurity among college students and implications for academic institutions. *American Journal for Health Promotion, 32*(2).

Pearon, M., Gaines, K., Pati, D., Colwell, M., Motheral, L., & Adams, N.G. (2019). The physiological impact of window murals on pediatric patients. *Health Environment Research & Design Journal, 12*(2), 116-129.

Perry, G., Taylor, N.W., Bothwell, P.C., Milbourn, C.C., Powell, G., & Singh, K.D. (2020). The gamma response to colour hue in humans: Evidence from MEG. *PLoS ONE, 15*(12).

Pfefferle, P.I., Keber, C.U., Cohen, R.M., & Garn, H. (2021). The hygiene hypothesis: Learning from but not living in the past. *Frontiers in Immunology, 12.*

Pinsonnault-Skvarenina, A., Carrier, M., Bockstael, A., Gagne, J.-P., & Leroux, T. (n.d.). Perception of noise mitigation approaches along a major highway construction site. *Transportation Research Part D: Transport and Environment, 104.*

Plascak, J.J., Llanos, A.A., Qin, B., Chavali, L., Lin, Y., Pawlish, K.S., . . . Bandera, E.V. (2021). Visual cues of the build environment and perceived stress among a cohort of Black breast cancer survivors. *Health & Place, 67.*

Repova, K., Baka, T., Krajcirovicova, K., Stanko, P., Axiriova, S., Reiter, R.J., & Simko, F. (2022). Melatonin as a potential approach to anxiety treatment. *International Journal of Molecular Sciences, 23*(24).

Roster, C.A., & Ferrari, J.R. (2019). Does work stress lead to office clutter, and how? Mediating influences of emotional exhaustion and indecision. *Environment and Behavior, 52*(9), 923-944.

Rudolph, K.E., Shev, A., Paksarian, D., Merikangas, K.R., Mennitt, D.J., James, P., & Casey, J.A. (2019). Environmental noise and sleep and mental health outcomes in a nationally representative sample of urban US adolescents. *Environmental Epidemiology, 3*(4).

Sandel, M., Cook, J., Poblacion, A., Sheward, R., Coleman, S.M., Vivieros, J., & Sturtevant, L. (2016). Housing as a health care investment: Affordable housing supports children's health. *National Housing Conference and Children's HealthWatch.*

Sansone, R.A., & Sansone, L.A. (2013). Sunshine, serotonin, and skin: A partial explanation for seasonal patterns in psychopathology. *Innovations in Clinical Neuroscience, 10*(7-8), 20-24.

Science for Environmental Policy. (2016). *Links between noise and air pollution and socioeconomic status.* Retrieved from http://ec.europa.eu/science-environment-policy

Scott, T.L., Masser, B.M., & Pachana, N.A. (2020). Positive aging benefits of home and community gardening activities: Older adults report enhanced self-esteem, productive endeavors, social engagement, and exercise. *SAGE Open Medicine, 8.*

Shirzadfar, H., & Sheikhi, K. (2020). An introduction on different types of phototherapy devices to cure neonatal jaundice: Internal structure of light sources & protection system. *Journal of Clinical and Translational Neonatology, 1*(1).

Singh, A., Daniel, L., Baker, E., & Bentley, R. (2019). Housing disadvantage and poor mental health: A systematic review. *American Journal of Preventive Medicine, 57*(2), 262-272.

Smiley, A., Ramos, W.D., Elliott, L.M., & Wolter, S.A. (2020). Association between trail use and self-rated wellness and health. *BMC Public Health, 20*(1).

Smith, D.G., Martinelli, R., Besra, G., Illarionov, P.A., Szatmari, I., Brazda, P., . . . Lowry, C.A. (2019). Identification and characterization of a novel anti-inflammatory lipid isolated from Mycobacterium vaccae, a soil-derived bacterium with immunoregulatory and stress resilience properties. *Psychopharmacology, 236*(5), 1653-1670.

Storoni, M. (2018, January 2). *Is too much light making us sick, sad, and stressed?* Retrieved from www.psychologytoday.com/us/blog/the-stress-proof-life/201801/is-too-much-light-making-us-sick-sad-and-stressed

Suli, D.P., Aini, N., & Prasetyo, Y.B. (2020). The effect of green color breathing therapy towards reduction of stress levels in hemodialized patients. *Journal Keperawatan, 10*(2).

Sun, L., Zhao, Y., Zhang, J., Chen, D., & Zhang, X. (2021). Research and application of noise barriers in highway construction. *2nd Annual Academy Exchange Conference on Science and Technology Innovation, 233.*

Swanson, H.L., & Ferrari, J R. (2022). Older adults and clutter: Age differences in clutter impact, psychological home, and subjective well-being. *Behavioral Sciences, 23*(5).

Thomson, E.M. (2019). Air pollution, stress, and allostatic load: Linking systemic and central nervous system impacts. *Journal of Alzheimer's Disease, 69*(3), 597-614.

Wang, X., Shi, Y., Zhang, B., & Chiang, Y. (2019). The influence of forest resting environments on stress using virtual reality. *International Journal of Environmental Research and Public Health, 16*(8).

Xiao, Q., Gee, G., Jones, R.R., Jia, P., James, P., & Hale, L. (2020). Cross-sectional association between outdoor artificial light at night and sleep duration in middle-to-older aged adults: The NIH-AARP Diet and Health Study. *Environmental Research, 180,* 108823.

Yin, J., Yuan, J., Arfaei, N., Catalano, P.J., Allen, J.G., & Spengler, J.D. (2020). Effects of biophilic indoor environment on stress and anxiety recovery: A between-subjects experiment in virtual reality. *Environment International, 136.*

Yoo, J.Y., Groer, M., Dutra, S.V., Sarkar, A., & McSkimming, D.I. (2020). Gut microbiota and immune system interactions. *Microorganisms, 8*(10).

Young, D.R., Hong, B.D., Lo, T., Inzhakova, G., Cohen, D.A., & Sidell, M.A. (2022). The longitudinal associations of physical activity, time spent outdoors in nature and symptoms of depression and anxiety during COVID-19 quarantine and social distancing in the United States. *Preventive Medicine, 154.*

Zaman, M., Muslim, M., & Jehangir, A. (2022). Environmental noise-induced cardiovascular, metabolic and mental health disorders. *Environmental Science and Pollution, 29*(51), 76485-76500.

Zarei, M., Wikramanayake, T.C., Falto-Aizpurua, L., Schachner, L.A., & Jimenez, J.J. (2016). Low level laser therapy and hair regrowth: An evidence-based review. *Lasers in Medical Science, 31*(2), 363-371.

Zhang, Y.-L., Byeon, H.-S., Hong, W.-H., Cha, G.-W., Lee, Y.-H., & Kim, Y.-C. (2021). Risk assessment of asbestos containing materials in a deteriorated dwelling area using four different methods. *Journal of Hazardous Materials, 410.*

## Chapter 10

Bernstein, D., Borkovec, T., & Hazlett-Stevens, H. (2000). *New directions in progressive relaxation training.* Greenwood Publishing Group.

Brauninger, I. (2012). Dance movement therapy group intervention in stress treatment: A randomized controlled trial. *The Arts in Psychotherapy*, 443-450.

Braus, M., & Morton, B. (2020). Art therapy in the time of COVID-19. *Psychological Trauma: Theory, Research, Practice, and Policy, 12*(S1), S267-S268.

Bryant, E.F. (2017). *Bhakti yoga: Tales and teachings from the Bhagavata Purana.* North Point Press.

Carpena, M.X., Souza Tavare, P., & Menezes, C.B. (2019). The effect of a six-week focused meditation training on depression and anxiety symptoms in Brazilian university students with 6 and 12 months of follow-up. *Journal of Affective Disorders, 246*, 401-407.

Chui, P.L., Wai, S., Lai, L.-L., See, M.H., & Tan, S.B. (2021). Mindful breathing. *Clinical Journal of Oncology Nursing, 25*(2), 174-180.

Cleveland Clinic. (2022, March 30). *Diaphragmatic breathing*. Retrieved from https://my.clevelandclinic.org/health/articles/9445-diaphragmatic-breathing

Drigas, A., & Karyotaki, M. (2018). Mindfulness training & assessment and intelligence. *International Journal of Recent Contributions from Engineering, Science, & IT, 6*(3), 70-84.

Drigas, A., & Mitsea, E. (2021). Metacognition, stress-relaxation balance & related hormones. *iJES, 9*(1).

Du, J., Huang, J., An, Y., & Xu, W. (2018). The relationship between stress and negative emotion: The mediating role of rumination. *Clinical Research and Trials, 4*.

Farokhi, M. (2011). Art therapy in humanistic psychiatry. *Procedia - Social and Behavioral Sciences, 30*, 2088-2092.

Goldstein, M.R., Lewin, R.K., & Allen, J.J. (2019). Improvements in well-being and cardiac metrics of stress following a yogic breathing workshop: Randomized controlled trial with active comparison. *Journal of American College Health, 70*(3), 918-928.

Hamasaki, H. (2020). Effects of diaphragmatic breathing on health: A narrative review. *Medicines, 7*(10).

Harne, B.P., Tahseen, A.A., Hiwale, A.S., & Dhekekar, R.S. (2019). Survey on Om meditation: Its effects on the human body and Om meditation as a tool for stress management. *Psych Archives, 12*(1).

Hopper, S., Murray, S.L., Ferrara, L.R., & Singleton, J.K. (2019). Effectiveness of diaphragmatic breathing for reducing physiological and psychological stress in adults: A quantitative systematic review. *JBI Database of Systematic Reviews and Implementation Reports, 17*(9), 1855-1876.

Janjhua, Y., Chaudhary, R., Sharma, N., & Kumar, K. (2020). A study on the effect of yoga on emotional regulation, self-esteem, and feelings of adolescents. *Journal of Family Medicine and Primary Care*, 3381-3386.

Joshi, S.P., Wong, A.-K.I., Brucker, A., Ardito, T.A., Chow, S.-C., Vaishnavi, S., & Lee, P.J. (2022). Efficacy of transcendental meditation to reduce stress among health care workers. *Journal of the American Medical Association, 5*(9).

Kaimal, G., Carroll-Haskins, K., Mensinger, J.L., Dieterich-Harwell, R.M., Manders, E., & Levin, W.P. (2019). Outcomes of art therapy and coloring for professional and informal caregivers of patients in a radiation oncology unit: A mixed methods pilot study. *European Journal of Oncology Nursing, 42*, 153-161.

Kaimal, G., Ray, K., & Muniz, J. (2016). Reduction of cortisol levels and participants' responses following art making. *Journal of the American Art Therapy Association, 33*(2), 74-80.

Kaur, I. (2021). Study of physiological and psychological of Pranayama. *International Journal of Physical Education, Sport, and Health, 8*(6), 77-79.

Kearney, D.J., Malte, C.A., Storms, M., & Simpson, T.L. (2021). Loving-kindness meditation vs. cognitive processing therapy for posttraumatic stress disorder among veterans: A randomized clinical trial. *JAMA Network Open, 4*(4).

Kocjan, J., Adamek, M., Gzik-Zroska, B., Czyzewski, D., & Rydel, M. (2017). Network of breathing. Multifunctional role of the diaphragm: A review. *Advance Respiratory Medicine*, 224-232.

Koncz, A., Demetrovics, Z., & Takacs, Z.K. (2021). Meditation interventions efficiently reduce cortisol levels of at-risk samples: A meta-analysis. *Health Psychology Review, 15*(1).

Kudesia, R.S. (2019). Mindfulness as metacognitive practice. *Academy of Management Review, 44*(2), 405-423.

Kuppusamy, M., Kamaldeen, D., Pitani, R., Amaldas, J., & Shanmugam, P. (2018). Effects of Bhramari pranayama on health: A systematic review. *Journal of Traditional and Contemporary Medicine, 8*(1), 11-16.

Lith, T.V. (2016). Art therapy in mental health: A systematic review of approaches and practices. *The Arts in Psychotherapy*, 9-22.

Liu, H., Wiedman, C.M., Lovelace-Chandler, V., Gong, S., & Salem, Y. (2023). Deep diaphragmatic breathing: Anatomical and biomechanical consideration. *Journal of Holistic Nursing*.

Luberto, C.M., Shinday, N., Song, R., Philpotts, L.L., Park, E.R., Fricchione, G.L., & Yeh, G.Y. (2018). A systematic review and meta-analysis on the effects of meditation on empathy, compassion, and prosocial behaviors. *Mindfulness, 9*, 708-724.

Ma, X., Yue, Z.-Q., Zhang, H., Gong, Z.-Q., Shi, Y.-T., Wei, G.-X., & Li, Y.-F. (2017). The effect of diaphragmatic breathing on attention, negative affect and stress in healthy adults. *Frontiers in Psychology, 8*.

Marshall, M., McClanahan, M., Warren, S.M., Rogers, R., & Ballmann, C. (2020). A comparison of the acute effects of different forms of yoga on physiological and psychological stress: A pilot study. *International Journal of Environmental Research and Public Health*.

Martin, L., Oepen, R., Bauer, K., Nottensteiner, A., Mergheim, K., Gruber, H., & Koch, S.C. (2018). Creative arts interventions for stress management and prevention: A systematic review. *Behavioral Science, 8*(2).

McNair, D. (2020). Flipping the creative switch using the 4, 7, 8 breathing technique. In E. Maisel (Ed.), *The creativity workbook for coaches and creatives*. Routledge.

Naik, G.S., Gaur, G.S., & Pal, G.K. (2018). Effect of modified slow breathing exercise on perceived stress and basal cardiovascular parameters. *International Journal of Yoga, 11*(1), 53-58.

Neyaz, O., Sumila, L., Nanda, S., & Wadhwe, S. (2019). Effectiveness of Hatha yoga versus conventional therapeutic exercises for chronic nonspecific low-back pain. *The Journal of Alternative and Complementary Medicine, 25*(9).

Norelli, S.K., Long, A., & Krepps, J.M. (2021). *Relaxation techniques*. StatPearls.

Norian, T., & McLaughlin, M.P. (2021). *Tantra yoga: Journey to unbreakable wholeness*. Ashaya Yoga.

Om, C. (2020). *The holy science of yoga*. BookBaby.

Pallathadka, L.K., Pallathadka, H., & Devi, T.B. (2022). An empirical study on the importance of karma yoga in modern society. *Integrated Journal for Research in Arts and Humanities, 2*(6), 99-106.

Pandekar, P.P., & Thangavelu, P.D. (2019). Effect of 4-7-8 breathing technique on anxiety and depression in moderate chronic obstructive pulmonary disease patients. *International Journal of Health Sciences and Research, 9*(5).

Pankhania, J. (2005). Yoga and its practice in psychological healing. In R. Moodley & W. West (Eds.), *Integrating traditional healing practices into counseling and psychotherapy.* Sage Publications.

Patel, N.K., Nivethitha, L., & Mooventhan, A. (2018). Effect of a yoga based meditation technique on emotional regulation, self-compassion, and mindfulness in college students. *Explore*, 443-447.

Phuphanich, M.E., Droessler, J., Altman, L., & Eapen, B. (2020). Movement-based therapies in rehabilitation. *Physical Medicine and Rehabilitation Clinics of North America*, 577-591.

Pozuelos, J.P., Mead, B.R., Rueda, M.R., & Malinowski, P. (2019). Short-term mindful breath awareness training improves inhibitory control and response monitoring. *Progress in Brain Research, 244*, 137-163.

Ray, A. (2010). *OM chanting and meditation.* Inner Light Publishers.

Reddy, J.S., & Roy, S. (2019). Understanding meditation based on the subjective experience and traditional goal: Implications for current meditation research. *Frontiers in Psychology, 10.*

Rosen, R., & Fraley, K. (2002). *The yoga of breath: A step-by-step guide to pranayama.* Shambhala.

Russo, M.A., Santarelli, D.M., & O'Rourke, D. (2017). The physiological effects of slow breathing in the healthy human. *Breathe, 13*(4), 298-309.

Schwind, J.K., McCay, E., Beanlands, H., Schindel Martin, L., Martin, J., & Binder, M. (2017). Mindfulness practice as teaching-learning strategies in higher education: A qualitative exploratory pilot study. *Nurse Education Today, 50*, 92-96.

Smalley, S., & Winston, D. (2022). *Fully present: The science, art, and practice of mindfulness.* Hatchette Go.

Song, W.J., & Park, J.W. (2019). The influence of stress on internet addiction: Mediating effects of self-control. *International Journal of Mental Health and Addiction*, 1063-1075.

Sruthi, M., Mishra, A.K., & Harti, S.S. (2022). Yoga and its path to spirituality: A review article. *International Journal of Alternative and Complementary Medicine*, 26-29.

Thibodeaux, N., & Rossano, M.J. (2018). Meditation and immune function: The impact of stress management on the immune system. *OMB Integrative and Complementary Medicine, 3*(4).

Tong, J., Qi, X., He, Z., Chen, S., Pedersen, S.J., Cooley, P.D., ... Zhu, Z. (2020). The immediate and durable effects of yoga and physical fitness exercises on stress. *Journal of American College Health*, 675-683.

Tripathi, M.N., Kumari, S., & Ganpat, T.S. (2018). Psychophysiological effects of yoga on stress in college students. *Journal of Education and Health Promotion, 7*(1), 43.

Vaartio-Rajalin, H., Santamaki-Fischer, R., Jokisalo, P., & Fagerstrom, L. (2021). Art making and expressive art therapy in adult health and nursing care: A scoping review. *International Journal of Nursing Sciences, 8*(1), 102-119.

Vierra, J., Boonla, O., & Prasertsri, P. (2022). Effects of sleep deprivation and 4-7-8 breathing control on heart rate variability, blood pressure, blood glucose, and endothelial function in healthy young adults. *Physiological Reports, 10*(13).

Vivekananda, S. (2015). *Raja yoga.* CreateSpace Independent Publishing Platform.

Wang, F., & Szabo, A. (2020). Effects of yoga on stress among healthy adults: A systematic review. *Alternative Therapies, 26*(4).

Witkiewitz, K., Roos, C.R., Colgan, D.D., & Bowen, S. (2017). *Mindfulness.* Hogrefe.

Yakobi, O., Smilek, D., & Danckert, J. (2021). The effects of mindfulness meditation on attention, executive control and working memory in healthy adults: A meta-analysis of randomized controlled trials. *Cognitive Therapy and Research, 45*, 543-560.

Yang, E., Schamber, R.M., Meyer, L., & Gold, J.I. (2018). Happier healers: Randomized controlled trial of mobile mindfulness for stress management. *The Journal of Alternative and Complementary Medicine*, 505-513.

Zeidan, F., & Vago, D. (2016). Mindfulness meditation-based relief: A mechanistic account. *Annals of the New York Academy of Sciences*, 114-127.

## Chapter 11

Barratt, J.M., & Duran, F. (2021). Does psychological capital and social support impact engagement and burnout in online distance learning students? *The Internet and Higher Education, 51.*

Bettinger, E.P., Fox, L., Loeb, S., & Taylor, E.S. (2017). Virtual classrooms: How online college courses affect student success. *American Economic Review, 107*(9), 2855-2875.

Biedermann, D., Schneider, J., & Drachsler, H. (2021). Digital self-control interventions for distracting media multitasking: A systematic review. *Journal of Computer Assisted Learning, 37*(5), 1217-1231.

Bratterud, H., Burgess, M., Fasy, B.T., Millman, D.L., Oster, T., & Sung, E.C. (2020). The Sund Diagram: Revitalizing the Eisenhower Matrix. *Diagrammatic Representation and Inference, 11*, 498-502.

Britt, S.L., Ammerman, D.A., Barrett, S.F., & Jones, S. (2017). Student loans, financial stress, and college student retention. *Journal of Student Financial Aid, 47*(1).

Broadbent, J., & Poon, W.L. (2015). Self-regulated learning strategies & academic achievement in online higher education learning environments: A systematic review. *Internet Higher Education, 27.*

Bryant, J., Bolt, R., Botfield, J.R., Martin, K., Doyle, M., Murphy, D., ... Aggleton, P. (2020). Beyond deficit: 'Strength-based approaches' in Indigenous health research. *Sociology of Health & Illness, 43*, 1405-1421.

Cadaret, M.C., & Bennett, S.R. (2019). College students' reported financial stress and its relationship to psychological distress. *Journal of College Counseling, 22*(3), 225-239.

Cho, M.H., & Yoo, J.S. (2017). Exploring online students' self-regulated learning with self-reported surveys and log files: A data mining approach. *Interactive Learning Environments, 25*(8), 970-982.

Howard, Z.L., Evans, N.J., Innes, R.J., Brown, S.D., & Eidels, A. (2020). How is multi-tasking different from increased difficulty? *Psychonomic Bulletin & Review*, 937-951.

Ismail, N.M., Putri, Z., & Noviyanti, A. (2022). Pomodoro technique analysis in Zoom-based classrooms. *Journal of English Education and Linguistic Studies, 9*(1), 75-96.

Luis, E., Bermejo-Martins, E., Martinez, M., Sarrionandia, A., Cortes, C., Oliveros, E.Y., . . . Fernandez-Berrocal, P. (2021). Relationship between self-care activities, stress and well-being during COVID-19 lockdown: A cross-cultural mediation model. *BMJ Open, 11*.

Mensah, A., & Adjei, N.K. (2020). Work-life balance and self-reported health among working adults in Europe: A gender and welfare state regime comparative analysis. *BMC Public Health, 20,* 1052.

Monsalve, E.M., Navarro, R., Cruz, S.J., Develles, J.R., Espartiro, C., & Tamon, C.-J. (2020). Assessment on effectiveness of Eisenhower Matrix in improving time management of selected grade 12 ABM students. *Ascendens Asia Singapore-Bestlink College of the Philippines Journal of Multidisciplinary Research, 2*(1).

Nayak, S.G. (2018). Time management in nursing: Hour of need. *International Journal of Caring Sciences, 11*(3).

Nikolaev, B. (2016). Does higher education increase hedonic and eudemonic happiness? *Journal of Happiness Studies, 19*, 483-504.

The Ohio State University. (2016). *National Student Financial Wellness Study*. Office of Student Life: College of Education and Human Ecology.

Osborne, R.H., Cheng, C.C., Nolte, S., Elmer, S., Besancon, S., Budhathoki, S.S., . . . Wahl, A. (2022). Health literacy measurement: Embracing diversity in a strengths-based approach to promote health. *BMJ Global Health, 7*(9).

Pattnaik, T., Samanta, S.R., & Mohanty, J. (2022). Work life balance of health care workers in the new normal: A review of literature. *Journal of Medicinal and Chemical Sciences*, 42-54.

Rapp, C.A., Saleebey, D., & Sullivan, W.P. (2005). The future of strengths-based social work. *Advances in Social Work, 6*(1), 79-90.

Saville, B.K., Bureau, A., Eckenrode, C., & Maley, M. (2018). Passion and burnout in college students. *College Student Journal, 52*(1), 105-117.

Somerville, L.H., Van Bavel, J.J., Lewis, N.A., Gruber, J., & Cunningham, W.A. (2021). Learn when—and how—to say no in your professional life. *Science*.

Substance Abuse and Mental Health Services Administration. (2021). *Key substance use and mental health indicators in the United States: Results from the 2020 National Survey on Drug Use and Health*. Center for Behavioral Health Statistics and Quality.

Tolkien, J.R.R. (2012). *The Hobbit*. New York: HarperCollins.

# INDEX

*Note:* The italicized *f* and *t* following page numbers refer to figures and tables, respectively.

# ABOUT THE AUTHOR

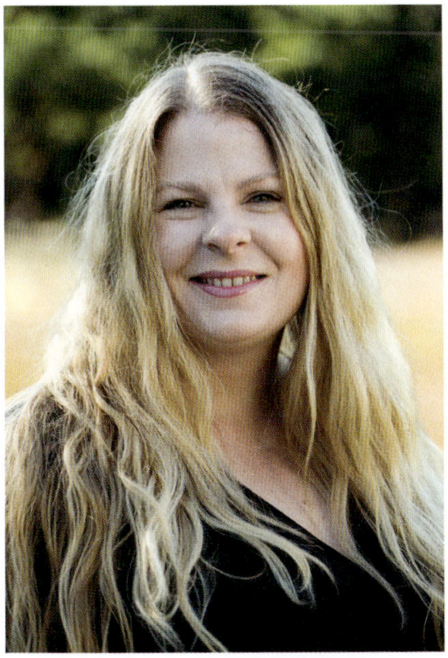

**Pardess Mitchell, EdD, MCHES**, is a professor at Harper College in Palatine, Illinois, where she also serves as department chair. She teaches a variety of courses, including health, women's health, community health, drugs in our culture, and public health, all of which cover the topic of stress management.

Pardess Mitchell recently coauthored *Drugs Across the Spectrum, Ninth Edition* (Cengage, 2024) and has contributed to other textbooks, including *Access to Health* and *Health: The Basics* (both from Pearson). She received her bachelor's degree in health education from the University of Maryland, her master's degree in health education from Southern Illinois University, and her doctorate in education, curriculum, and instruction from Northern Illinois University.

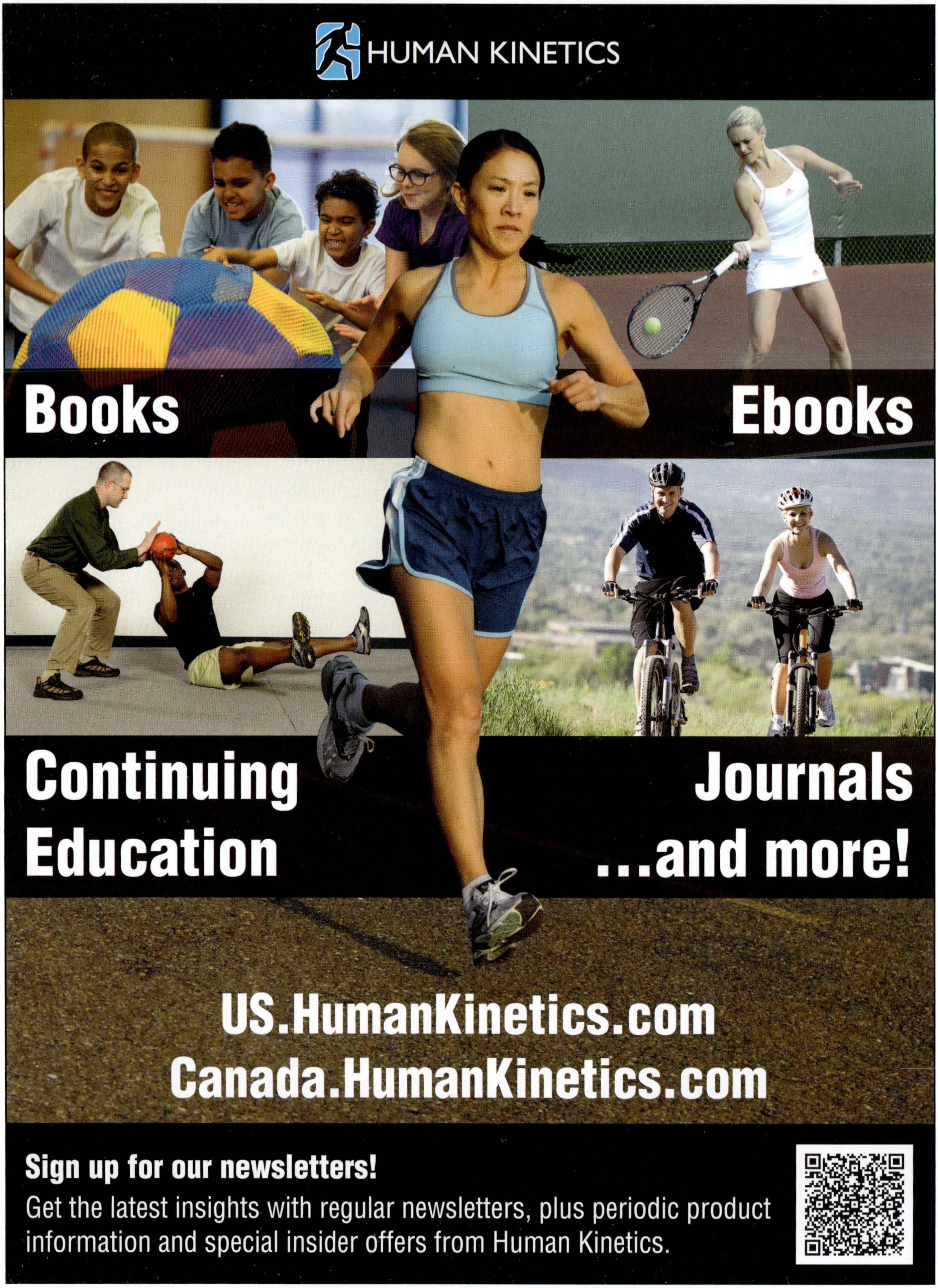
HUMAN KINETICS
Books
Ebooks
Continuing Education
Journals
...and more!
US.HumanKinetics.com
Canada.HumanKinetics.com
Sign up for our newsletters!
Get the latest insights with regular newsletters, plus periodic product information and special insider offers from Human Kinetics.